The Evolution of Forensic Psychiatry

The Evolution of Forensic Psychiatry

History, Current Developments, Future Directions

EDITED BY

Robert L. Sadoff, M.D.

OXFORD
UNIVERSITY PRESS

OXFORD
UNIVERSITY PRESS

Oxford University Press is a department of the University of Oxford. It furthers the University's objective of excellence in research, scholarship, and education by publishing worldwide.

Oxford New York
Auckland Cape Town Dar es Salaam Hong Kong Karachi
Kuala Lumpur Madrid Melbourne Mexico City Nairobi
New Delhi Shanghai Taipei Toronto

With offices in
Argentina Austria Brazil Chile Czech Republic France Greece
Guatemala Hungary Italy Japan Poland Portugal Singapore
South Korea Switzerland Thailand Turkey Ukraine Vietnam

Oxford is a registered trademark of Oxford University Press in the UK and certain other countries.

Published in the United States of America by
Oxford University Press
198 Madison Avenue, New York, NY 10016

Library of Congress Cataloging-in-Publication Data
The evolution of forensic psychiatry : history, current developments, future directions / edited by Robert L. Sadoff.
p. ; cm.
Includes bibliographical references and index.
ISBN 978-0-19-939343-5 (alk. paper)
I. Sadoff, Robert L., 1936- , editor.
[DNLM: 1. Forensic Psychiatry—trends. 2. Forensic Psychiatry—history. W 740]
RA1151
614'.15—dc23
2014040352

9 8 7 6 5 4 3 2 1
Printed in the United States of America
on acid-free paper

This book, which contains contributions from so many and such diverse professions, is dedicated to my mentors and teachers, to my esteemed and cherished colleagues, to my students, both current and past, and to the people we have served over the years, all of whom have taught me so much that has led to the ideas formulated in this volume.

Contents

Preface: How We Got to Where We Are and Where We Are Going

At the annual meetings of the American Psychiatric Association there was regularly a meeting of the Section of Psychiatry and the Law. (The APA was structured with "sections" at that time and each section met at the annual meeting.)

I attended my first annual meeting in 1953 in St. Louis, Missouri. Dr. Manfred Guttmacher, who was Chief Medical Officer of the Supreme Bench of Baltimore (later the Circuit Court for Baltimore City), my mentor, invited me to come to the meeting, where I met the forerunners of today's "Forensic Psychiatry." Henry Davidson, Colonel Albert Glass, John Ordway, Seymour Pollack, Saleem Shah, and others. I was welcomed warmly and even asked my opinion about several of the issues discussed. I was also invited to the lounge for a drink after the meeting, where I heard many stories about interesting cases and testimony. I think this warm reception convinced that this is where I wanted to be.

Subsequently I attended every APA Annual Meeting and the meetings of the Psychiatry Law Section. In 1959 I was appointed Court Psychiatrist to the Circuit Court for Baltimore County, where I established one of the first "forensic" fellowship programs with a grant from the NIMH-Crime & Delinquency Section. There were five grants available and Seymour Pollack at USC also had one. I had one fellow the first year and used subsequent grant funds to teach law & psychiatry to residents at all of the areas residency programs.

I don't recall when the word *forensic* came into being. It may have come from the American Academy of Forensic Sciences, which had a section of Law and Psychiatry. Eventually this term, forensic psychiatry, became associated with those psychiatrists who devoted a part of their professional time to the broad field of Law and Psychiatry.

At the APA meetings the group attending the Psychiatry and Law section grew to include Melvin Heller, Bob Sadoff, Seymour Halleck, Louis McGarry, John Torrens, Erwin Perr, Emmanuel Tanay, Herb Thomas, Joe Satten, and others. As the group grew larger it became too big for informal meetings in hotel lounges, so by 1968 we asked the APA to give us a room of our own after the official program was over for the day. I had a portable bar (it looked like a microscope case), which I dutifully brought along to help us relax. By this time, everyone attending had established various types of programs in their communities associated with the courts. We shared our experiences, making suggestions to each other to help us strengthen our role at the courts and residency programs. This "cross-pollination" was the beginning of the growth of our field.

Finally at the group's meeting at the APA's annual meeting in May, 1969 in Miami, we decided that we should establish a formal organization. After much discussion we settled on the American Academy of Psychiatry and the Law (AAPL). We decided to have our first meeting the third weekend in October in the Baltimore–Washington area and I was asked to organize the meeting.

The AAPL's inaugural meeting was held at the Friendship International Hotel (Friendship Airport) in October 1969 and was attended by about 35 psychiatrists who devoted a part of their practices to legal issues. Forensic psychiatry was a subspecialty for us. However, we knew that there were many psychiatrists who occasionally testified in court, who needed guidance and would welcome a chance to learn more.

The following May, the APA met in Washington, DC and AAPL shared a booth with the Patuxent Institution in Jessup, Maryland (a special institution designated to treat "defective delinquents"). We energetically recruited members to "this organization for those who do some psychiatric-legal consultations or who work in correctional institutions." We knew that much of this work was being done by the average psychiatrist, who was eager to gain some special knowledge so his or her contacts with the law would be better informed. We also believed that the AAPL should become the "school" for the future teachers of forensic psychiatry and the place where ideas could be exchanged.

Since then, the AAPL has grown to the premier organization for those who labor at the interface of psychiatry and the law. It is interesting to note that the AAPL's membership has stabilized over the years at about 2000. That seems to be the saturation point for forensic psychiatrist in Canada and the United States. Eventually fellowship programs in forensic psychiatry were established at almost every residency program and a Certification Board was established.

The AAPL and forensic psychiatry have continued to grow as exemplified by the various authors of the sections that Dr. Sadoff has included in this textbook, *Evolution of Forensic Psychiatry: History, Current Developments, Future Directions*. Dr. Sadoff has recruited leaders in most of the fields that impinge on this broad field as well as many of the directors of fellowship programs, each of whom has his or her own way of teaching forensic psychiatry. Just as the laws vary from state to state, so do the ways different psychiatrists view each issue.

Every breakthrough in science impinges on our field. Will the genome reveal who is going to become a "law-breaking dangerous psychopathic killer?" Will genetic tinkering allow us the change some of that behavior? Will new enhanced brain studies enable us to predict who might be dangerous? Despite these developments, "the law" is very cautious, as it should be, in immediately accepting every new scientific development as an explanation of certain behavior and, therefore, an "excuse" for it.

This is what makes forensic psychiatry so exciting. Stay tuned.

—Jonas R. Rappeport, M.D.

Acknowledgments

I am deeply indebted to all who have contributed to this volume, which contains diverse ideas from many professions and from all subspecialties of psychiatry. Forensic psychiatry is a growing field that has embraced other subspecialties of psychiatry as well as many professions and separate schools within the university. The practice of forensic psychiatry has outgrown its traditional bounds of forensic examination, report writing, and expert testimony. It includes consultation with many subspecialties of medicine and psychiatry and many other academic professions, including psychology, criminology, law, nursing, bioethics, social work, neuroscience, and communications. Forensic psychiatrists frequently consult with judges and legislators in formulating legal decisions and judicial opinions. The teaching of forensic psychiatry must include these other specialties and professions in order to provide the student and practitioner with current information and cases that not only reflect our current developments, but also predict the complexities of future forensic issues.

All of the contributors to this volume are experts in their particular professions, and the forensic psychiatrists are the leaders of the field in America. I am greatly indebted to all of them for bringing together diverse knowledge, experience, and teaching in one volume. It is our hope that the integration of this knowledge will light the way to the future for students, researchers, and practitioners in many scientific fields, and particularly for those specializing in forensic psychiatry.

I am indebted to the publishers at Oxford University Press for having the foresight to accept this challenging view of forensic psychiatry.

Finally, I am deeply indebted to my dear family, my parents who encouraged me to study both medicine and law, my children who endured my absences, and mostly my wonderful wife, Joan, who has been my muse, my inspiration, and my partner for all these years, and who has encouraged and supported the work that I do. To all of you, I am eternally grateful.

List of Contributors

Kenneth L. Appelbaum, M.D.
Clinical Professor of Psychiatry
Director, Correctional Mental Health Policy and Research
Center for Health Policy and Research, Commonwealth Medicine;
University of Massachusetts Medical School
Worcester, Massachusetts

Steven Berkowitz, M.D.
Clinical Assistant Professor of Psychiatry
Perelman School of Medicine
University of Pennsylvania
Philadelphia, Pennsylvania

Stephen Bates Billick, M.D.
Clinical Professor of Psychiatry
New York University School of Medicine
New York, New York

Kathleen Brown, R.N. Ph.D.
Associate Practice Professor
University of Pennsylvania
School of Nursing
Philadelphia, Pennsylvania

NiaLena Caravasos, Esquire
Law Office of NiaLena Caravasos, LLC
Philadelphia, Pennsylvania

J. Richard Ciccone, M.D.
Professor of Psychiatry
University of Rochester
Rochester, New York

George Cronin, Ph.D.
Pennsylvania State Police

Frank M. Dattilio, Ph.D., ABPP
Department of Psychiatry
University of Pennsylvania
Philadelphia, Pennsylvania; and
Department of Psychiatry
Harvard Medical School
Boston, Massachusetts

Joseph N. DiGiacomo, M.D.
Clinical Professor of Psychiatry
Perelman School of Medicine
University of Pennsylvania
Philadelphia, Pennsylvania

Danielle M. Dorn, M.S.
Clinical Research Coordinator
Perelman School of Medicine
University of Pennsylvania
Philadelphia, Pennsylvania

Eric Y. Drogin, Ph.D., J.D., ABPP
Harvard Medical School
Department of Psychiatry
Program in Psychiatry and the Law
Beth Israel Deaconess Medical Center
Boston, Massachusetts

Laurentine Fromm, M.D.
Clinical Associate, Department of Psychiatry
Perelman School of Medicine
University of Pennsylvania
Philadelphia, Pennsylvania

Yu Gao, Ph.D.
Assistant Professor, Department of Psychology
Brooklyn College
Brooklyn, New York

Richard J. Gelles, Ph.D.
Joanne and Raymond Welsh Chair of Child Welfare and Family Violence
School of Social Policy and Practice
University of Pennsylvania
Philadelphia, Pennsylvania

Andrea Glenn, Ph.D.
Assistant Professor, Department of Psychology
University of Alabama
Tuscaloosa, Alabama

Oren M. Gur, Ph.D.
Department of Criminology, Law and Justice
University of Illinois at Chicago
Chicago, Illinois

Ruben C. Gur, Ph.D.
Professor of Psychology in Psychiatry
Perelman School of Medicine
Brain Behavior Laboratory
University of Pennsylvania
Philadelphia, Pennsylvania

Thomas G. Gutheil, M.D.
Professor of Psychiatry and Co-founder, Program in Psychiatry and the Law
Department of Psychiatry
Beth Israel-Deaconess Medical Center and Massachusetts Mental Health Center
Harvard Medical School
Boston, Massachusetts

Alisa R. Gutman, M.D., Ph.D.
Attending Psychiatrist, Philadelphia VA Medical Center
Clinical Associate, Perelman School of Medicine
University of Pennsylvania
Philadelphia, Pennsylvania

Melvin S. Heller, M.D. (Retired)
Clinical Professor of Psychiatry and Lecturer in Law
Co-Director, Unit in Law and Psychiatry
Temple University Schools of Law and Medicine
Philadelphia, Pennsylvania

Joshua C. W. Jones, M.D.
Clinical Assistant Professor of Psychiatry
University of Rochester Medical Center
Medical Director, Peninsula Behavioral Health
Port Angeles, Washington

William S. Laufer, Ph.D., J.D.
Julian Aresty Professor
Professor of Legal Studies and Business Ethics, Sociology and Criminology
Director, Carol and Lawrence Zicklin Center for Business Ethics Research, The Wharton School
University of Pennsylvania
Philadelphia, Pennsylvania

Richard F. Limoges, M.D.
Clinical Associate Professor of Psychiatry
Perelman School of Medicine
University of Pennsylvania
Philadelphia, Pennsylvania

Catherine Mao, J.D.
Private Practice of Law
Certificate in Neuroscience
University of Pennsylvania
Philadelphia, Pennsylvania

Hon. Robert J. Matthews, J.D.
Senior Judge, First Judicial District of Pennsylvania

Jeffrey L. Metzner, M.D.
Clinical Professor of Psychiatry
University of Colorado School of Medicine
Denver, Colorado

Stephen J. Morse, Ph.D., J.D.
Ferdinand Wakeman Hubbell Professor of Law and
Professor of Psychology and Law in Psychiatry
Associate Director, Center for Neuroscience and Society
Diplomate, American Board of Professional Psychology (Forensic)
University of Pennsylvania Law School
Philadelphia, Pennsylvania

Kajal R. Patel, M.D.
Practicing Psychiatrist
Atlanta, Georgia

Michael L. Perlin, J.D.
Director, International Mental Disability Law Reform Project
Director, Online Mental Disability Law Program
New York Law School
New York, New York

Claire Pouncey, M.D., Ph.D.
Private Practice of Psychiatry
Chair, Section on Medicine, Ethics and the Law
College of Physicians of Philadelphia
Philadelphia, Pennsylvania

Mark R. Pressman, Ph.D., D.ABSM
Adjunct Professor of Law, Villanova University School of Law
Clinical Professor, Lankenau Institute for Medical Research
Clinical Professor of Medicine, Jefferson Medical College
Director Emeritus, Sleep Medicine Services, Lankenau Medical Center
Wynnewood, Pennsylvania

Adrian Raine, D.Phil.
Richard Perry University Professor
Departments of Criminology, Psychiatry and Psychology
University of Pennsylvania
Philadelphia, Pennsylvania

Jonas R. Rappeport, M.D.
Clinical Professor of Psychiatry, University of Maryland Medical School
Associate Professor of Psychiatry (part-time-retired) Johns Hopkins School of Medicine
Baltimore, Maryland

Phillip J. Resnick, M.D.
Professor of Psychiatry, Case Western Reserve University of Medicine
Cleveland, Ohio

Richard Rosner, M.D.
Clinical Professor, Department of Psychiatry and
Department of Child and Adolescent Psychiatry
New York University School of Medicine
New York, New York

Susan Rushing, M.D., J.D.
Clinical Assistant Professor of Psychiatry
Perelman School of Medicine
University of Pennsylvania
Philadelphia, Pennsylvania

Robert L. Sadoff, M.D.
Clinical Professor of Psychiatry
Perelman School of Medicine
University of Pennsylvania
Philadelphia, Pennsylvania

Robert A. Schug, Ph.D.
Assistant Professor of Criminal Justice and Forensic Psychology
School of Criminology, Criminal Justice, and Emergency Management
California State University, Long Beach, California

Charles L. Scott, M.D.
Chief, Division of Psychiatry and the Law
Professor of Clinical Psychiatry
Department of Psychiatry & Behavioral Sciences
University of California, Davis Medical Center
Sacramento, California

Rachel Shmuts, D.O.
Fellow in Psychosomatic Medicine
Hospital of the University of Pennsylvania
Philadelphia, Pennsylvania

Annie Steinberg, M.D.
Clinical Professor of Psychiatry
Perelman School of Medicine
University of Pennsylvania
Philadelphia, Pennsylvania

Joel E. Streim, M.D.
Professor of Psychiatry, Geriatric Psychiatry Section
Department of Psychiatry, Perelman School of Medicine
University of Pennsylvania and
Philadelphia Veterans Affairs Medical Center
Philadelphia, Pennsylvania

Robert L. Trestman, Ph.D., M.D.
Professor of Medicine, Psychiatry and Nursing
Executive Director, Correctional Managed Health Care
University of Connecticut Health Center
Farmington, Connecticut

Clarence Watson, J.D., M.D.
Clinical Assistant Professor of Psychiatry
Perelman School of Medicine
University of Pennsylvania
Philadelphia, Pennsylvania

Robert M. Weinrieb, M.D.
Director, Psychosomatic Medicine and Psychosomatic Medicine fellowship, Perelman School of Medicine
University of Pennsylvania
Philadelphia, Pennsylvania

Kenneth J. Weiss, M.D.
Clinical Professor of Psychiatry
Perelman School of Medicine
University of Pennsylvania
Philadelphia, Pennsylvania

Debra Schilling Wolfe, M.Ed.
Executive Director, Field Center for Children's Policy, Practice and Research
University of Pennsylvania
Philadelphia, Pennsylvania

Yaling Yang, Ph.D.
Department of Pediatrics, Children's Hospital Los Angeles
USC Keck School of Medicine
Los Angeles, California

Introduction

Forensic psychiatry is a subspecialty of psychiatry that deals with people who are involved in legal matters, both criminal and civil. That is the simple definition that I usually give when asked on the witness stand. The authors of the ethics guidelines for the practice of forensic psychiatry for the American Academy of Psychiatry and the Law have defined forensic psychiatry in a more elaborate manner:

> Forensic psychiatry is a subspecialty of psychiatry in which scientific and clinical expertise is applied in legal contexts involving civil, criminal, correctional, regulatory, or legislative matters, and its specialized clinical consultations in areas such as risk assessment or employment.[1]

Forensic psychiatry was not always so precise in its definition. The early forensic psychiatrists were called *alienists* because they worked with people who were deemed to be "alien to society." (Some critics even thought that psychiatrists appeared to be "alien to society.") Psychiatry was not always a major specialty of medicine, and forensic psychiatry has only recently become a major subspecialty of psychiatry.

As Benjamin Rush is considered to be the father of American psychiatry, so Isaac Ray is known as the father of forensic psychiatry in the United States. His contributions, as noted by historian forensic psychiatrist, Dr. Kenneth Weiss, in his chapter are progressive and timeless.[2] However, there could be a gap in professional recognition from the time of Isaac Ray in the late nineteenth century until mid-twentieth century when people such as Gregory Zilboorg, the great psychiatric historian, took center stage. Doctors Andrew Watson, Richard Lonsdorf, Jonas Robitscher, Jay Katz, and Alan Stone, began teaching, not only in medical schools, but also in law schools. Psychiatrists such as Dr. Robitscher, gained law degrees to bolster their credibility and their credentials for teaching the courses in law and psychiatry. Others, such as Dr. Melvin Heller and Professor Samuel Polsky, started the

Unit in Law and Psychiatry at Temple University in the 1950s. Dr. Jonas Rappeport, considered the father of modern forensic psychiatry, developed his clinic in psychiatry and law in Baltimore and taught both at the University of Maryland and at Johns Hopkins.

It was Dr. Rappeport, with several others, who initiated the modern era of rapid growth and proliferation of the field of forensic psychiatry by beginning the American Academy of Psychiatry and the Law (AAPL) in 1969. Dr. Rappeport called together several teachers of forensic psychiatry in order to organize, as a scholarly group, to promote the field of forensic psychiatry, and to aid in the teaching of this growing subspecialty. Three of the original group comprised the membership committee, Doctors Seymour Halleck, Ames Robey, and Robert Sadoff, meeting in 1969, listed 100 potential candidates for membership in the AAPL. Not surprisingly, all 100 agreed and the organization grew exponentially from that point to the present time, at which there are now well over 2500 members worldwide. The newsletter of the AAPL was developed as well as the bulletin of the AAPL, which later became the journal (JAAPL). Other journals, such as *The Journal of Psychiatry and Law*, *The Journal of Forensic Psychiatry*, and *The International Journal of Law and Mental Health* began to publish articles from contributors from around the world.

There have been at least two other organizations of medical/legal interest that preceded the AAPL. One was the American College of Legal Medicine (ACLM) in which the fellows had to be dually degreed both in medicine and law, and consisted primarily of pathologists and other non-psychiatric physicians who had law degrees. The other organization was the American Academy of Forensic Sciences (AAFS), which included members from various medical, legal, and scientific disciplines: forensic odontology, forensic pathology, questioned documents, jurisprudence, and a small group of psychiatrists led by Drs. Meier Tuchler, Seymour Pollack, and Bernard Diamond.

Through the leadership of Dr. Richard Rosner, of New York University, came the development of fellowship training in forensic psychiatry at various university medical centers. Dr. Rosner, through the AAFS and AAPL, coordinated the efforts and initiated the accrediting committee that visited various programs to ensure high quality of training and compliance with required curriculum. Dr. Rosner also led the way to formal examinations of forensic psychiatrists with the inauguration of the American Board of Forensic Psychiatry (ABFP) in the late 1970s. That board certified several scores of forensic psychiatrists until 1994, when its sun set in favor of board certification through the American Board of Psychiatry and Neurology (ABPN). Subspecialty board examinations had been resisted by the American Psychiatric Association until the mid-1990s, when several subspecialty board examinations arose, including that for forensic psychiatry, which became a 10-year certification rather than lifelong as is the certification for general psychiatry.

Scholarly programs that were developed in various institutions became more formalized under the guidance of the Accreditation Council for Graduate Medical Education (ACGME). Currently there are about 40 accredited fellowship training programs in forensic psychiatry throughout the United States. The number of fellows in each program ranges from one to four, and about 75 individuals are trained each year in forensic psychiatry and thus become eligible to take the board certification examination.

Many of the fellowship programs have attorneys on the faculty and are affiliated with law schools in which mental health law or mental disability law is taught. The fellows are expected to know the landmark cases that are developed through the Supreme Court of the United States and other major courts where policy is determined. For example, historically, the concept of the right to treatment, initiated by Dr. Morton Birnbaum in his seminal article, "The Right to Treatment"[3] led to cases such *Donaldson v. O'Connor* (1968)[4] that mandated the right to adequate treatment for those individuals who were involuntarily committed for psychiatric treatment. Other cases followed, including *Washington v. Harper* (1990)[5] and *Sell v U.S.* (2003),[6] which authorized treatment for those criminal defendants who were deemed incompetent to stand trial and who were believed to be able to become competent with appropriate treatment.

Experienced forensic psychiatrists are seen almost daily in news articles about prominent criminal cases in which they testify about the mental state of the defendant at the time of the commission of the charged offense. Forensic psychiatrists have commented on a number of issues facing the community at large, including gun control, torture of terrorist suspects, and death penalty cases. The development of biomedical ethics within forensic psychiatry has also become a major field in which the practice has been regulated through ethical considerations. Issues such as confidentiality, privileged communications, privacy, and informed consent are important, as is the concept of "wearing two hats," in which the treating psychiatrist, in most cases, should not testify as the expert witness for his or her patient.[7] Various textbooks have emerged from both law professors as well as professors of psychiatry and from practicing psychiatrists, and are listed in the Suggested Reading of this book. This book is not a textbook of how to conduct forensic psychiatry, but rather an historical development of the growth and evolution of the field within psychiatry and medicine and how it has been influenced by, and also influenced other subspecialties in psychiatry and other disciplines of scholarly endeavors, such as law, psychology, criminology, nursing, social work, and bioethics.

The past half century has witnessed the burgeoning of forensic psychiatry from the status of "alienism" to that of multidisciplinary science, in which, increasingly, scientific techniques such as neuroimaging and psychological testing have influenced juries in a number of cases. To illustrate not only the growth of forensic psychiatry within medicine and law, but the breadth of its influence spreading to various other fields, this book has authors of chapters from subspecialties in medicine and psychiatry to non-physician specialists who work with forensic psychiatrists in various cases. Perhaps the most common discipline working with the forensic psychiatrist is the forensic psychologist, who often complements the opinions given in particular cases through his or her work conducting interviews as well as a battery of appropriate psychological tests, which are regularly updated and modernized.

Within the psychiatric profession, there are subspecialties that are both paramount to forensic psychiatry but also dovetail and intersect with this growing subspecialty. These include child psychiatry, geriatric psychiatry, social and community psychiatry, correctional psychiatry, addiction psychiatry, consultation and liaison psychiatry, psychosomatic medicine, psychopharmacology, sleep medicine and, most recently, neuroimaging.

Specifically, a psychiatrist specializing in consultation and liaison psychiatry may be asked to examine a person who refuses lifesaving surgery for reasons that appear to be irrational or are based on excessive fear rather than reality. Whether that person is competent to refuse treatment and requires a guardian to make decisions for him, is one that the consultation and liaison psychiatrist is often called upon to make on the surgical floor. The evaluation of competency is clearly a forensic issue and consultation with a forensic psychiatrist may be necessary in some cases. However, many psychiatrists working in consultation and liaison psychiatry have training in forensic issues regarding the assessment of competency. Psychopharmacology is another area of psychiatry that often depends on forensic issues such as malpractice, when improper medication is combined and damage results. Competency determination is also a major concern for the geriatric psychiatrist when dealing with older folks who have dementia and other serious illnesses. Clearly, there is a link between addiction medicine and forensic psychiatry since many of the individuals charged with crime also have serious substance abuse problems. There are also behavioral addictions that require forensic assessment since many become involved in criminal cases.[8] Correctional psychiatrists also have training in forensic work since they obviously come in contact with those who have been charged and convicted of criminal behavior. Perhaps the most common subspecialty of psychiatry that is linked with forensic issues is that of child and adolescent psychiatry. There are now special training programs in forensic psychiatry for the child and adolescent psychiatrist.

One of the purposes of this book is to illustrate how forensic psychiatrists can teach other subspecialists in psychiatry and can learn from them as well. It is the reciprocal education the forensic psychiatrist receives in that he or she learns from each of his colleagues in various subspecialties.

Similarly, forensic psychiatry has had an impact on various other schools of education, including psychology, criminology, law, nursing, social work, and bioethics. This book also contains chapters by specialists in each of these fields illustrating the integrative education and research that occurs between and among these various schools of thought and forensic psychiatry. Finally, translating the research in teaching of the integrative programs at any university, specifically at the University of Pennsylvania, is the application to the criminal justice system and to the civil courts as well. The main goal is to improve the justice system with the integrative knowledge that has been obtained through research, practice, and experience in forensic psychiatry by many other educational programs.

Practicing attorneys, both defense and prosecution, and judges, have also contributed to the education of the forensic psychiatrist. In addition, the same individuals reciprocally have learned from psychiatric experts while working with them in various cases. Through the affiliation of the AAFS, forensic psychiatrists often work with criminalists and crime scene investigators. Pennsylvania State Corporal, George Cronin, Ph.D., presents a chapter in this book on the coordinated efforts of the police investigation team with forensic psychiatric experts.[9]

In keeping with the professional growth of the field, a number of experts in neuroscience elaborate on the utilization of neuroimaging in various aspects of civil and criminal cases. Specifically, brain scans (positron emission tomography and functional magnetic resonance imaging) have been introduced in criminal cases, death penalty cases, and other cases in which violent behavior has occurred.

Thus, the forensic psychiatrist learns from various disciplines and other specialties of psychiatry. In addition, the forensic psychiatrist teaches the same people from whom he learns and there is a reciprocal educational component to the work of the forensic psychiatrist. Several of the outstanding teachers in forensic psychiatry present their work in several chapters of this book. For example, Dr. Philip Resnick from Case Western University teaches the board review course every year at the annual AAPL meetings for fellows and others to strengthen their intellectual background on questions that are likely to be asked on board examinations. Dr. Resnick has given this course and many other courses at the American Psychiatric Association and at the AAPL for many years and is considered the teachers' teacher of forensic psychiatry.

Dr. Thomas Gutheil from Harvard University has been an outstanding teacher, giving many lectures, assisting Dr. Resnick in the board review course and publishing various practical guides for residents in psychiatry and fellows in forensic psychiatry.[10,11] He has also written with Dr. Paul Appelbaum, from Columbia University, textbooks of forensic psychiatry.[12] Dr. Richard Ciccone initiated the Board Review Course and has written on the forensic psychiatrist as teacher.[13] Dr. Charles Scott, has prepared a curriculum for the child forensic psychiatrist which appears in the appendix of this book.[14] He presents the program that he has developed at the University of California-Davis in one of the chapters.

My Training and Teaching in Forensic Psychiatry

My training in forensic psychiatry began in my residency program at UCLA when I was privileged to hear a lecture by one of the pioneers in forensic psychiatry, Dr. Seymour Pollack, who taught at USC. In furtherance of my training, I would travel across town from UCLA to USC to hear him present to his students and residents and also to observe competency examinations that he supervised.

Following my 3 years of training in psychiatry I was inducted in the United States Army as a psychiatrist at Fort Dix, New Jersey, where I was in charge of stockade and courts martial psychiatry from 1963 to 1965. During those 2 years that I was at Fort Dix, I traveled to Temple University in Philadelphia in the evening to the law school to learn how lawyers think about mental health issues. I was privileged to work with Dr. Melvin Heller and Professor Samuel Polsky, who ran the Unit in Law and Psychiatry. Professor Polsky taught courses in mental health law, disability law, and criminal law and psychiatry. I also took courses from other professors on jurisprudence, legal history, conflicts in law, and other courses to support my education in the law. I also worked one half day per week in the Unit in Law and Psychiatry until I was discharged from the army, at which time I took a fellowship year in forensic psychiatry with Dr. Heller and Professor Polsky. During my fellowship year I had the opportunity to conduct research on dangerousness and to publish professional papers.

Following that year, I was named as the first director of the State Maximum Security Forensic Diagnostic Hospital at Holmesburg Prison in Philadelphia. There I was in charge of conducting forensic assessments on individuals confined to the detention center for competency and criminal responsibility. Following those 2 years, I started a private practice of forensic psychiatry and continued teaching law and psychiatry at Temple University until 1972, at which time I transferred to the Villanova University School of Law, where I taught for 13 years, until 1985. I also transferred to the University of Pennsylvania School of Medicine, where I began as a clinical assistant professor of psychiatry and director of the Center for Studies in Social-Legal Psychiatry that had been started by Dr. Jonas Robitscher, a lawyer/psychiatrist who had been named to the first endowed chair in forensic psychiatry: The Henry Luce Chair at Emory University in Atlanta, Georgia.

My course at the Villanova University Law School began as a seminar limited to 25 students so that we could have interactional dialogue and a seminar atmosphere. Because of the popularity of the course, it rose to well over 100 students by the time I finished teaching at Villanova and it became more of a lecture classroom.

I started my work at the University of Pennsylvania Medical School in 1972, I was fortunate to have a fellow in forensic psychiatry come from the United States Naval Base in Philadelphia, taking a full year off in order to study forensic psychiatry. He was followed by two others who worked full-time in conducting research, teaching, and clinical experience in forensic work. We were fortunate to receive grant money for our research and clinical experience from the National Institute of Mental Health and the National Institute of Justice. We developed a forensic psychiatry clinic at Penn where we examined people at the request of the public defender and the Legal Aid Society.

Just as forensic psychiatry has evolved into a major subspecialty of psychiatry with roles in many areas of civil and criminal law, so too did the program at the University of Pennsylvania grow and develop into a major section in the Department of Psychiatry. We were very fortunate to have outstanding students at Penn who maintained an interest in and a commitment to forensic psychiatry. Dr. Annie Steinberg, a pediatrician and child psychiatrist, has worked diligently in forensic child and adolescent psychiatry for several decades and is currently heading our subdivision of child and adolescent forensic psychiatry, a growing program in which we train child and adolescent psychiatrists as well as adult forensic psychiatrists. Dr. Kenneth Weiss, who had studied with us several decades ago, continued his teaching at Penn and is currently associate director of the Forensic Psychiatry fellowship Program. Dr. Henry Bleier, an outstanding teacher at Penn, affiliated with the VA Hospital in consultation and liaison psychiatry, has continued his interest and teaching in forensic psychiatry and heads our subdivision of Consultation and Liaison Forensic Psychiatry. Several other outstanding students who took residency in psychiatry at the University of Pennsylvania went on to distinguish themselves as forensic psychiatrists in other parts of the country, developing their own forensic psychiatry fellowship programs and teaching in others.

Much of the early teaching of forensic psychiatry was through mentoring. I was mentored by Dr. Melvin Heller and I was fortunate enough to mentor such distinguished forensic psychiatrists as Dr. Stephen Billick, currently one of the leading child and adolescent forensic psychiatrists teaching in the fellowship programs at New York University, Columbia University, and New York Medical School. Dr. Billick in turn mentored Dr. Zachary Torry, who later became one of our forensic psychiatry fellows and is now working as a forensic psychiatrist on the west coast.

The training involved clinical examinations of criminal and civil cases, some involving traveling long distances where we conducted "traveling seminars" while driving to and from various institutions where people were examined under supervision.

One of the other major teaching experiences for medical students, psychiatry residents, and fellows in forensic psychiatry, has been the seminar "Practical Applications of Forensic Psychiatry" that has now been ongoing for more than 30 years and provides category one credits to a number of psychiatrists practicing in the Philadelphia area who participate in the seminar. Currently, that seminar is an interdisciplinary mode of teaching that includes professors from various schools within the university, including the law school, psychology, criminology, bioethics, nursing, social policy and practice, and neuroscience. Private attorneys are also guest lecturers as well as judges and colleagues from around the country.

Since the advent of the forensic psychiatry fellowship programs that began many years ago, we have considered beginning a program at the University of Pennsylvania and were successful in launching the program with one fellow in 2009. We now have three fellows in forensic psychiatry, one a fully trained child and adolescent psychiatrist. In addition to the didactic and academic work, the clinical experience is obtained through affiliation with various institutions in the community including the Philadelphia Court Clinic that was initiated by Dr. Melvin Heller several decades ago. The fellows obtain experience in conducting short-term competency examinations on defendants brought to the clinic for evaluation. The fellows also find clinical experience with juveniles at the Youth Study Center and at Family Court. The affiliation with the Joseph J. Peters Institute offers clinical experience in evaluating sex offenders and victims of sexual violence. Dr. Steven Berkowitz, a prominent child psychiatrist specializing in child trauma, trains our fellows at the Pennsylvania Hospital in evaluating juvenile trauma. The program has an affiliation with two major forensic psychiatric centers: The Delaware Psychiatric Center where Dr. Clarence Watson, a prominent lawyer/psychiatrist, directs the training and mentors the fellows in Wilmington, Delaware. The other forensic center is the Ann Klein Forensic Center in Trenton, New Jersey, where Dr. Elizabeth Hogan and other psychiatrists and forensic psychiatrists train our fellows. It is significant to note that at least two of our former fellows are now full-time faculty at the Ann Klein Forensic Center. The fellows also affiliate with the Veteran's Administration Hospital where Dr. Henry Bleier, one of the outstanding teachers in the Department of Psychiatry, mentors our fellows in consultation and liaison psychiatry and the treatment of veterans who return from combat with post traumatic stress disorder.

The fellows also take courses at the law school, primarily the course of Professor Stephen Morse and are also trained by Professor Michael Perlin from New York Law School, one of the most prolific authors on mental health law.

In addition to the extensive clinical experience, the fellows are also given lectures by many of our faculty and from faculty members of different schools within the university, including law, nursing, psychology, criminology, biomedical ethics, social policy and practice, and neuroscience. There are psychiatrists and lawyers on the faculty who train the fellows in the significance of legal cases and the landmark cases in forensic psychiatry.

Plans are underway to develop a Center for Forensic Psychiatry at the University of Pennsylvania that will include many of the schools outside of psychiatry, including medicine, law, psychology, criminology nursing, biomedical ethics, social policy and practice, communications, and neuroscience. The integration of various schools with forensic psychiatry will enable interdisciplinary research and teaching among the schools and also provide translational consultation to the criminal and civil court system in the community in order to improve the quality of justice. The fellows have been involved in evaluating cases under *Miller vs. Alabama*,[15] which has been successful in keeping juveniles from a sentence of life without parole. We have also consulted with school systems to prevent violence by students or faculty. We are also concerned about suicide among the students at various schools and have provided consultation and guidance to the providers of care in order to prevent further self-destructive behavior.

In summary, this book illustrates the evolution of forensic psychiatry to the point where the forensic psychiatrist is involved in a number of different subdivisions of psychiatry and in other specialties that involve legal proceedings. The teaching of forensic psychiatry must include a vast number of specialties. The future of forensic psychiatry will include the use of newer technology such as videoconferencing, telemedicine, and neuroimaging. The forensic psychiatrist has evolved from the "alienist" to a multidisciplinary scientist. Education, training, and clinical experiences will need to keep pace with the ever-growing and expanding subspecialty if effective consultation with the justice system is to occur. The American Academy of Psychiatry and the Law will continue to serve as a national resource center for education and interdisciplinary communication to strengthen the profession.

—Robert L. Sadoff, M.D.

References

1. American Academy of Psychiatry and the Law, Ethics Committee. (2005). Bloomfield, CT.
2. Weiss K. (2015). American forensic psychiatry begins: Setting standards. In RL Sadoff (Ed.), *Evolution ofForensic psychiatry: history, current developments, future directions*. New York: Oxford University Press.
3. Birnbaum M. (1960). The right to treatment. *Amer Bar Assoc J*, *46*, 499–505.
4. *Donaldson v. O'Connor*. (1974). 493 F. 2d 507.
5. *Washington v. Harper*. (1990). 494 U. S. 210, 110 S. Ct. 1028.
6. *Sell v. U.S.* (2003). 123 S. Ct. 2174.
7. Strasburger L, Gutheil TG, & Brodsky A. (1997). On wearing two hats: role conflict in serving as both psychotherapist and expert witness. *Am J Psychiatry*, 154, 448–456.
8. Sadoff RL, Drogin EY, & Gurmu S. (2014). Forensic implications of behavioral addictions. In M Ascher, & P Levounis (Eds.), *The behavioral addictions casebook*. Washington, DC: American Psychiatric Press.
9. Cronin G. (2015). Forensic psychiatry in law enforcement: A practitioner's perspective. In RL Sadoff (Ed.), *Forensic psychiatry: Historical review, current developments, future directions*. New York: Oxford University Press.
10. Gutheil TG. (1998a). *The psychiatrist as expert witness*. Washington, DC: American Psychiatric Press.

11. Gutheil TG. (1998b). *The psychiatrist in court: A survival guide.* Washington, DC: American Psychiatric Press.
12. Gutheil TG, & Appelbaum P. (2008). *Clinical handbook of psychiatry and the law* (3d ed.). New York: McGraw-Hill.
13. Ciccone JR, & Jones JCW. (2012). The teaching roles of the forensic psychiatrist. *J Psychiatry Law, 40,* 167–184.
14. Scott C. (2011). The child and adolescent track in the forensic fellowship. *Child Adolesc Psychiatric Clin North Am, 20,* 565–575.
15. *Miller v. Alabama.* (2012). 132 S. Ct. 2455.

SECTION ONE

History

1

American Forensic Psychiatry Begins

Setting Standards

Kenneth J. Weiss

How did forensic psychiatry begin in America? What are its roots and who drafted the blueprint? Was its inception a wholesale import of European ideas or minted from fresh local sources? In this magnificent volume, Dr. Sadoff and colleagues have traced the evolution of psychiatry's often uncomfortable but decidedly necessary fellowship with the law. There is consensus that the signal event propelling forensic psychiatry into the forefront of psychiatry was the publication of Isaac Ray's *A Treatise on the Medical Jurisprudence of Insanity* in 1838.[1] This was several years before M'Naghten's trial at The Old Bailey in London (1843) and the founding of the Association of Medical Superintendents of American Institutions for the Insane (AMSAII, the forerunner of the American Psychiatric Association [APA]) in 1844 in Philadelphia. Oddly, Ray, untrained in the law, had yet to obtain employment as an asylum doctor, which he did in Augusta, Maine in 1841.

To say that he was a savant and ahead of his time barely captures the fact that he set the table for an agenda that still preoccupies our profession. In his review of legal aspects of psychiatry for the hundredth anniversary of the APA, Zilboorg speaks reverentially of Ray's qualities.[2] At the same time, it is apparent that Ray did not forge forensic psychiatry alone. His work was shaped by dialectics that continue to render expert witnesses uneasy in their chairs: the natural tension between the aims of medicine and the law, the degree to which medicine can improve jurisprudence, the ethics of practice, and the ambiguity present in psychiatric concepts. In this brief introduction, I will highlight a few key concepts introduced in the nineteenth century that formed the basis for contemporary forensic psychiatry.

American Psychiatry and the Law: Homegrown or European Import?

While the 30-year-old Isaac Ray was composing his remarkable compendium from remote Eastport, Maine, there was little American case law and virtually no guidance from the medical profession. Luckily, Eastport, the easternmost town in America, was convenient for receiving shipments of materials from Boston and across the Atlantic. Ray was eager to present the panorama of psychiatric relations to the law, pressing on colleagues to send him the latest examples of the jurisprudence of insanity.[3] Not only did he do so, he organized the history of the jurisprudence of psychiatry and presented current nomenclature. In short, Ray drew the blueprint for forensic psychiatry before he had seen his first case. Zilboorg, writing in 1944, observed of the *Treatise*, "The spirit of the work, the general attitude of the psychiatrist toward the prevailing legal traditions in relation to the mentally ill, seem not only familiar to the present-day psychiatrist but even at times contemporary—all this despite the fact that the book was written by a young general medical man over one hundred years ago" (Ref. 2, p. 547).

Causes of Insanity in the Organs of the Mind

It had been increasingly apparent to scientists since the late eighteenth century that the brain was somehow responsible for human behavior. Although the flawed pseudoscience of phrenology failed to provide a meaningful basis for jurisprudence,[4] Ray was captivated by its compatibility with a materialist philosophy that linked mental disease and behavior.[5] In his *Treatise* he melded his trust in science to discover the medical bases of mental disease with the European idea that any "organ" of the mind could become deranged, thereby producing insanity. If insanity could take various forms, it might best explain otherwise culpable behaviors to juries and judges. Here is an example of Ray's appeal to common sense in appreciating the varieties of mental derangement:

> No inconsiderable portion of the insane know perfectly well when they do wrong, and may be deterred therefrom by the fear of punishment or deprivation of privileges. Ask a patient, after recovery, if he did not know at the time, that certain acts of his were wrong, and often the answer will be "yes." "Did you then feel constrained by an irresistible impulse to act in spite of your convictions?" "No. I acted as I did, because it gave me pleasure; I suppose the devil was in me." When will the world recognize the truth, as well established as any in nature, that insanity not only impairs the intellectual or reasoning power, but perverts the moral faculties, vitiating the tastes and sentiments, and furnishing strange motives and impulses,—in one word, transforming the man into a fiend. (Ref. 1, p. 460)

Ray was convinced that derangements of emotion were on par with those of reason, a definite European import. Thus, whereas delusions could produce insane acts, as Ray knew from England's *Hadfield* case of 1800, so too could overwhelming passions. The latter, "moral insanity," strongly supported by Ray, was vigorously debated in America.[2] Its principal opponent, Dr. John Purdue Gray, longstanding editor of the *Journal of Insanity*, viewed Ray as a nemesis.[7] The battle of these titans could have taken place during the trial of Charles Guiteau, President Garfield's assassin, in 1881 and 1882. But Ray died earlier in 1881, leaving the battle to others who ultimately failed to convince the jury that Guiteau, while able to reason, was otherwise insane.[8]

Ray's *Treatise*, the first American textbook of forensic psychiatry, was an instant success. It was promptly republished in Edinburgh, Scotland, a bastion of phrenology, where Benjamin Rush had received his medical education. There had been celebrated trials in London in which insanity had been considered in relation to acts of high treason against royalty.[9] By the time of the *Treatise*'s Edinburgh publication in 1839, there was much concern about the legal standard for acquittal by reason of insanity. Within the British justice system there was room for both delusional and moral insanity as grounds for acquittal. The pendulum had swung from the restrictive "wild beast test"[10] to more liberal interpretations of insanity. Accordingly, when Glaswegian Daniel M'Naghten shot and killed the English Prime minister's secretary under the influence of mental disease, his lawyer, Alexander Cockburn, used Ray's *Treatise* as an authority on jurisprudence.[11] In the book, Ray laid out his analysis of the famous insanity trials in England to date: Arnold in 1724, Ferrers in 1760, Hadfield in 1800, and Bellingham in 1812.[11] In his book, Ray made it clear that tests for insanity were clinical matters for medical types to define, not legislators. For further scholarly treatment of the development of tests for criminal responsibility, the interested reader is directed to Diamond and Platt's review through mid-twentieth century and to Perlin's comprehensive work.[12,13]

Cockburn's arguments, detailed in Diamond's analysis,[11] were quite successful from an advocacy viewpoint. Two neutral experts hearing the medical testimony and observing M'Naghten in court but, like Ray, not having personally examined him, agreed with the defense arguments and informed the court; there was no opposing testimony. Lord Chief Justice Tindal was sufficiently impressed to halt the proceedings: "We feel the evidence, especially of the last two gentlemen who have been examined, and who are strangers to both sides, and only observers of the case, to be very strong, and sufficient to induce my learned brother and myself to stop the case" (Ref. 11, p. 654). The jury returned a verdict of "not guilty, on the ground of insanity."

M'Naghten's acquittal, while a boon to Cockburn's career (he was knighted in 1850 and in 1859 elevated to Lord Chief Justice of the Queen's Bench), ignited a firestorm of what Diamond considered "totally unjustified criticism" in the press.[11] Queen Victoria herself wrote to Prime Minister Peel (M'Naghten's intended victim) in protest.[11] The residual effect of the verdict was the formulation by the House of Lords of M'Naghten's Rules, the most famous of which is the standard for insanity acquittal. The standard restricts its focus to a cognitive test, whether the accused knew the nature and quality of the act or that it was wrong. One could say, without blaming Isaac Ray, that the repercussions of M'Naghten's acquittal solidified the use of the cognitive test in America.[2] Some version of the test had been used in American courts since 1816,[12] but it would take decades before Isaac Ray was able to reinsert moral insanity into the range of options for jurors—at least those in New Hampshire.[14]

Writing in 1956, Diamond surveyed the landscape of jurisprudence in criminal matters and the significance of Ray's early work:

> It is safe to say that never since, in an English or an American courtroom, has a scientific work by a psychiatrist been treated with such respect as was The Medical Jurisprudence of Insanity. Out of the public and parliamentary indignation over M'Naghten's acquittal came the celebrated opinion of the Judges, and the resulting so-called M'Naghten Rules superseding all earlier legal tests, have, since 1843, constituted the essential criteria for determining criminal responsibility or irresponsibility in all English-speaking countries. Of late they have been brought under considerable criticism, especially in the United States. (Ref. 11, p. 655)

By the time of publication of Diamond's historical note, the matter of changing the test for insanity had been answered in federal jurisdiction via Judge Bazelon's decision in *Durham v. U.S.*[15] That decision, which remained in effect until 1972, permitted broad analyses of mental states, such that insanity could be proved if the criminal act in question had been the product of mental disease or defect. This was similar to the New Hampshire standard Ray helped Judge Doe to craft. As Perlin observed, *Durham* represented a "no rule" standard, giving rise to interpretation of "product." This ambiguity led to its being superseded by a more definite standard in *U.S. v. Brawner*,[16] specifically the two-pronged American Law Institute test for insanity, in 1972. Containing both a *cognitive* and a *volitional* prong, the *Brawner* standard was replaced in 1984 by the Insanity Defense Reform Act (for the federal jurisdiction) after President Reagan's near-assassination.

M'Naghten and Forensic Standards

Many readers will be in *M'Naghten* jurisdictions. The debates about the standard's utility and conformity to science continue, as Morse[17] has observed: "Much scholarly ink has been spilled and many pixels illuminated about specific issues within *M'Naghten* and its variants...." (p 927). Some principles emerge from *M'Naghten's Case* that will be familiar to today's practitioners. The first is that, no matter how much maligned a legal standard may be, jurisprudence in the corresponding jurisdiction must follow. Perlin[13] compiled a list of critical comments on the rule: "'untrustworthy,' a 'façade,' 'absolutist,' an illustration of 'a fiction being a fetish,' 'an absurd dictum which has long been discredited by medical science,' and 'outmoded and unrealistic'" (p 81). Nevertheless, if the expert witness believes that the defendant was suffering from a mental disease that produced an irresistible impulse to kill, for example, such testimony must be reserved for mitigation. The testimony, if offered at trial, will be barred; or worse, the defendant will have been led down a garden path to peril. Isaac Ray was aware that medical testimony in mitigation is often the most helpful placement, when he tried to delay the hanging of a convict with epilepsy.[18]

Second, while Ray preferred the French justice system to the English,[2] we can see that M'Naghten's trial avoided a battle of the experts—remarkable, given the publicity of the case. Instead, the jury heard medical testimony on the question of insanity, the judge deferred to two impartial experts, and the prosecutor acquiesced. American jurisprudence has never adopted a style of medical evidence that is nonpartisan in nature, despite serious attempts at reform.[19] Yet, the template was available but the road not taken.

Third, public outcry among citizens to eliminate "getting away with murder," followed by legislative crackdowns to restrict or eliminate the insanity defense, run counter to legal traditions and in America may represent a violation of due-process rights.[20] Whenever practicable, then, forensic psychiatrists have an obligation to follow Isaac Ray's lead and promote the introduction of science into the dialog about criminal responsibility. However, our enthusiasm must be tempered by the reality, as Morse[20] notes, "Causation is not *per se* an excusing condition in criminal law."

Forensic Principles Appear in Print

Before Isaac Ray graduated from medical school in Maine in 1827, medical jurisprudence was already a topic worthy of attention in America. Gold observed that, by 1840, most American medical schools had courses in medical jurisprudence, and that nearly all of the courses addressed insanity.[21] Dr. T. Romeyn Beck undertook to summarize knowledge in a massive work first published in 1823: *Elements of Medical Jurisprudence*.[22] Beck, teaching at the medical school in Geneva, New York, was later persuaded to become the second editor of the *Journal of Insanity* in 1849 after the death of its founder, Amariah Brigham.[23] Not a psychiatrist, Beck had great respect for the importance of mental life in the adjudications of age-old legal problems. Gold quoted his comment on experts: "It need hardly be suggested that in many instances, a legal decision depends on the testimony of medical witnesses" (Ref. 21, p. 19).

Beck remained editor of the *Journal* until 1854, when John P. Gray began his tenure of 32 years. Meanwhile, Beck's *Elements* enjoyed a long life as the first American text on the subject. Ray referred to the 1823 book in his 1838 *Treatise*, noting Beck's opinion on the relationship of voluntary intoxication to criminal culpability. In a parallel development from the legal side, Francis Wharton, a legal scholar in Philadelphia, with the help of physician Dr. Moreton Stillé, published a *Treatise on Medical Jurisprudence* in 1855.[24] Of interest is that their first section was on mental unsoundness. Wharton, who respected the importance of mental states in legal matters, was a leading thinker in matters such as involuntary confessions[25] and culpability of persons during sleep[26] and, like Ray, remains vital.[27]

It was not simply a matter of Beck's *Elements* being first; his subject matter took an unflinching look at humanity and the sordid predicaments brought to justice. Looking at the contents of the 1825 second edition,[28] the following stand out: feigned diseases, impotence and sterility, doubtful sex, rape, infanticide, legitimacy, and mental alienation (insanity). Taking his simplified nomenclature from Esquirol (Mania, Melancholia [or Monomania], Dementia, and Idiocy), he divided the jurisprudence of insanity into categories that will appear familiar: (1) The symptoms that constitute a state of insanity; (2) of feigned and concealed insanity; (3) of the legal definition of a state of mental alienation, and the adjudications under it; (4) of inferior degrees of diseased mind; (5) of the state of mind necessary to constitute a valid will; and (6) of the deaf and dumb—their capacity, and the morality of their actions (Ref. 28, p. 227).

Beck based the diagnosis of *insanity* (then a medical determination, whereas now a purely legal term) on observed behaviors and physical findings. For example, he cited Benjamin Rush's correlations of medical findings to mania: "Dr. Rush mentions, that Dr. Moore, at his request, examined the maniacs in the Pennsylvania Hospital, with reference to this symptom [nasal mucus], and found it present in two-thirds of them.... Maniacs also endure a degree of heat and cold, which to a sane person would be inconvenient and even distressing" (Ref. 28, p. 229). More to the issue of delusions and behavior, Beck relied on the observations of Dr. John Haslam, who had written about English medical jurisprudence in 1817.[29]

> Haslam observes, that he scarcely recollects an instance of a lunatic becoming blind, but numbers are deaf; and those who are not deaf, are troubled with difficulty of hearing, and tinnitus aurium. It is from the disorder of this organ, and which is referable to the original diseased action of the functions of the brain, that many maniacs derive the delusion under which they labour. The commission which they suppose themselves to receive from some superior being, is given by the ear—they imagine it is constantly repeated. They are thus, they imagine, urged to its performance, and, in too many cases, murder or self-destruction is the unhappy result. (Ref. 28, p. 229)

It is of interest to note here that Beck was following a tradition of being mindful of persons feigning insanity, a topic later continued by Ray and that has been a perennial concern to forensic experts and attorneys. In his 1838 Sixth Edition,[30] Beck displayed his insight: "The medical witness is often required to decide on the actual existence of insanity, and it, therefore, behooves him to be well acquainted with its actual symptoms" (Ref. 30, p. 405). A partial list of "symptoms" to rule out malingering included:

> Insanity is seldom sudden in its attacks.... With the feigned... they are sudden, abrupt, and violent.... The deception is not maintained when the pretenders are alone and unwatched—the assumed malady then disappears.... Pretenders will often outstrip madness itself.... They overdo their part.... Real lunatics, at the period of remission, are desirous of being deemed free of their malady.... The feigned never desire to conceal their condition.... The physician should endeavor to obtain from the individual, a history of himself (Ref. 30, pp. 405–406).

Beck endorsed the teachings of Pinel and Esquirol. By adhering to the French nomenclature, as Ray would do too contemporaneously, Beck endorsed partial insanity or monomania, as well as conditions of mania that might tend to excuse criminal behavior. These conditions represented mental states of unclouded consciousness but with intense feelings and urges, such as those possessed by M'Naghten. As noted earlier, the moral insanity argument was quashed by Dr. Gray, who was Beck's successor at the Utica-based *Journal*. Because standards for insanity adjudications vary by jurisdiction, it behooves expert witnesses to be familiar with them in each case.[31]

In the civil domain, Beck discussed testamentary capacity, urging careful and comprehensive clinical assessment: "The symptoms—the state of the individual, his conversation and actions, should all be canvassed, and from them an opinion must be formed" (Ref. 30, p. 464). He linked unsoundness of mind with physical illnesses, in addition to drunkenness and idiocy; for example, "Among the diseases which incapacitate an individual from making a valid will, or at least render his rationality doubtful, may be enumerated the following: lethargic and comatose affections... an attack of apoplexy... phrenitis, delirium tremens... typhoid fever... [and] phthisis pulmonalis" (Ref. 30, pp. 463–464). The emerging standard of establishing causal links between demonstrable diseases and specific functional capacities has persisted and evolved.

Psychiatry Stakes a Claim

How did American psychiatrists regard forensic matters in the nineteenth century? One need look no further than the first volume of the *American Journal of Insanity* in 1844 to find an agenda for forensic psychiatry. In an article entitled *Medical Jurisprudence of Insanity*, Coventry sketched applications for expert testimony and published answers of the 15 English judges to the questions posed by the post-*M'Naghten* House of Lords, all in 11 pages.[32] Coventry, like Beck, taught medical jurisprudence in Geneva, New York. In an otherwise anecdotal and uninspired article, lacking Ray's gravitas (and failing to mention his colleague), the author lists four areas of concern for potential expert witnesses: (1) criminal responsibility: "The plea of insanity as a bar to punishment in criminal prosecution"; (2) civil commitment: "The propriety of confinement when danger to the individual himself or to others is apprehended"; (3) general civil competency: "The capacity and right of an insane person, or one supposed to be insane, of managing his own affairs"; and (4) testamentary capacity: "The state of mind necessary to constitute a valid will" (p 134).

It is no exaggeration to state that psychiatry's agenda was tightly bound to jurisprudence in the early days of the superintendents' Association. The adjudication of disputes and conflicts had long required expert knowledge. And since human qualities and capacities were often at issue—for example, whether a person was culpable under the law—early psychiatrists were forced to learn that their diagnoses and testimony played a role in the resolution of the situation without invading the domain of the jury or judge. Looking at the application of psychiatric testimony to the criminal law, Zilboorg identified the core issues in the structure of justice:

> The history of this conflict is the history of the medical jurisprudence of insanity, for it is around this conflict that we find all the constellations of psychological, scientific, sociological, and cultural contradictions which have accumulated through the

> ages of human social life, all the isomeres of prejudice and bigotry and hate which are brought into play when man becomes a felon, and finally all the anxiety which society experiences when scientific knowledge calls upon man to be objective in the face of the most destructive aspects of human nature. Society seems to be afraid even to forgive a sin, particularly when science declines to accuse. (Ref. 2, p. 514)

Returning to Coventry's four agenda items, we see that, whereas the first deals with criminal responsibility, the others cover civil areas. In the third issue of the *Journal*, Dr. Buttolph reported on the 1844 murder trial of Abner Rogers, Jr.;[33] concurrently, Isaac Ray, a witness in the case, reported his findings in a law journal.[6] In the same issue there was a discussion of presenting postmortem findings, based on an understanding of physiology, in a proper way for court.[34] The following conveys the degree of sophistication in medical jurisprudence in 1844 and the seriousness of forensic considerations among AMSAII members.

> *The Abner Rogers Trial:*[33] The defendant was a repeat offender confined to the State Prison in Massachusetts, where, in 1843, he killed the warden by stabbing. The prison doctor testified that Rogers was a malingerer and that he had tried to deceive the doctor into thinking he was mentally ill. In the four months before the homicide, Rogers came to the infirmary 12 times. Within three days of the incident, he appeared agitated, possibly delusional, and hearing voices. That day he made repeated requests to see the warden.
>
> Dr. Luther Bell, superintendent of McLean Asylum and AMSAII founder, examined Rogers two days after the incident, and four times more. He documented many psychotic symptoms, including bizarre phrasing, delusions, and derogatory auditory hallucinations. He attended the trial and heard the evidence. Beforehand, he would have thought the killing was done by an ordinary person. Now, he believed that this was a form of insanity that was well known, but not to the general public and, therefore, not easily feigned.
>
> Dr. Samuel B. Woodward of Worcester, another AMSAII founder, also heard the testimony and testified. He said the defendant was insane, a case of monomania arising from hallucinations, difficult to feign. His formulation was that when he saw the victim with a stranger he imagined that his time had come for punishment. Then he "felt an irresistible impulse to the homicidal act. My experience would lead me to think that all his thoughts were engrossed by this one act of punishment, and that his other controlling motives, for the time being, ceased to act." (Ref. 33, p. 267)
>
> Dr. Ray of Maine, also an AMSAII founder, heard the testimony and testified. He said: "... I believe the defendant was insane at the time of the homicide. I have not heard a single fact testified to in regard to him, during the week of the homicide, which I consider incompatible with his insanity. [Another fact] struck me forcibly: that there seemed to be no constant effort on his part to convey the impression that he was insane. In regard to the physical symptoms, I should say that these showed that something was the matter with the man. The state of

> his pulse, his coated tongue, and shrunken features, plainly showed that he was diseased in some way. I think I never saw, heard, or read, of a case of simulation of this kind. It would be extremely difficult to counterfeit it so as not to be detected." (Ref. 33, pp. 267–268)
>
> The judge's charge to the jury is interesting, including this clarification of the experts' role: "The opinions of professional men on a question of this description are competent evidence, and in many cases are entitled to great consideration and respect. The rule of law, on which this proof of the opinion of witnesses, who know nothing of the actual facts of the case, is founded, is not peculiar to medical testimony, but is a general rule, applicable to all cases, when the question is one depending on skill and science, in any peculiar department" (Ref. 33, p. 270). The jury found Rogers insane and he was committed to the hospital in Worcester, where he died a violent death months later. In Ray's account, he doubted that the judge had been aware of the M'Naghten Rule, which would have limited the testimony to the defendant's knowledge of the wrongfulness of his actions.[6] Instead, the test in Massachusetts was a mélange of commonsense operational definitions of lack of culpability: "A person is not responsible for any criminal act he may commit, if by reason of mental infirmity he is incapable of distinguishing between right and wrong in regard to the particular act, and of knowing that the act itself will subject him to punishment; or, has no will, no conscience, or controlling, mental power; or, has not sufficient power of memory to recollect the relations in which he stands to others and in which they stand to him; or, has his reason, conscience and judgment so overwhelmed by the violence of the disease, as to act on an irresistible, uncontrollable impulse." (Ref. 6, pp. 459–460)

The question of rights of the individual, when well or incapacitated, was very much on the minds of our founders, as Coventry pointed out. Although space limitations prevent a full treatment of civil commitment and capacities, it is worthwhile to outline the developments of these areas within forensic psychiatry, discussed at length by Zilboorg.[2] The nineteenth century witnessed a growing industry of psychiatrists analyzing the state of mind in will contests. The practice of judging testamentary capacity produced newsworthy material when large sums were at stake. Expert reports on the issue could occupy hundreds of pages,[35] and were among the favorite activities of Isaac Ray.[2] Summarizing his thoughts on the importance of expert scrutiny of claims of senility toward the end of his career, Ray cautioned against equating aging with senility and promoted science over legal tradition in adjudicating such matters.[2,36]

The question of the rights of the mentally ill, especially civil commitment, is "intimately woven into the history of psychiatry" (Ref. 2, p. 528). Psychiatry was as interested in the matter in the mid-nineteenth century as it was a century later. The interested reader is referred to Albert Deutsch's classic *The Mentally Ill in America*.[37] As now, there were stakeholders who were often at odds: patients, their families, doctors, asylums, state legislatures, and rights advocates, for example. The basic premises have not changed: a mentally ill and dangerous person can be deprived of freedom under the law. However, medical paternalism should not trump civil rights; nor should the domination of wives by husbands or the powerless by the greedy. Isaac Ray, for example, in his tireless campaign to reform civil commitment, would put medical judgment ahead of the wishes of other stakeholders and believed that it was a mistake to construct civil proceedings as if they were criminal. Having proposed a scheme for commitment procedures (among other things) to AMSAII in 1850,[38,39] it took many years for his "project" to get out of committee.[40] Ray's 1850 proposal was a more efficient scheme than that proposed by the English:

> In England the Lord Chancellor appoints a committee of five persons, one of them, a barrister at law, with whom is associated a jury of twelve men summoned by the sheriff. The jury hear the evidence and render their verdict to the commissioners who sit as a court, by whom the proceedings are reported to the chancellor. This certainly is too cumbersome and expensive a proceeding for this country, while it is quite probable that the rights of individuals would be as well protected by a more summary process. I would propose a commission of not less than four nor more than six persons, one of them a lawyer and another a physician, for the purpose of giving a suitable direction to the inquisition, who should have the party brought before them, hear the testimony, and render a decision accordingly. (Ref. 40, p. 223)

Ray's recommendations for civil commitment built in more protections for citizens than did older customs of commitment via a doctor's or spouse's say-so. Suspicion surrounding the circumstances of commitment and the potential for abuse had been growing.[2] Several years before Ray's project, the case of Morgan Hinchman, a patient at the Friends Asylum in Philadelphia brought attention to the commitment process and rights of the individual. In the *Hinchman* case, brought to[41] life by D'Antonio, the patient sued his family, friends, and doctors for false imprisonment. Admitted after his family got a physician who had not seen him for a year, Hinchman was essentially railroaded into the asylum, where he complained that his family was robbing him. His lawsuit brought out the truth of his claims and he won a judgment against his family, whereas the doctors were not liable.

While Ray's project was dormant in the superintendents' Association, the case of Elizabeth P.W. Packard was prominent. She had been confined from 1860 to 1863 at the Illinois State Hospital by her husband on what turned out to be flimsy grounds. When her husband threatened to move her out of state, she brought a legal action via habeas corpus and had a trial in 1864.[42] Testifying that she was never insane, the jury agreed and the taint of insanity was removed. Afterward, she continued her campaign to change the law of Illinois (and elsewhere) in the direction of having trials for anyone "accused" of being insane. The legislature complied and enacted a law in 1867 ostensibly to protect women and the insane from nefarious acts. As Deutsch observed, however, "the remedy proved worse than the condition it was supposed to cure" (Ref. 37, p. 307). The law, which left commitment decisions to lay juries, had a chilling effect on families' decisions to seek treatment for mentally ill relatives—not to mention the scorn of the psychiatric community.[2,37]

In terms of setting standards, Isaac Ray was once again at the forefront. Although he respected the rights of individuals, some of his attitudes ran counter to those of other stakeholders. Distrustful of judges and jurors, who knew little about psychiatry, Ray wanted minimal input from legal types while opposing a system of railroading citizens into asylums. He definitely opposed Mrs. Packard, who was distrustful of doctors and used her own trial as a template for civil commitment proceedings. In retrospect, Mrs. Packard did much to draw attention to a form of women's oppression that was condoned by doctors, whereas her model of adjudication was too problematic. Ray despised the habeas corpus solution to patients' rights and made it clear that physicians were uniquely qualified to judge sanity.[3] Nevertheless, we can see from the scenarios from mid-nineteenth century that psychiatry and the legal system struggled uncomfortably to meld their goals and methods.

General and Forensic Psychiatry Go to School Together

As Gold pointed out, the basis of forensic psychiatry is general psychiatry.[21] As noted, the AMSAII members' agenda, reflected in the *Journal of Insanity*, included in-depth discussions of trials and applications of psychiatry to jurisprudence. Although AMSAII appeared in 1844, medical jurisprudence had already made its way into medical education; for example, via Beck and others. Indeed, Beck reviewed several books on medical jurisprudence over two issues of the *Journal* in 1845.[43] Looking at the contents of the January 1846 issue, it is apparent that the editors placed medicolegal education well within general psychiatry. Topics included brain physiology and pathology, the authority to restrain the insane, and homicidal insanity.

Beck also introduced synopses of legal decisions into the *Journal*; for example, in an 1853 issue.[44] The first case, from New York State involved testamentary capacity and undue influence. The court ruled that state of mind could be inferred from competently given lay testimony. The second, a Mississippi case, asked whether a woman was insane when she entered into a marriage. Again, no expert witnesses were required, and lay testimony proved she was sane. The third, a Maryland case of a man with religious eccentricities, inquired of his testamentary capacity. Some of his actions, lay witnesses said, had been animated by the voice of God telling him to do various things with his possessions. Although the court found him of sound mind, Beck commented on an apparent disparity between what might be considered insanity in civil versus criminal cases:

> With all due humility, we ask this question: if whether John Townshend had killed a person, his *sanity*, would with the above testimony, have ever been acknowledged? Certainly not. And here, as we have elsewhere remarked, there is a remarkable distinction taken between civil and criminal cases in this respect. Still the decision is usually with juries, and of course we can only anticipate a continuance of the diversity (Ref. 44, p. 183).

It is safe to conclude that Beck, like Ray, appreciated the capriciousness of the jury system—perhaps all the more reason for early psychiatrists to support the use of expert testimony in technical matters.

About 20 years after AMSAII formed in Philadelphia, at least one medical school could boast a dedicated curriculum in mental disorders. Pliny Earle, addressing the Berkshire Medical Institute in 1863,[45] noted misconceptions that had kept the subject from prominence: the ideas that insanity was rare and that a general practitioner would never have occasion to encounter a patient with it. Waging what amounted to a military assault against ignorance, he was ready to claim victory:

> True, some three or four raids, in the shape of summer or sub-courses of lectures upon mental disorders, have been made upon them by the physicians; but, in every instance, the invading party was so weak that a retreat was soon ordered, and the territory was again abandoned to its position of neutrality. But... in the autumn of 1863, the Berkshire Medical College came manfully from its stronghold, and surrendered unconditionally without a battle. (Ref. 45, p. 5).

After congratulating Berkshire on its forward thinking and refuting the notion that knowledge of "craziness" was self-evident and unworthy of study, Earle turned to the application of psychiatry to legal settings. In this passage, he predicted dicey outcomes when ill-prepared witnesses come to court:

> [I]n trials for homicide, where the plea of insanity has been raised in favor of the prisoner at the bar, many physicians who had neither studied the subject in the schools nor had any considerable practical acquaintance with it, and, doubtless, in some instances, without having read a treatise upon it, have been called, as experts, to hear the testimony and give an opinion deduced therefrom. Strange enough, those physicians, thus inadequately prepared, have obeyed the summons; and some of them have even sought it. The result has been that a few of them, sagacious men, of sound judgment and some practical experience, have passed the ordeal with credit to themselves and no detriment to the profession;... while but too many others, supplying their deficiency of knowledge by a complement of confidence, have tied themselves to the Promethean rock with a cord of blunders, and the lawyers have torn from them, strip by strip, their bleeding flesh, until nothing was left but dry and disjointed bones, dangling and rattling in the wind. Were psychological medicine properly taught in the schools, such mistakes, which bring odium upon the profession, would not be likely to occur. (Ref. 45, p. 19)

As convincing as Earle's arguments may be, the battle for parity in medical education would continue throughout the nineteenth century. Even in Philadelphia, where Benjamin Rush had taught his "observations" in late eighteenth and early nineteenth centuries,[46] Jefferson Medical College agreed to have Isaac Ray deliver a series of lectures on insanity in the early 1870s—in the summer sessions.[47] About the same time, physicians in Edinburgh resolved to incorporate psychiatry into the medical curriculum. In accord with Earle, Ray, who completed his career in Philadelphia, assumed that psychiatry would be relevant to all practitioners. A 1-year course in nervous and mental disease appeared again at Jefferson in

1883, and a formal department was created under Dr. F.X. Dercum in 1892.[47] Of interest is Dr. Dercum's weighing in on the standards for expert testimony. In an 1898 article for the *Albany Law Journal*,[48] he decried the misuse of experts by lawyers and the need for strict standards on the conduct of witnesses, who are bias prone. In a comical coda to his otherwise sober approach, Dercum recalled the case of a will contest, in which the testator's sanity was questioned. After eminent experts testified that the decedent had been insane, the family physician was called to the stand. Making the point that the practice of hypothetical questions was flawed, Dercum recounted the following:

> [T]he family physician, although himself not an expert, being called to the stand by counsel for the will, declared the testator sane, and then, on cross-examination, being asked the rather improper question as to how it was that he, not being an expert, opposed his opinion to the distinguished physicians who had testified before him, he answered: "Yes, Drs. So and So," naming the experts, "are able men—there are none better—but in the present instance their opinion is worthless, as they never saw the patient." How strongly such a common-sense answer appeals to the average lay mind needs no comment. (Ref. 47, p. 15)

Isaac Ray's course at Jefferson and the emergence of a formal department there provide documentation that forensic teaching was present from the inception of psychiatric education. Because there is a record of Ray's lectures, we can see that the subject matter included much forensic material. Using the nomenclature adapted from the French, among his lectures was one on moral insanity. The following is his rationale for the doctrine:

> There is no reason to suppose that the affective powers are exempt from the visitation of disease. That a material organ, the brain, is as necessary for their manifestation, as for that of the intellect proper, no one can doubt; and if there is a material organ in the case, a thing of flesh and blood, then of course, we may have disease. And surely we are not prepared to make a man responsible for the effect of disease—not even when the disease is seated in viscera remote from the head. When a patient suffering under the torments of the gout or dyspepsia vents his spleen upon every living thing within reach, even to the infliction of a blow, we scarcely blame him, though it is not pretended that his reason is disordered. (Ref. 47, p. 1050)

Other topics included the legal consequences of epilepsy, dementia, general paralysis (syphilis), and the insanity of seduced or deserted women. Commenting on testamentary capacity, Ray was clear that clinical determinations were within the general practitioner's domain: "The civil acts of very old persons are often disputed on the ground of mental incompetency, and their wills especially, have been a fruitful source of litigation. The family physician's testimony is necessarily called for, and it is entitled to great consideration" (Ref. 47, p. 1051).

Interest in legal matters continued during the Gray years at the *Journal* (1854–1886). For example, in an account of a trial for a murder in 1871, questions arose as to the trajectory of insanity adjudications.[49] Dr. Clarke, who listened to the testimony and then testified for the defense, posed these questions for the education of the readers: What is mania transitoria? Who are liable? How should it affect jurisprudence? He wrote:

> The writer of this article, having been called by the defence to listen to all the testimony in the case, after careful examination of the authorities, aided by his somewhat limited experience, endeavored to answer the first and second of these questions, upon the witness stand; and, believing other cases will, and ought to be influenced by this one, desires to present the principles evolved, in a permanent and convenient form, and to answer the last question. (Ref. 49, pp. 399–400).

The significant point here is about the *Journal*'s content—that in 1872 it would deem significant publication of an article on how psychiatric evidence was presented and why that would be important to practitioners. The pinnacle of the trend occurred in 1882, when the *Journal* published an account of the trial of Charles Guiteau, President Garfield's assassin.[50] Several physicians testified that the defendant was (medically) insane at the time of the shooting. The account included lengthy colloquies between attorneys and Dr. Gray, chief witness for the prosecution. Here we see all the elements of forensic psychiatry laid bare: the tactics of defense and prosecution in selecting experts, the exposition of the state of the art in psychiatry, and the way in which different witnesses applied their findings to the question of legal insanity. In the end, Gray, taking the other witnesses to school, as it were, prevailed. Guiteau was convicted and executed, still manifestly mentally ill on the gallows.

Forensic Psychiatry: It Was Always There

The birth of psychiatry as a specialty of sorts (asylum medicine), attended by 13 "midwives" in Philadelphia in 1844 was a splendid event. Like the founders of the United States a few decades earlier, the group of asylum superintendents did not wholly invent a model structure. The English courts had been actively struggling with the question of criminal responsibility since 1800, and the French had reconceived the place of the mentally ill in society at around the same time. At the dawn of the nineteenth century, America had much work to do in claiming moral care of citizens. Unlike European models such as the one in Gheel, Belgium,[51] where the disabled were woven into the fabric of society, America's "out of sight, out of mind" traditions needed to be dismantled. Patient-rights advocates, led by Dorothea Dix, forced the issue of freeing the mentally ill from jails and almshouses many years after Pinel's geste in Paris. Afterward, the rush to build asylums created the next wave of transinstitutionalization, with abuses not envisioned by Dix.[37] The next wave of patient-rights advocates blamed the doctors for abuses and imprisonment.[3] Thus, by the time AMSAII formulated its agenda, the superintendents already had full plates of issues: the rights of patients cared for by the state, pursuing moral care of the insane, and helping courts to understand the relationship of pathological psychology to deviant or incompetent behaviors. Psychiatry was born forensic.

There were no psychiatric subspecialties in 1844, let alone identified forensic experts. Several of the AMSAII founders mentioned here took a keen interest in medicolegal matters, as did practitioners in other areas of medicine. Medical superintendents were called upon to attend trials and give testimony. As noted, "medical jurisprudence" had already been established, and it was not a huge conceptual leap to codifying the jurisprudence of insanity. We are fortunate that Isaac Ray failed at general practice in Maine and took the time to collate the world's literature on insanity (the medical term) and the law.[52] He deserves the lion's share of the credit for founding forensic psychiatry in America, although his efforts over the ensuing decades were fraught.[2,52,53] Ray still had to deal with the realities that remain familiar today: that judges, juries, and legislatures—not doctors—make legal decisions; that there were no unified standards of conduct for expert witnesses; that the adversarial system of justice could foster corruption; and that the tests for insanity were flawed and capricious.

Many of the standards for today's practice were forged in the nineteenth century, as a scientific approach to mental illness took shape. A review of Isaac Ray's advice to forensic practitioners, commemorating his 200th birthday, concluded that his observations retain great vitality.[54] This can be seen in his comments in an 1851 *Journal of Insanity* article.[55] Let us close with a few of his "hints."

> [T]he duty of an expert is very different from those which ordinarily occupy our attention....
>
> [U]nless the whole ground is carefully surveyed, [the medical witness is susceptible to] *breaking down* [italics original] on the witness stand.
>
> [The main resource a witness needs] is a well-ordered, well-digested, comprehensive knowledge of mental phenomena, in a sound as well as unsound state. The question which, in one shape or another, is presented to the witness, is, whether certain mental phenomena indicate mental unsoundness.
>
> [The expert] is, in form at least, the party's witness, engaged by him, and by him made acquainted with all that he knows respecting the merits of the case. The consequence of such a relation is that he can scarcely help testifying under a bias.
>
> [To a lawyer:] I will make the examination, or hear the evidence in the case, if you wish it, and if the conclusions to which they lead me, will serve your client, you are at liberty to call me, but otherwise you had better not place me on the stand.
>
> [A]bove all things [the expert witness] should be cool and quiet, and never be provoked into a sharp reply or a cutting retort.... He must make up his mind to have his sentiments travestied and sneered at, his motives impugned, and pitfalls dug in his path, with the same kind of indifference with which he would hear the maledictions of an excited patient.[55]

References

1. Ray I. (1838). *A treatise on the medical jurisprudence of insanity.* Boston: Little, Brown & Co.
2. Zilboorg G. (1944). Legal aspects of psychiatry. In JK Hall, G Zilboorg, & HA Bunker (Eds.), *One hundred years of American psychiatry* (pp. 507–584). New York: Columbia University Press.

3. Weiss KJ. (2013). Isaac Ray, malpractice defendant. *J Am Acad Psychiatry Law, 41*(3), 382–390.
4. Weiss, KJ. (2007). Isaac Ray at 200: Phrenology and expert testimony. *J Am Acad Psychiatry Law, 35*(3), 339–345.
5. Weiss KJ. (2006). Isaac Ray's affair with phrenology. *J Psychiatry Law, 34*(Winter), 455–494.
6. Ray I. (1845). Trial of Abner Rogers. *The Law Reporter, 7*(10), 449–460.
7. Belkin GS. (1996). Moral insanity, science and religion in nineteenth-century America: The Gray-Ray debate. *Hist Psychiatry, 7*, 591–613.
8. Rosenberg CE. (1968). *The trial of the assassin Guiteau: Psychiatry and the law in the gilded age.* Chicago: University of Chicago Press.
9. Eigen JP. (1995). *Witnessing insanity: Madness and mad-doctors in the English court.* New Haven, CT: Yale University Press.
10. Platt AM, & Diamond BL. (1965). The origins and development of the "wild beast" concept of mental illness and its relation to theories of criminal responsibility. *J Hist Behav Sci, 1*(4), 355–367.
11. Diamond BL. (1956). Isaac Ray and the trial of Daniel M'Naghten. *Am J Psychiatry, 112*(8), 651–656.
12. Diamond BL, & Platt A. (1966). The origins of the "right and wrong" test of criminal responsibility and its subsequent development in the United States: An historical survey. *Cal L Rev, 54*, 1227–1260.
13. Perlin ML. (1994). *The jurisprudence of the insanity defense.* Durham, NC: Carolina Academic Press.
14. Quen, JM. (1983). Isaac Ray and the development of American psychiatry and the law. *Psych Clin N Amer, 6*(4), 527–537.
15. Durham v. United States. 214 F.2d 862 (D.C. Cir. 1954).
16. United States v. Brawner. 471 F. 2d 969 (D.C. Cir. 1972).
17. Morse SJ. (2011). Mental disorder and criminal law. *J Crim L Criminol, 101*(3), 885–968.
18. Weiss KJ. (2008). Epilepsy and homicide: Isaac Ray on mitigation. *J Psychiatry Law, 36*(Summer), 171–209.
19. Weiss KJ, & John H. (2014). Wigmore on the abolition of partisan expert witnesses. *J Am Acad Psychiatry Law*, 2015, *43*(1), 21–31.
20. Morse SJ, & Bonnie RJ. (2013). Abolition of the insanity defense violates due process. *J Am Acad Psychiatry Law, 41*(4), 488–495.
21. Gold LH. (2010). Rediscovering forensic psychiatry. In RI Simon, & LH Gold (Eds.), *The American psychiatric publishing textbook of forensic psychiatry* (2nd ed., pp. 3–41). Washington, DC: American Psychiatric Press, Inc.
22. Beck TR. (1823). *Elements of medical jurisprudence.* Albany, NY: Websters and Skinners.
23. Van Deusen EH. (1856). *A biographical sketch of T. Romeyn Beck, M.D., L.L.D.* New York: Holman & Gray.
24. Wharton, F, & Stillé M. (1855). *A treatise on medical jurisprudence.* Philadelphia: Kay & Brother.
25. Wharton F: (1861). Involuntary confessions. *Am J Insanity, 17*(3):250–296.
26. Weiss KJ, & del Busto E. (2011). Early American jurisprudence of sleep violence. *Sleep Med Clin, 6*, 49–482.
27. Weiss KJ. (2012). Classics in psychiatry and the law: Francis Wharton on involuntary confessions. *J Am Acad Psychiatry Law, 40*(1), 67–80.
28. Beck TR. (1825). *Elements of medical jurisprudence* (2nd ed.). London: John Anderson.
29. Haslam J. (1817). *Medical jurisprudence as it relates to insanity, according to the laws of England.* London: C. Hunter.
30. Beck TR, & Beck JB. (1838). *Elements of medical jurisprudence* (6th ed.). London: Longman, Orme, et al.
31. Ciccone JR. (1992). Murder, insanity, and medical expert witnesses. *Arch Neurol, 49*, 608–611.
32. Coventry CB. (1844). Medical jurisprudence of insanity. *Am J Insanity, 1*(2), 134–144.
33. Buttolph HA. (1845). Medical jurisprudence of insanity. *Am J Insanity, 1*(3), 258–274.
34. Davis NS. (1845). The importance of a correct physiology of the brain, as applied to the elucidation of medico-legal questions; and the necessity of greater accuracy and minuteness in reporting post mortem examinations. *Am J Insanity, 1*(3), 235–243.

35. Weiss KJ, Wettstein RM, Sadoff RL, Silva JA, & Norko MA. (2011). History and function of the psychiatric report. In A Buchanan, & M Norko (Eds.), *The psychiatric report* (pp. 11–21). Cambridge, UK: Cambridge University Press.
36. Ray I. (1886). Testamentary capacity (1877). In *Papers read before the Medico-Legal Society of New York, from its organization, Third Series, 1875 to 1878* (pp. 421–440). New York: The Medico-Legal Society.
37. Deutsch A. (1949). *The Mentally ill in America* (2nd ed.). New York: Columbia University Press.
38. Kirkbride TS. (1850). Proceedings of the fifth annual meeting of the Association of Medical Superintendents of American Institutions for the Insane. *Am J Insanity, 7*(1), 75–88.
39. Ray I. (1851). Project of a law for determining the legal relations of the insane. *Am J Insanity, 7*(3), 215–234.
40. Ray I. (1869). Project of a law for determining the legal relations of the insane. *Quart J Psychol Med Med Jurisprudence, 3*, 495–505.
41. D'Antonio P. (2006). *Founding friends. families, staff, and patients at the friends asylum in early nineteenth-century Philadelphia*. Bethlehem, PA: Lehigh University Press.
42. Packard EPW. (1873). *Modern persecution, or married woman's liabilities, as demonstrated by the action of the Illinois legislature* (Vol. II). Self-published in 1873 and reprinted in facsimile edition by the University of Michigan Scholarly Publishing Office.
43. Beck TR. (1845/1846). Bibliographical notices. *Am J Insanity, 2*(1), 80–89 and 2(3), 267–284.
44. Beck TR. (1853). Law cases bearing on the question of insanity. *Am J Insanity, 10*(2), 179–184.
45. Earle P. (1867). *An address delivered before the Berkshire Medical Institute, November 24, 1863*. Utica, NY: Roberts.
46. Carlson ET. (1977). Benjamin Rush and mental health. *Ann NY Acad Sci, 291*(1), 94–103.
47. Weiss KJ. (2012). Psychiatry for the general practitioner: Isaac Ray's Jefferson lectures, 1871 to 1873. *J Nerv Ment Dis, 200*(12), 1047–1053.
48. Dercum FX. (1898). Expert evidence from the standpoint of a witness. *Albany Law J, 57*(14), 215–220.
49. Clarke ST. (1872). Case of Pierce.—Plea insanity. *Am J Insanity, 28*(3):399–409.
50. Anonymous. (1882). The Guiteau trial. *Am J Insanity,38*(3):303–448.
51. Anonymous. (1848). A village of lunatics. *Am J Insanity, 4*(3):217–222.
52. Quen JM. (1974). Isaac Ray: Have we learned his lessons? *Bull Am Acad Psychiatry Law, 2*(3), 137–147.
53. Hughes JS. (1986). *In the law's darkness: Isaac Ray and the medical jurisprudence of insanity in nineteenth-century America*. New York: Oceana Publications.
54. Weiss KJ. (2007). Isaac Ray's advice to medical witnesses: Still relevant? *Am J Foren Psychiatry, 28*(2), 35–49.
55. Ray I. (1851). Hints to the medical witness in questions of insanity. *Am J Insanity, 8*(1):53–67.

2

Development of Forensic Psychiatry Training at Temple University and Services in Philadelphia and Pennsylvania

A Memoir

Melvin S. Heller

This chapter was written by Dr. Melvin Heller and edited by Dr. Robert Sadoff. Dr. Melvin Heller and Dr. Samuel Polsky co-directed the first Unit in Law and Psychiatry at Temple University in late 1950s. Dr. Heller gives the following account.

A Call From Temple University

About a year after I completed my child psychiatry fellowship and personal training analysis, Professor English's secretary phoned me from Temple and said that he would like me to meet a young professor, one Samuel Polsky, LLD, PhD, from Temple's Law School. And so we met in Dr. English's office and hit it off almost immediately. Dr. English explained what Sam Polsky already knew, namely that Dean Robert Bucher of Temple's Medical School and Dean Benjamin Boyer of Temple's Law School, were desirous of establishing an Institute of Law and the Health Sciences at Temple, beginning with a Unit in Law and Psychiatry.

Dr. Polsky summarized: "Dr. English and Dean Boyer think that you and I would be highly qualified to embark on this initial interdisciplinary effort as the Co-Directors of Temple's Unit in Law and Psychiatry." Well, I was flattered, and inwardly more thrilled because I had immediately sensed that Sam Polsky was my kind of a guy, to put it mildly. Professor Polsky, who insisted that I call him Sam, was a brilliant young lawyer only 2 years older than I, with an already tenured faculty position as Associate Professor at Temple University Law School.

Sam had obtained scholarships to Penn and then Harvard Law School where he excelled both academically and in debating. This was followed by a Rockefeller Fellowship at Scotland's University of Edinburgh, where he obtained his Ph.D. in Legal Medicine. Sam Polsky and I ended up working together for some 20 years and becoming best friends. During our time together, before his untimely death in October 1974, we succeeded in building the best interdisciplinary training facility in Law and Psychiatry in the area. Following Sam's death, Law Professor William Traylor and I continued our interdisciplinary Law and Psychiatry course re-titled as Mental Health Law until our retirement in 1990.

Drs. Heller and Polsky as Co-directors of Temple's Unit in Law and Psychiatry

Although we had the blessings and backings of our two Deans, and a nice office with an impressive sign on the door that read Temple Unit in Law and Psychiatry, the Deans had no money to stake us. Funding our Unit wasn't that easy back then. Sam started the ball rolling by getting our new Law and Psychiatry program a $3,000 grant from the Legal Aid Society of Philadelphia, providing we matched it. We were then able to convince the Mental Health Association of Southern PA to provide the matching grant. So with that $6,000 and a bit of friendly persuasion, we were able to hire a smart and polite young secretary.

Sam and I were eager to teach, and learn from each other, as much as we could about key concepts, professional language, terms, methods and procedures of our two professions, long and separately concerned with what psychiatry largely labeled as mentally disordered behaviors that were prohibited by law as disorderly, unacceptable, and criminal acts. In trying to share with each other the essence of what we had learned, Sam and I became not only each other's private tutors, but prize students as well. It has been said that the best way to learn is to teach.

Our Research on the Legal Interview

Sam and I had applied for a research grant to study the initial fact gathering, office or bedside interviews used by lawyers and doctors when focusing on the presenting problem of their clients or patients. Sam and I boldly undertook our 3-year Temple study of the legal interview, borrowing lavishly on the generosity of many volunteers among the students, psychiatric residents, faculty, colleagues, as well as interested and willing friends in our nearby legal and medical professions.

Our supporters included Deans Benjamin Boyer and Robert Bucher of schools of law and medicine respectively, Dr. O. Spurgeon English, Chairman of the Department of

Psychiatry, and Robert D. Abrahams, Chief Counsel of the Philadelphia Legal Aid Society, and many faculty members too numerous to list here. The 3-year study was subsequently presented at the annual meeting of the National Legal and Defender Association and published by them as a 42-page monograph in 1960 entitled *An Introduction to Legal Interviewing* by Heller, Polen, and Polsky.

Some Further Thoughts on Law and Psychiatry

As I look back on my body of work, my 32 years of co-teaching our third-year elective law school courses in Law and Psychiatry, subsequently renamed as Mental Health Law, provided one of the most privileged and gratifying experiences and opportunities of the many that came my way during a long professional career.

How was it that co-teaching a law school course involving merely the part-time effort of a few hours each week per semester was so important to me, especially during what had very often been my 60-hour working week back then? There were reasons. First, I had come to feel rather deeply that teaching this course in Law and Psychiatry to a future generation of lawyers could be meaningful to society or "socially significant" in my father's words of long ago. Where did I get that idea? Well to begin with, when I looked at the nature and makeup of our community's civic organizations and our local governments, lawyers seemed to be fully if not overly represented in leadership positions, and pretty influential, in comparison with school teachers, college professors, and medical doctors, for example.

Among our law students would be our future judges, and very likely a large percentage of state legislators, corporate law firm partners, business executives, and other influential movers and shakers in civic affairs. Teaching these lawyers-to-be the practical and applicable aspects of what I had labored long to learn as a clinical psychiatrist would constitute a most worthy part of my "body of work," especially while they were still a group of reachable and motivated students, amenable to new ideas.

The Law's Focus on State of Mind

We proceeded for an entire semester each year, with Sam discussing the legal issues and landmark cases encountered in mental health law while I introduced our class to the main clinical categories and psycho-pathological concepts of mental disorders they might encounter in legal cases presenting problems at the juncture of the mental health and justice systems.

Each semester it seemed that Sam could hardly wait for my description of the psychotic disorders so that he could then launch into his discussion of the insanity defense, called exculpatory insanity in legal terms. Exculpatory insanity regards a defendant to be without blame because of severe mental impairment at the time of the crime. The underlying moral and philosophical problem is whether a severely deranged person who was still able to plan and carry out a homicide, for example, can be held without blame and declared "not guilty by reason of insanity." Or should a young child or early juvenile who planned and purposely committed a murder be held responsible for it—and at what age should that kick in? These are still pressing questions that different societies, cultures, and legal codes have addressed since ancient times.

Sam came up with the astonishing idea that we could do an interdisciplinary research study, and exploratory review by university lawyers and psychiatrists, of our federal insanity procedures in order to identify existing problems and potential remedies. Teaching and research went hand in hand, he reasoned. Of course I agreed with him, but asked how could we get a practical handle on this issue. Sam replied that because we had already done a reasonably successful interdisciplinary study of the legal interview and presented our findings and recommendations at the annual meeting of the National Legal Aid and Defender Association, why not apply for an NIH research grant to do a study of our Insanity Procedures Under Federal Law?

We received Research Grant OM 366 in 1958, and began our long study of Insanity Procedures Under Federal Law. This turned out to be an even larger undertaking than we had anticipated; a magnum opus involving a substantial number of our faculty colleagues, professional associates, and senior students at Temple Medical and Law schools who volunteered to serve, along with secretaries and nurses as "mock jurors" in reviewing the mental health testimony and legal arguments in actual trial transcripts.

We submitted our NIMH report and findings in a 308-page volume in 1965 as Temple University Research Studies in Law and Medicine, entitled *Insanity Procedures Under Federal Law* by Heller and Polsky.

The first hundred or more pages of our report are essentially Sam's singular contribution based on his scholarly grasp of "the problem of insanity" as he called it. Let me quote a few introductive lines of his perceptive writing from page 1 of our report.

> The problem of insanity as a legal defense has long been the subject of much discussion, but the object of few investigative studies. This is a matter of little surprise since the subject constantly borders on the essentially meta-psychological and philosophical problems of free will versus unconscious psychic determination and mental illness. For purposes of scientific study, such concepts elude attempts at objective definition.... The concepts of absent or diminished moral responsibility in the face of mental illness are in part psychiatric, in part legal, and partly ethical-cultural. The approach (to the problem) cannot be that of mental illness alone by specialists in that field.... On the other hand can there continue to be successful adjudication on the basis of two hundred year old concepts that were only partly accepted even before the development of modern psychiatry?

As for the basic data of our study, Sam wrote,

> The data which one seeks to acquire in the present study does not lend itself to the typical experimental model of isolation of factors and ordinary comparison with so-called control data. The trial, pre-trial considerations, post-trial disposition are

all regarded in this study as integral parts of a single context. Indeed, the context of the trial cannot be completely separated from the emotional climate of the society, culture or subculture in which the trial takes place.

How We Proceeded

A number of psychiatrists and lawyers among our faculty colleagues were interested in the legal, medical, and philosophical problems that the insanity defense entailed. They, along with selected psychiatric residents in our newly established forensic fellowship program, assisted us immeasurably in studying the official transcripts of some 47 federal trials in which insanity was raised as a defense. We understood that lawyers and psychiatrists would observe an exculpatory insanity trial from different perspectives, but that neither would have the same impressions as juries comprised of lay persons.

Where would we find an interested pool of persons whom we would recruit as mock jurors? We had an abundance of volunteers among first-year medical and law students, as well as secretaries and nurses who provided their responses as lay persons to materials recorded in the trial transcripts. One question we put to our mock jurors was whether the psychiatrist made a significant difference in the disposition of each case and if so, how? In our preliminary instructions to our mock jury, the lay observers were encouraged to report any stimuli or impressions from the transcript materials that registered upon them to influence their feeling that the defendant was or was not insane in the legal sense.

Our analyses of the trial transcripts by our consulting lawyers and psychiatrists, and the responses of our mock jurors in follow-up interviews and questionnaires identified a number of reasons why the insanity defense is so problematical to lawyers, psychiatrists, juries, courts, and the public at large.

Our Findings

First, the insanity defense was not used as intended. Such concepts as the "nature and quality" of an act, or whether the act is a "product" of a mental disorder fail to provide sufficiently useful, clear, and effective guidelines that lay jurors can apply with confidence in assessing the legal evidence and psychiatric testimony on which they must decide whether or not a defendant was so mentally disordered at the time of the crime as to be legally insane.

Our findings also indicated that the underlying prospect of capital punishment would lay heavily in the latent agendas and consciences of insanity defense jurors. That issue was further complicated by courts in allowing testimony about a defendant's dangerousness during insanity defense trials. Added to these findings were the matter of conflicting expert testimony, the time delay between the crime and the expert's examination, and finally the jurors' own preconceptions of "insane" as "crazy" in everyday, ordinary use as a familiar and common term.

Unfortunately, insanity defense jurors were not provided with the court's instructions concerning the legal definitions of insanity until after they had heard all the evidence. This required jurors to then try to unlearn what they always knew about insane or crazy people and try to re-approach the evidence they had heard in accordance with the court's new instructions. Given these multiple and distinct findings, there was no way we could avoid concluding that jurors' decisions in insanity defense trials were based more on the individual juror's emotional responses and attitudes about the defendant's "viciousness," the victim's vulnerability and the circumstances of the crime rather than to the adversary opinions of the prosecution and defense attorneys, and testimony of their respective mental health experts.

Our study of the insanity defense, which took so much of our research time, was mainly of academic rather than clinical interest to me back then. I had regarded the insanity defense as a relatively low-frequency event, pumped up to importance in the media. There are far more legally "sane" but clinically psychotic inmates currently incarcerated in our state penitentiaries and local prisons than the relatively few but highly publicized insanity cases.

To expose and train our psychiatric residents and forensic fellows, Sam and I knew that we needed to somehow link up with public-sector forensic facilities in courts and corrections which could provide our law and forensic psychiatry students with real-time clinical experiences by participating in the actual work of courts and prisons with real prosecutors, defense lawyers, and justice system personnel.

Evaluation of Untried Defendants and Assessing for Dangerousness

Because there was a recurrent shortage of beds in a locked psychiatric ward at Philadelphia General Hospital, a large number of mentally ill persons who had been declared incompetent to stand trial while facing criminal charges were being detained in Philadelphia's County Prison instead of a mental hospital.

Untried defendants are supposed to be "presumed innocent" until tried and proven guilty. My evaluation of these individuals was required to determine whether or not the defendant was currently so impaired by mental illness as to be unable to understand the charges, proceedings, and nature of the trial and, therefore, could not really assist counsel in his defense.

The first question I needed to address was whether or not the untried defendant was still mentally ill, and if so, was the defendant so mentally ill that he presented such a risk of harm to himself or others that he required custodial supervision and safe management in a secure environment.

That psychiatrists were called on to make such assessments raised many proper questions as to whether or not a psychiatrist, or any other specialist, can reliably predict the future dangerousness of another human being. From my prior work with offenders, I have learned that the short answer is, "No." But because the question of these defendants' future dangerousness was either implied or openly raised by the court, I had learned to proceed both cautiously and humbly with my clinical prognoses and predictions of future risk.

How I Evaluated Risk of Violence in Prisoners

Here is how I went about it. I looked casually, but constantly, at the individual's physical behavior during the interview, including his so-called "body language." I listened even more carefully to how he related to me as a person. In addition to his thought content and actual words, I made note of his ongoing feelings and mood during the interview. And mine as well. Was I having a hard time finding something to like about him? If so, why? Did his feelings seem overly depressed on the one hand, or unduly elated on the other? His vocabulary and word choice alone would tell me something about his verbal IQ even without a formal intelligence test, which could be subsequently performed if needed.

In my former experiences as a prison psychiatrist, I had found that the offender's past history and record of prior violent behavior was the most important predictor of future violent behavior. There were no blood studies, litmus tests, or other measures for the reliable prediction of future violent behaviors in individuals, and there still are none. The best we could do was to look at the individual's track record.

What was the inmate's past track record? What has been the condition of his environment or "track" so to speak? What kind of inner circumstances and personal load of stress will he likely be carrying on release from custody? What are his relationships with others likely to be on release from custody? Will he likely be returning to a slipperier, risky, or "muddy" track as a recurrent alcohol or substance abuser? Does he have an emotionally supportive family? These to me were the right questions to ask myself about him. If I put them all together, in professional language and terms, I found that I could often provide the court with a carefully considered clinical opinion that was explainable and reasonably helpful, if not sufficiently or biblically prophetic. It was that kind of practical working approach that had often put me on the same page in conversations with parole officers and others in the criminal justice systems who sought my opinion.

The Pennsylvania Prison Society

In seeking to extend our community outreach, I met with persons from the Pennsylvania Prison Society. The Pennsylvania Prison Society was allegedly the oldest nonprofit agency in the United States, founded in 1787 "to diminish the excessive and undue misery of prisons." In due course I was invited to join their Board of Directors and had the privilege of working with a number of truly remarkable persons.

Years of postdoctoral training and clinical experience provided me with a very practical background and desirable resume for the work that Sam Polsky and I had undertaken. My clinical background as a Yale-trained psychiatrist, Board certified in both Adult and Child Psychiatry, with the unusual professional experience of 2 years and the full-time, chief psychiatrist for an 1,100 bed maximum security federal penitentiary made me a relatively rare commodity in the mental health employment market of the 1950s. And so, my phone rang with repeated calls from the nearby and conveniently located Eastern State Penitentiary in Philadelphia.

I had known that Eastern State Penitentiary was no ordinary prison, but had once been Pennsylvania's renowned and quite famous "Prison at Cherry Hill." It had dated back to 1829 and was still standing solidly where it was built at its original place that subsequently became 22nd Street and Fairmount Ave. in contemporary Philadelphia.

The old prison had been the subject of much interest to early penologists both here and abroad, not only for its novel "wheel-spoke" architecture in which cell-blocks radiated out from a central security station or hub, but for its radical provision for the single cell housing of inmates in order to encourage solitary reflection and deep personal penitence. Hence, it was viewed and named as a "penitentiary" rather than a prison, but, as a rose is a rose by any other name, it was prison to those who experienced the unyielding enclosure of its bars that was so unlike the sweet beauty of a rose.

Pennsylvania's new prison had been visited by the likes of Alexis de Tocqueville and Charles Dickens in their day, and had housed numerous felons including Al Capone and Willie Sutton among its more infamous guests. Remarkably, it still remained uniquely useful well into the twentieth century as an advantageously located, well-functioning and much-needed maximum security facility in unusually close proximity to Philadelphia's courts, numerous universities, and the visitation needs of a number of its inmates whose families resided in Philadelphia's inner-city population centers.

Developing Further Clinical Facilities: a Contract with Eastern State Penitentiary

Sam and I knew that Warden William Banmiller and Dr. Michael Morello needed to find better ways to provide psychiatric services at Eastern State Penitentiary, and we came up with an idea. We knew that our supervised senior Residents and Forensic Fellows could provide the best available services, and that a working relationship with Eastern State would reward our Temple Unit in Law and Psychiatry with a unique, nearby, and much needed additional clinical facility for training our residents and Fellows in forensic psychiatry. Sam and I knew that very few people, including psychiatrists, have the endurance, motivation, and sheer will to study real prisoners and their keepers in an actual maximum security penitentiary environment. In this instance Mike Morello and Warden Banmiller needed psychiatric services for Eastern State, and lawyer Sam was ready to present and close our deal. I can still remember to this day almost his exact words. Our proposal was straightforward and in Sam's words went pretty much as follows.

"Mel and I want to interest and train more psychiatrists in Forensic Fellowship programs. We need forensic facilities to train such residents. Mike, and Warden Banmiller, if we set up a program to do this at Eastern State Penitentiary we can give you better than Mel. We can give you double Mel."

And then very quickly, Sam laid out our plan for Temple's Unit in Law and Psychiatry to provide the services of supervised residents and fellows in forensic psychiatry that would be selected from well trained and highly qualified, licensed psychiatrists who were interested in obtaining subspecialty experience in forensic psychiatry. Eastern State Penitentiary's proposed salary for highly qualified, full-time academic psychiatrists such as Dr. Heller would be paid to Temple's Unit in Law and Psychiatry and divided to cover the modest annual stipends of several full-time psychiatrists in Temple's forensic fellowship program at its then major clinical facility, Eastern State Penitentiary.

Seeing great interest on the part of Warden Banmiller, Sam added that we had already checked this all out with Temple's administration as well as with Dean Boyer at the Law School and with Dr. English, Chairman of Temple's Psychiatry Department at the Medical school. The package was quickly sewn up when Sam assured Warden Banmiller that Temple's plan was for Professor Heller to personally supervise the forensic fellows as part of his academic duties, adding that they would meet in regular group sessions, which would be held in our modestly renovated clinical facility to be established on 3 Block at Eastern State Penitentiary. And we could start almost right away.

Three weeks later the contract was signed and we embarked on the very first university-based forensic psychiatry fellowship program in the tri-state area—or anywhere else that we knew of at the time.

The Citizens Crime Commission

Also welcome were calls I received from Ephraim Gomberg, Executive Director of the Citizens Crime Commission of Philadelphia. The Citizens Crime Commission invited me to attend a meeting of their Board of Directors and present a brief talk about my former experiences with mentally ill offenders among federal prison inmates.

In the early 1960s, the Citizens Crime Commission of Philadelphia sponsored a series of judicial seminars on sentencing. Based on my experiences with the Federal Bureau of Prisons and sentenced prisoners in the US penitentiary in Terre Haute, I was asked to participate on the panel of speakers.

It was following one of these seminars at which I spoke that the Hon. Vincent Carroll, President Judge of the Philadelphia Court of Common Pleas, approached me most cordially saying with a smile that he had heard "mostly good things" about me, and wanted to know if I would be personally interested in reorganizing and providing psychiatric services for the Court. With the concept and model of the contract that had been arranged between Temple University and Eastern State Penitentiary, and desiring to further develop the best clinical facilities for training psychiatric residents and fellows in forensic psychiatry, I suggested that Temple's Unit in Law and Psychiatry could supervise our senior residents with special interests in forensic psychiatry and forensic fellows to supply diagnostic and clinical evaluation services to the Court of Common Pleas.

Temple's Diagnostic Services to the Court of Common Pleas

President Judge Carroll and the Board of Judges were most enthusiastic and arranged a contract with Temple's Unit in Law and Psychiatry to provide psychiatric evaluations of defendants and presentence offenders for Philadelphia's Courts of Common Pleas. This contract was adjusted according to the Court's increasing caseload and renewed annually for an additional twenty-some years.

The Children's Aid Society

Along the way in my child psychiatric private practice, I encountered several couples who became involved in legal adoption issues. In the course of working with one of them, I met with Dr. Elizabeth Lawder the Director of the Children's Aid Society (CAS), which was then the Commonwealth's largest adoption and foster care agency. Dr. Lawder and her staff were extremely knowledgeable about adoption and foster care. Foster care had been a prominent feature in the backgrounds of juvenile and young adult offenders with whom I had been working in the correctional system. Knowing that foster care and adoption involved child psychiatric concerns that were replete with legal issues, I had applied to work with CAS to gain more direct clinical experience with foster child and family forensic issues such as the birth mother's informed consent when giving up her child for adoption, as well as adverse child developmental matters connected with physical, emotional, and sexual abuse in foster care.

Dr. Guy and Our Psychiatric Services at Philadelphia's County Prison System

We were very much in need and fortunate in recruiting a well-trained and unusually capable psychiatrist from another medical center across the city. He was about my own age, and was looking for "a change of scene—a new job, a new neighborhood, new associates, and a new start." And so, Sam Polsky and I met Dr. Edward Blair Guy who turned out to be one of our most valued forensic colleagues and good friends.

Sam Polsky and I rapidly oriented Ed Guy to the newly developing field of forensic psychiatry. We familiarized him to the basic issues, and then simply introduced and exposed him to the enormous challenges and needs of so-called "correctional psychiatry." I eagerly shared with Ed what I could of my own prison experiences to speed him on his way to becoming one of the most capable and dedicated psychiatrists whom I have been privileged to bring into this professionally challenging field of forensic psychiatry, and prison work in particular. For many years, Dr. Guy served us and Philadelphia's County Prisons admirably as the Chief Psychiatrist under our Temple University contract to supply mental health services to the county prison system, which grew to include the State Maximum Security Forensic Diagnostic Hospital at Holmsburg Prison.

Temple University Fellowships in Forensic Psychiatry

Drs. Norman Anderson and Fred Herring III were among the very first of our own psychiatric residents who signed on eagerly for our new forensic psychiatry fellowship program at Temple. Additional candidates soon followed. I shall mention only a number of the many fine persons who came to study forensic psychiatry with Sam Polsky and me when few if any other forensic psychiatry fellowships with extensive clinical and academic facilities were being offered in the late 1950s and 1960s. Some of our very brightest and well-trained psychiatrists were from abroad. Such doctors as Brij Sethi from India, and Juan Pedro from Puerto Rico enhanced our perspectives about comparable mental health laws and procedures in their own countries.

With our several state and county service contracts we had ample funds to add two additional forensic fellowships for child psychiatrists whose clinical time was divided between the Children's Aid Society and Temple's forensic facilities. In successive years we gained two of our mostly worthy and interesting forensic fellows. These were Drs. Paul McQuaid from Ireland and Dr. Martin Gay from Scotland. Drs. McQuaid and Gay added more than their distinctive accents and professional viewpoints as we compared aspects of our various American and British Mental Health Acts and legal procedures.

In due course, experienced forensic fellows also provided opinion testimony when requested by the court on an individualized case-by-case basis. Their testimony remained structured and formal even during highly adversary, and sometimes heated, cross-examinations when our second-year fellows had been taught, prepared, and sometimes even rehearsed by Dr. Polsky or me to defend their opinions and stand their ground. There were few cross-examination questions that Professor Polsky or I could not anticipate.

Although our forensic fellows had substantial clinical experience with patients during their prior residency training, working with defendants in courts and prisons was different than seeing patients in one's private office or public sector clinic. In matters of competency and presentence examinations, as well as probation and parole evaluations, our forensic fellows and their patients needed to understand that third parties were involved—namely justice system personnel as elected or appointed representatives of the public. And so we discussed and hashed out these crucial exceptions and limits to our traditional concepts of doctor–patient relationships and privacy.

Psychiatric Residents and Forensic Fellows Who Worked with Us at Temple

Forensic fellows who subsequently continued to include the practice of forensic psychiatry in their careers included Drs. Arthur Boxer, Edward Guy, Norman Jablon, Larry Rotenberg, Robert Sadoff, and Ralph Wolf to mention but a few of the "old originals" who worked with our Temple Unit back then on Block 3 of Pennsylvania's Eastern State Penitentiary more than 50 years ago. I am very proud and gratified at having introduced so many fine physicians directly and indirectly to forensic psychiatry and to the ongoing need for mental health professionals to work in the criminal justice system's courts and correctional facilities.

Mentoring in Forensic Psychiatry

Traditionally, mentoring was the major educational experience forensic psychiatrists had before the development of fellowships and formal training programs. I have been fortunate to mentor a number of young forensic psychiatrists who went on to develop their own programs and to mentor future generations of forensic psychiatrists. What greater reward and pleasure can teachers have than to be succeeded by truly productive and highly regarded scholars to carry on the profession?

3

The Modern Era of Forensic Psychiatry

Richard Rosner and Robert L. Sadoff

As noted by Dr. Kenneth Weiss in his chapter on The History of Forensic Psychiatry, the profession was a relatively esoteric one, with individual teachers and a limited number of students. The modern era began in 1969, when Dr. Jonas R. Rappeport called together eight teachers of forensic psychiatry to Baltimore to inaugurate the American Academy of Psychiatry and the Law (AAPL). There had been individual institutions in which forensic psychiatry was taught and practiced. For example, see Dr. Melvin Heller's chapter on his development of the Unit in Law and Psychiatry at Temple University. He refers to his experience as a student at Yale, where there was a Unit in Law and Psychiatry in the 1950s. Early leaders in the field included Drs. Bernard Diamond and Seymour Pollack in California, Joseph Satten at the Menninger Clinic, Ames Robey in Michigan, Jay Katz at Yale, Jonas Robitscher at the University of Pennsylvania, and Jonas Rappeport at the University of Maryland. In some institutions, forensic psychiatry was taught as part of community and social psychiatry and did not emerge as a clear subspecialty of psychiatry until the 1970s.

Before the inauguration of AAPL, there were two other national organizations in which psychiatrists participated: The American College of Legal Medicine (ACLM) in which the fellows were required to have both law and medical degrees and consisted primarily of forensic pathologists and other nonpsychiatric physicians. The American Academy of Forensic Sciences (AAFS) was the leading national organization in which forensic psychiatrists participated with many other forensic scientists, including lawyers, criminalists, forensic odontologists, forensic pathologists, and questioned document experts. The psychiatric leaders within AAFS included Dr. Diamond, Dr. Pollack, and Dr. Meier Tuchler. Neither ACLM nor AAFS had a major impact on forensic psychiatry until the 1970s.

As AAPL grew and became a major national organization of forensic psychiatrists, individuals such as Dr. Richard Rosner, from New York University, decided that there needed to be specialized training for forensic psychiatrists. As an active member of both AAPL and AAFS, Dr. Rosner brought together the leaders of both organizations to initiate a fellowship program in forensic psychiatry that had standards for teaching and clinical experiences in order to qualify as an accredited fellowship. Dr. Rosner published four seminal articles relating to fellowship programs from 1981[1]o 1983.[2] His paper, "Accreditation of fellowship programs in forensic psychiatry: A preliminary report," was published in the Bulletin of the American Academy of Psychiatry and the Law in 1981 documenting the programs as he envisioned them and as they developed.

Before the development of the standards, psychiatrists would enroll in programs that were diverse, some being partial programs with little clinical experience, and others more comprehensive programs with both clinical and didactic experiences. At that time, the term *fellow* was not universally accepted, because there was no core content to the programs nor a standard curriculum. Some fellows had spent 1 day per week "shadowing" a senior forensic psychiatrist. Other fellows had spent a part of a fourth year of a general psychiatry residency in an elective in forensic psychiatry. It was rare that some persons had spent a postresidency full year in forensic psychiatry training with multiple supervised forensic experiences in a structured didactic program.

Dr. Richard Rosner, who was active in both AAFS and AAPL, called for an organizing meeting for a Joint Committee to develop standards for postgraduate fellowship training programs in psychiatry and the law. At that meeting, under Dr. Rosner's leadership, different senior psychiatrists, directing different "fellowship" programs, undertook to develop proposals for minimal core content of each component of a 1-year postresidency fellowship in forensic psychiatry. Dr. Rosner subsequently received, collated, and edited the proposals into a report on Standards for Fellowships in Forensic Psychiatry. The report was submitted and approved both by AAFS and AAPL, and published both in the Journal of Forensic Sciences and the Bulletin of AAPL.

Dr. Rosner described the Committee to Develop Standards for Post-Graduate Fellowship Training Programs in Psychiatry and the Law that was composed of 18 experienced forensic psychiatry educators from both the United States and Canada, with individuals from both AAPL and the Psychiatry Section of the AAFS.

Dr. Rosner indicated that there would be three steps to any formal accreditation effort:

> First, uniform standards would have to be developed for all aspects for Fellowship Training in Psychiatry and the Law. The standards would have to be reviewed, revised and accepted both by AAPL and AAFS.
>
> Second, the final standards would have to be considered, perhaps revised, and endorsed by the American Board of Forensic Psychiatry.
>
> Third, a formal accreditation system would have to be developed so that the Fellowship Programs could apply to AAPL and AAFS for official review of their programs, and obtain a Certificate of Accreditation.

Dr. Rosner then discussed Board Certification by the American Board of Forensic Psychiatry (ABFP): "The American Board of Forensic Psychiatry has no means of assessing the credentials of persons who claim to be graduates of Fellowship Programs and who request two years' credit (toward the five year experience requirement of the Board) for one year of fellowship training. There is no shared understanding as to what should be in an adequate Forensic Psychiatry Fellowship." Dr. Rosner noted that initially each of the fellowship programs "has its own unique qualities, both in assets and liabilities, and there is no uniform set of criteria against which the various programs can be measured." Further, he states, "In theory, almost any group of psychiatrists could set up a program, calling it a Post-Graduate Fellowship, and be in business." In order to take the Board examination, the candidate must show that he/she has had an accredited training program in forensic psychiatry. That means the program must have met the standards developed by the Committee.

With respect to Board Certification in Forensic Psychiatry, the following are historical facts: The ABFP was created by the Forensic Science Foundation (FSF) and AAFS, utilizing money that was obtained by a grant to the Forensic Science Foundation from the National Institute of Justice. Dr. Meier I. Tuchler, President of AAFS, attended an AAPL general business meeting and explained to the members of AAPL the purpose of the ABFP. He invited AAPL to co-sponsor with AAFS and FSF, the ABFP. With Dr. Rappeport's leadership, the AAPL membership voted to co-sponsor the ABFP.

Following the inauguration of the ABFP, the Credentials Committee of the ABFP received and largely granted requests for 2-years' credit toward the experience requirement for 1 year of fellowship in forensic psychiatry from applicants who claimed they had taken a "fellowship" in forensic psychiatry.

The following year, Dr. Rosner published "Standards for fellowship programs in forensic psychiatry: The report of the Joint Committee on Accreditation of Fellowships in Forensic Psychiatry." In that paper, he discusses the several subcommittees of the Committee on Accreditation, as follows:

1. The subcommittee on core curriculum was chaired by Dr. Howard V. Zonana from the Yale University Forensic Psychiatry Program. The Committee divided the material into the following five areas:
   A. Forensic Psychiatry—The use of psychiatric concepts and expertise to resolve legal issues
   B. Legal Regulation of Psychiatry—The legal definition of the rights and responsibilities of patients, practitioners and hospitals
   C. Special Psychiatric and Legal Literature—Those areas of the legal psychiatric literature that indirectly relate to the specific issues in A and B, but which form the core material that a psychiatrist working in this area should be familiar with
   D. Basic References—General texts and journals
   E. Updated lists of legal cases listed by the American Board of Forensic Psychiatry
2. The subcommittee on clinical experiences, headed by Dr. J. Richard Ciccone from the Rochester Medical School Forensic Psychiatry Program. He notes, "The fellowship program should be able to build on skills and abilities which have developed during the

completion of an approved residency program in psychiatry.... Among the psychiatrist's skills which can be further developed during the fellowship are the following":

A. Conducting the clinical interview
B. Clinical reasoning
C. Mature clinical judgment and decision-making

He notes that, ideally, all clinical experiences must be supervised by an experienced forensic psychiatrist. He also recommends a second forensic psychiatry teacher to diminish "the fellows emerging from his training with a singular view of how to proceed as a forensic psychiatrist."

3. The subcommittee on faculty qualifications jointly headed by Dr. Robert L. Sadoff of the University of Pennsylvania Forensic Psychiatry Program and Dr. Phillip J. Resnick of the University of Cleveland's Forensic Psychiatry Program. They recommended the director of the fellowship program should be an experienced forensic psychiatrist and be certified by the American Board of Forensic Psychiatry and that additional members of the faculty include an experienced forensic psychologist, an attorney, and a child psychiatrist. At a minimum, the director should be a member of the senior faculty of a medical school's department of psychiatry.
4. The subcommittee on library resources jointly headed by Dr. Jonas R. Rappeport of the University of Maryland's Forensic Psychiatry Program, and Dr. Park E. Dietz, of the Harvard University Forensic Psychiatry Program, have developed a core library list of 13 essential textbooks, 12 basic reference books, and 13 fundamental research monographs.
5. The subcommittee on Legal Aspects of Training was headed by Dr. James Cavanaugh of the Rush-Presbyterian-St. Luke's Medical Center's Forensic Psychiatry Program. His report, in cooperation with Barbara A. Weiner, J.D., notes, "At a minimum, any fellowship program should have an attorney as a very active part of the program. The attorney should meet on a formal basis with a fellow to discuss the legal issues." They state the following exposures are essential to a well run, broad program:
   A. Courses at a law school. Courses in criminal law, mental health law, and negligence would be very desirable.
   B. Participating in the trial advocacy course of the law school...
   C. Speakers' program: law, like medicine, is filled with many specialties. Having practicing attorneys speak on criminal law, malpractice, workers' compensation, personal injury, etc., is more useful than any courses from the law school.
   D. Formal affiliation, which will give the fellow court experience: and a program should be designed so the fellow will be given the opportunity to do court ordered evaluations and to testify. This exposure should be in the civil as well as the criminal area.
6. The subcommittee on research training, headed by Dr. Park E. Dietz of the Harvard University Forensic Psychiatry Program, notes that the minimal criteria for accreditation should include:
   A. Accessibility to a major medical library
   B. Accessibility to a major law library

C. Accessibility to at least one of the following: behavioral science research resources:
   (1) Computer processing
   (2) Programmable calculator
   (3) One way mirror observation room
   (4) Videotape equipment
   (5) Endocrine assays
   (6) Psychotropic drug assays
   (7) Electroencephalography
   (8) Computerized tomography
   (9) Calligraphy
   (10) Plethysmography
   (11) The medical examiner's office
   (12) A research requirement for the completion of the fellowship

7. The subcommittee on training in education, headed by Dr. David J. Barry of the University of Rochester's Forensic Psychiatry Program. He notes, "An essential component of any post-residency training program in forensic psychiatry is a continuing series of opportunities designed to foster the fellow's development as a teacher."
8. The subcommittee on the outcome of training was headed by Dr. Seymour Pollack at the University of Southern California's Forensic Psychiatry Program. He notes that, "The ideal outcome of the specialty education and training program in forensic psychiatry is, of course, a reflection of the philosophy of the specialty program and its values, insofar as these, themselves, reflect the operation or roles/function of the ideal forensic psychiatrist."
9. The subcommittee on training in the United Kingdom and Canada was jointly headed by Dr. Selwyn M. Smith and Dr. John M. Bradford of the Royal Ottawa Hospital's Forensic Psychiatry Program. They note, "The situation with regard to forensic psychiatry in Canada is not as well developed as in the United Kingdom. Academic centers of forensic psychiatry exist in Toronto, Ottawa, Montreal, Calgary and Vancouver. There is no recognized formal accredited training in forensic psychiatry and perhaps what is more disturbing is that... very few if any of the 'forensic psychiatrists' have undergone any formal academic training, but have built up their knowledge through experience in relation to the various positions that they hold."

With the development and publication of "Standards for Fellowship Programs in Forensic Psychiatry," Dr. Rosner proposed to both AAFS and AAPL that the Joint Committee on "Standards for Fellowship in Forensic Psychiatry" had completed its task and that it should be replaced by the Accreditation Council on Fellowships in Forensic Psychiatry (ACFFP); the new organization was co-sponsored by both AAFS and AAPL.

Historically, the Accreditation Council on Fellowships in Forensic Psychiatry was initially based at the central office of AAFS, which had more extensive staff and more space than AAPL's Baltimore, Maryland headquarters. When AAPL shifted its location to Hartford, Connecticut, the decision was made to move the ACFFP into AAPL's new office. The decision to move was financial: AAFS charged the ACFFP for its administrative support services, whereas AAPL offered to provide such services at no charge. Despite the change in geographic location, the ACFFP continued to be co-sponsored both by AAFS and AAPL.

In 1982,[3] the Joint Committee on Accreditation of Fellowship Programs in Forensic Psychiatry published a report establishing clear goals and objectives for forensic psychiatry fellowship programs and means for assessing outcome and effectiveness. The report included a didactic core curriculum with civil and criminal forensic psychiatry, correctional psychiatry, specific landmark cases, and supervised clinical experiences.

The two-step process for accreditation of Forensic Psychiatric Fellowship Programs included:

> Completion and submission of a detailed paper form describing the nature, scope, and content of the Forensic Psychiatry Training Program.
>
> A site visit by two senior forensic psychiatrists to evaluate the program, to make sure that the program did what it said it did and that it had what it said it had as resources for training.

The site visits were sometimes exhausting (as well as exhaustive). On one occasion, Dr. Abraham L. Halpern and Dr. Richard Rosner began the site visit at 8:00 a.m. and completed the visit at 10:00 p.m. All of the diverse clinical/experiential sites of the program were visited, interviews were held with the clinical directors of the program and of the separate sites, and detailed discussions were held with each of the trainees (outside of the presence of program staff). Other senior forensic psychiatrists who made site visits and accredited the training programs included Dr. Stanley Portnow, Dr. Jonas Rappeport, and Dr. Robert Sadoff.

In his presidential address, Dr. Rosner published his talk entitled *Forensic psychiatry: subspecialty* in the Bulletin of AAPL in 1989.[4] In that address, he summarizes the difficulties that forensic psychiatry has had in achieving recognition by the organized credentialing bodies in medicine and psychiatry. He notes that the American Psychiatric Association struggled to approve forensic psychiatry as a subspecialty. He also presents the Catch-22 of accreditation by noting that the Accreditation Council for Graduate Medical Education (ACGME) "declined to undertake the accreditation of Subspecialty Fellowships in Forensic Psychiatry because the field does not meet all of their prerequisites. For example, the ACGME only reviews programs in fields whose certifying Boards are recognized by the ABMS (the American Board of Medical Specialties)." However, he notes that the "American Board of Medical Specialties" has explained that, among other reasons, they have requirements for subspecialty certifying Boards with which forensic psychiatry does not currently comply. For example, candidates for a certifying board recognized by the ABMS must be graduates of an ACGME-accredited subspecialty fellowship. Thus, the ABMS requires forensic psychiatrists to first be graduates of an ACGME accredited fellowship program and the ACGME requires them to first be possessed of an ABMS-recognized certifying board. Dr. Rosner notes, "that there is something intrinsically impossible in these mutually incompatible prerequisites is recognized by all parties, but the policies are not readily modified."

The evolution of forensic psychiatry was strengthened in the 1990s when ACGME replaced the Accreditation Council of Fellowships in Forensic Psychiatry at the time when APA accepted forensic psychiatry as a subspecialty. The American Board of Psychiatry and Neurology then became the certifying Board, replacing the ABFP, which sunset in 1994. At that time, new board certification examinations were developed and were limited to 10 years, after which a re-examination was required to maintain one's board certification. Ten forensic psychiatrists prepared the board examination and took a separate examination prepared by a member of ABPN. There are now several scores of forensic psychiatrists who have been certified by ABPN, initially as Added Qualifications in Forensic Psychiatry and currently, Board Certification in Forensic Psychiatry.

At present, there are 40 ACGME Accredited Forensic Psychiatry Fellowship Training Programs in the United States. About 75 individuals are graduated each year from these programs, many of whom go on to take their board certification examinations by the ABPN and are certified in forensic psychiatry for 10 years. There is a maintenance of certification by the ABPN with requirements for self-assessment testing, personal patient programs and Category 1 credits in Continuing Medical Education in order to be eligible to retake the board examination after 10 years.

In 1999, the ACGME endorsed the initiation of core competencies in residency training in forensic psychiatry and other subspecialities. Core competency areas included the following:

- Patient care
- Medical knowledge
- Practice-based learning and improvement
- Interpersonal and communication skills
- Professionalism
- System-based practice

The following changes occurred when ACGME became the accrediting agency:

1. The cost of accreditation was substantially increased. Initially, the cost was held down in order to encourage institutions to develop competent forensic training programs.
2. Following the first accreditation by ACGME, the site visitors were no longer forensic psychiatrists.
3. The focus was shifted to documentation of the program's components and processes rather than in person, qualitative evaluation of the program. Assessment of the six major categories of training in the core curriculum were assessed on a regular basis by ACGME.

Dr. Debra A. Pinals notes that the following is required by forensic psychiatry fellows:

> The forensic psychiatrist must demonstrate the utmost professionalism along with an ability to communicate with each other, evaluees and other disciplines.

> The forensic psychiatrist must have a sound grasp of general psychiatry and psychiatric treatment and must have an understanding of systems of care, from acute psychiatric units to correctional settings. The forensic psychiatrist must be able to utilize evidence-based methods to prepare reports and offer testimony; and, of course, there must be a constant effort to improve practice to professional experiences and self education.[5]

Pinals documents the changes in the forensic psychiatry trainee shifting from general psychiatry to forensic psychiatry. She points out, in her fine article, the stages of development of a forensic trainee based on empirical observation of and reflection with forensic fellows on their experiences each year over the previous 10 years. She discusses various stages of development of the forensic psychiatry trainee beginning with transformation, the growth of confidence and adaptation, and identification and realization in Stage 3. She correlates the experience of the trainees to the learning objectives of ACGME. Her conclusions are worth repeating here:

> The profession demands high ethical standards and sophisticated knowledge of many aspects of psychiatry, law, ethics, and public policy. The responsibility of guiding trainees through learning stages is not to be taken lightly. . . . The task requires giving of oneself, allowing fellows to see supervisors as people with strengths and weaknesses, and helping them set realistic expectations for themselves that will last throughout their careers."

References

1. Rosner, R. (1981). Accreditation of fellowship programs in forensic psychiatry: A Preliminary Report. *B AAPL*, *8*(4), 381–386.
2. Rosner, R. (1982). Accreditation of fellowship programs in forensic psychiatry: The development of the final report on standards. *B AAPL*, *10*(4), 281–283.
3. Rosner, R. (1982). Standards for fellowship programs in forensic psychiatry: A report of the Joint Committee on Accreditation of Fellowship Programs in Forensic Psychiatry. *B AAPL*, *10*(4), 285–292.
4. Rosner, R. (1989). Forensic psychiatry: A subspecialty. The Presidential Address at the 19th Annual Meeting of the American Academy of Psychiatry and the Law. *B Am Acad Psych Law*, *17*(4), 323–333.
5. Pinals, D. (2005). Forensic psychiatry fellowship training: Developmental stages as an educational framework. *J AAPL*, *33*, 317–323.

SECTION TWO

Current Developments: Teaching Forensic Psychiatry

4

The Teaching Roles of the Forensic Psychiatrist

J. Richard Ciccone and Joshua C. W. Jones

> If [the teacher] is indeed wise he does not bid you enter the house of his wisdom, but rather leads you to the threshold of your own mind.
>
> Khalil Gibran

> The mediocre teacher tells. The good teacher explains. The superior teacher demonstrates. The great teacher inspires.
>
> William Arthur Ward

> A teacher affects eternity; he can never tell where his influence stops.
>
> Henry Adams

A great teacher is informative, generative, inspirational, and transformative. Of all the paths down which a subspecialty can shepherd the development of its physicians—as technicians, interventionalists, diagnosticians, healers, and so on—the archetypal role that the forensic psychiatrist plays in modern society is, put succinctly, that of a teacher.

Forensic psychiatry was born outside of the academic arena, spawning from necessity in the state hospitals during a time of rebalancing between the principles of *parens patria* and police powers in states' treatment of the mentally ill. Following World War II, there was also a dramatic increase in the number of departments of psychiatry in academic centers, and as the resources became available to expand the support of psychiatric subspecialties, forensic psychiatry, already growing, was welcomed into the ivory tower. These changes both expanded and focused the teaching roles and venues of the forensic psychiatrist.

Two important benchmarks for any subspecialty gaining acceptance in the academic world is the establishment of a professional organization and a mechanism for certification of competence. The American Academy of Psychiatry and the Law (AAPL), founded in 1969 by a collection of psychiatrists already teaching in medical centers and law schools, played a central role in the development of modern forensic psychiatry. The AAPL's primary mission was, and remains, education: providing forensic psychiatrists with opportunities to exchange ideas and experiences, developing standards for the practice of forensic psychiatry, and encouraging and supporting training programs. In the AAPL's formative years, there were few fellowship programs, so the efforts to educate practicing psychiatrists about forensic psychiatry provided the focus for the AAPL annual meeting. The AAPL meetings in the early 1970s had plenary sessions that dealt with topics vital to forensic psychiatry, including report writing and testifying.

In the mid-1970s, the National Institute of Justice (NIJ) requested proposals for the creation of a certification process in previously neglected areas of the forensic sciences. The Forensic Science Foundation (FSF) and the American Academy of Forensic Sciences (AAFS) invited the APPL to join their effort to answer the NIJ.[1] In June 1976, the American Board of Forensic Psychiatry (ABFP) was launched. The ABFP accepted the AAPL's invitation to have its office in the AAPL's headquarters.

In constructing the examinations, the ABFP decided the experience, clinical forensic skills, and knowledge necessary to be found competent in the subspecialty of forensic psychiatry. The ABFP required passing two examinations; the first examination was a 3-hour written examination. After passing the written test, the candidate was eligible to take the second examination, which consisted of three 1-hour oral exams. In 1979, in response to the board examination and the perceived need for preparation for the examination, one of the authors, (JRC), under the AAPL's auspices, founded the Forensic Psychiatry Course: Board Review and Update.

The teaching function of the forensic psychiatrist stems from the fact that in our view a forensic psychiatrist is first a psychiatrist; that is, a physician who specializes in the diagnosis and treatment of disorders of thinking, feeling, and behavior. At the core, then, a forensic psychiatrist applies that specialized knowledge to answer legal questions. Moreover, the forensic psychiatrist is uniquely qualified to provide expert treatment to individuals involved with the criminal justice system. In order to be a valued consultant, the forensic psychiatrist must first have excellent knowledge of psychiatry, and merge that expertise with knowledge of the system to which he or she is consulting. Usually, the psychiatric concepts that a forensic psychiatrist must apply to legal questions are foreign to the consulting party, but the opinions and/or recommendations that the forensic psychiatrist delivers are usually solely within the power of the consulting party to enact. As such, in order to be effective, the forensic psychiatrist must teach enough foreign concepts to the consulting party that it becomes obvious that the opinions and recommendations of the forensic psychiatrist are important and necessary. Frequently, the psychiatrist must teach psychiatry to the legal system; sometimes, the psychiatrist must teach forensics to the medical system.

As we have stated, the forensic psychiatrist is first a physician who specializes in psychiatry, and as such, reviewing the role of forensic psychiatrist as teacher first must begin at the most fundamental of teaching roles, that within the medical community.

Teacher in Medical Settings

Medical Students

Although sometimes removed from the fundamental teaching of base trainees, the forensic psychiatrist may have the opportunity to make important contributions to the education of the medical student. We would encourage forensic psychiatrists to take opportunities available to educate medical students—even those not obviously interested in psychiatry as their specialty—about psychiatry and the role of the forensic expert. Medical students are deeply immersed in learning the basics of the art of interviewing patients, regardless of what specialty they end up choosing. Forensic psychiatrists should see themselves as expert teachers in the art of interviewing patients. The interrogative techniques and detached-but-empathic stance needed to turn the difficult interview with the psychopathic criminal defendant into a useful information-gathering exercise is directly applicable to helping the young medical student interview the embarrassed and withholding psychiatric-, primary care-, or emergency-setting patient. Beyond information gathering, the expert establishment of rapport with the difficult patient can be modeled for and taught to the medical student.

Skills in clinical reasoning follow logically from skills in clinical interviewing. Again, the forensic psychiatrist is an expert at reasoning based on information gathered from interviews and reconciling that information with collateral sources. For the medical student, these collateral sources may be the patient's history, family input, and lab values. The forensic psychiatrist is used to explaining how the psychiatrist arrives at a particular decision, and this reasoning process is vital for the medical student to both observe and learn from in real time. It is also beneficial for the medical student to have guidance in feeling comfortable training and treating in jails and prisons, where inmates suffer from a variety of psychiatric and physical problems. In this context, the forensic psychiatrist can guide the trainees in identifying the psychosocial contributors to the inmates' illnesses and helping them gain a familiarity with the system that can allow the trainees access to an excellent source of training experiences and opportunities for rewarding interventions.

We would also be remiss if we did not mention the numerous anecdotes we have heard in which a medical student's interaction with a forensic psychiatrist was powerful enough to steer that student into a career in psychiatry and ultimately forensic psychiatry.

Psychiatric Residents

John Romano, M.D., one of the towering figures in American psychiatry in the twentieth century, and a powerful leader in psychiatric education stated "... few matters could be of more importance to the future of our profession than how its young are prepared.... Before World War II,... [t]here was no regular curriculum for psychiatric residents and periods of study and experience, following the internship, were usually one or two years."[2] These postinternship training programs were essentially apprenticeships. Romano pointed out that the enactment of the National Mental Health Law in 1946 led to a notable "increase in the number, the size, and in the diversification of function of our academic departments of psychiatry..." that was accompanied by a dramatic increase in psychiatric residency programs that provided more formal and structured education.[2]

The task of the psychiatric residency is to provide "a broad conceptual and therapeutic frame of reference involving biologic, intrapsychic and interpersonal systems-and interactions with one another, plus a developmental approach to such.... It would also require an ambiance of pluralism and an insistence of critical perceptiveness of data and openness to new information and experience."[3] The ability to conduct a psychiatric interview is central to being a psychiatrist, and therefore a vital skill for a forensic psychiatrist. As mentioned, the forensic psychiatrist is an expert in interviewing difficult subjects and thus being involved in teaching clinical interviewing is an appropriate role for the forensic psychiatrist. Along with honing interviewing skills, the psychiatric resident is developing the ability to synthesize the interview data with other gathered information and clinical knowledge, otherwise summarized as the skill of clinical reasoning. This clinical reasoning includes diagnostic formulation. Both in inpatient and outpatient settings, helping the psychiatric resident develop skills in diagnostic formulation is an important role for forensic psychiatrists within the setting of the psychiatric residency program. Forensic psychiatrists frequently must defend diagnoses against public scrutiny, and are therefore well suited to teach how to arrive at diagnoses and explain the underlying clinical reasoning. The cross-examination by a skilled attorney at trial resembles the Socratic questioning of a seasoned instructor at a case conference. Clinical reasoning naturally informs clinical decision making. In the forensic setting, clinical reasoning informs the opinion of the forensic psychiatrist. Of course, although we are drawing a bright line between clinical and forensic psychiatry for the purpose of illustrating the role of the forensic psychiatrist in teaching clinical skills to residents, that line is artificial and all clinical psychiatric practice includes some elements of forensic psychiatry, for example, treatment over objection cases, involuntary hospitalizations, risk assessments, and mandatory reporting requirements. The forensic psychiatrist is well suited to guide the psychiatric resident in developing the skills to navigate these potential pitfalls of psychiatric practice.

Not only is the teaching of psychiatric residents by forensic psychiatrists worthwhile, but some experience in forensic psychiatry also is required in residency education. The Accreditation Council for Graduate Medical Education (ACGME) requirements for Graduate Medical Education in Psychiatry, promulgated in July 2007, call for an experience in forensic psychiatry that exposes the residents to the evaluation of forensic issues such as risk assessment, competency to stand trial, criminal responsibility, and involuntary commitment. The ACGME also calls for the experience to include writing a forensic report and, where feasible, says that giving testimony in court is highly desirable.[4] Unfortunately, in many programs the ACGME's minimum requirements are only just met and the opportunity to use the forensic psychiatric faculty more broadly is lost.[5,6]

A resident in most programs today has the opportunity to be part of a rotating sampling of multidisciplinary service teams inside an academic setting, and in some instances, to function as a consultant outside the protective confines of the university hospital. One of these settings, in many programs, is in the court clinic.

Court clinics are, as Romano noted, a "portal of entry into the mental health care system for a group of patients, predominantly young, non-white males of low socioeconomic status. Many of these persons who otherwise would not receive psychiatric care can be identified and treated when the clinical services are located in close collaborative proximity with those who direct the criminal justice system."[2] The court clinics provide an opportune setting for residents to have supervised clinical experiences along with didactics on topics of special interest and knowledge to forensic psychiatrists. As Barry pointed out, "professional education is always influenced more directly by changes in the practice of the profession than by theoretical or basic science approaches. Thus, the resident in most programs today has the opportunity to be part of a multi-disciplinary service team... and in some instances, to function as a consultant, rather than service provider, outside the protective confines of the hospital."[7]

In the court clinic setting, the resident learns the course of a criminal trial and the roles of various individuals, from lawyers to judges to probation officers. In the pre-evaluation/referral conference, the resident can learn firsthand the lack of a common language between medicine and law and yet the value of working to understand what is being asked and how to phrase the answers in language that will be useful to the legal system.

Of course, in the court clinic setting, the goal of the psychiatric service is not always—and in fact is usually not—the provision of clinical treatment. When the resulting services have to do with more than the delivery of psychiatric treatment, the resident frequently confronts the dual agent task of answering questions from the criminal justice system. The resident is then thrust into unfamiliar terrain. Much has been written about different ideologies and basic assumptions of the medical system versus the criminal justice system and the problems related to the application of clinical knowledge to answer legal questions. Teaching psychiatric residents to translate psychiatric knowledge and skill into language that is both useful to and understood by the criminal justice system is essential. Preparing written reports for the court is an effective vehicle for the psychiatric resident to learn this translational skill. The forensic psychiatrist supervising the court clinic is advised to take extra time and pay special attention to teaching the written report because it is obviously vital to the court consultation and can be a transformational experience for the resident thinking about pursuing forensic psychiatry as a career.

In the setting of the court clinic, Barry noted that "The residents' initial bias to the population they encounter, reflected in the over diagnosis of antisocial personality disorder and no mental disorder, gives way to a better rounded understanding, and a better quality care, of the patient-defendant."[7] Although some patient–defendants go on to commit major crimes, the vast majority who commit additional crimes commit minor ones. If they commit additional crimes, they will remain involved with the criminal justice system; their mental health needs may bring them to the attention of the mental health system. This calls for the forensic psychiatrist to bring the two systems together for the benefit of both the individual and society. Lamberti and Weisman have written about the way in which their knowledge of the legal system joined together with their knowledge of psychiatry has enabled them to facilitate the two systems working together.[8] The forensic psychiatrist is uniquely qualified to instruct psychiatric residents on the care and treatment of this population.

Teaching residents in the court clinic should be more than experiential. Didactics, often on topics not presented elsewhere in training, are an essential part of the court clinic experience for the psychiatric resident. The list of didactic topics naturally includes seminars on competence to stand trial, competencies in civil settings, criminal responsibility, right to treatment, right to refuse treatment, involuntary civil commitment, and malpractice, among many others.

In the court clinic setting, skills learned on clinical rotations are reinforced and applied to a novel environment for psychiatric residents. The resident's skills in the clinical interview as a way to gather information is strengthened, and the necessity of reconciling the interview information with multiple sources of collateral information (e.g., family members, police reports, psychiatric history) becomes second nature. The importance of the forensic psychiatric report as the main vehicle of communication with the criminal justice system cannot be overestimated.

Forensic Psychiatry Fellows

The most obvious teaching role for the forensic psychiatrist is in the training of forensic psychiatry fellows, and the development of forensic psychiatry training programs. In May 1980 the Committee on Accreditation of Fellowship Programs in Forensic Psychiatry had an organizational meeting. By April 1981, the committee submitted its report to the AAPL executive committee and turned its attention to development and implementation of a formal accreditation process. Published standards for fellowship training programs in forensic psychiatry followed in 1982.[9,10] The Accreditation Council of Forensic Psychiatry Fellowships (ACFPF), jointly sponsored by the AAPL and AAFS, was founded in 1982 as a semi-autonomous component of AAPL. In 1988, the ACFPF began site visits to forensic psychiatric fellowship programs and accredited the first eight forensic psychiatry fellowships in 1989. The forensic psychiatrist as teacher developed standards and played a major role in the creation of the mechanism to accredit training programs in forensic psychiatry.

In 1992, at the request of AAPL and American Psychiatric Association (APA) and in light of evidence that there was a scholarly basis for, unique clinical skills inherent to, and significant interest in the field of forensic psychiatry, the American Board of Psychiatry and Neurology (ABPN) petitioned the American Board of Medical Specialties (ABMS) for authorization to offer a subspecialty examination in forensic psychiatry. The ABMS approved the request and the first ABPN examination in forensic psychiatry was administered in 1994.

The ABPN administration of the forensic psychiatry examination started a ticking clock of sorts, as guidelines of the day required that the ACGME approved accreditation standards for fellowships within 5 years of the first subspecialty board examination. In 1997, the ACGME accepted the accreditation of forensic psychiatry fellowships, and the first 11 forensic psychiatry fellowships were accredited by the ACGME in 1999. The ACGME requirements have continued to evolve and must be incorporated into the training of the forensic psychiatry fellow.[11,12]

Everything that is true about the psychiatric resident's experience in the court clinic is amplified and enhanced in both intensity and sophistication for the forensic psychiatric fellow. In addition, the forensic fellow is intensely involved in the forensic psychiatric hospital with evaluation and treatment of defendants found not competent to stand trial, and of acquittees found not guilty by reason of insanity. Many forensic psychiatry programs also involve the forensic fellow in evaluations for civil litigation, evaluations and treatment of sex offenders, and other forensic evaluations. The role of the teaching forensic psychiatrist here is obvious, including modeling for, instructing to, and supervision of the forensic fellow. Expanding the forensic fellow's view of data gathered during the interview of a subject beyond trusting the subject's words in making a clinical judgment to trusting but verifying with record reviews and psychological testing in forming a forensic opinion captures the role of the teaching forensic psychiatrist at the fellowship level. Perhaps the most vital teaching function for the forensic psychiatrist in the fellowship setting is in the tutelage of the fellow's communication with the courts. Testimony skills, report writing including structure and content, and fostering the relationships with the court and its officers that helps sustain a forensic psychiatric practice are all paramount skills that a forensic psychiatrist should impart to fellows. Additionally, for several years, some forensic psychiatry fellowship programs have added a special focus or an identified training track for psychiatrists who have completed a child and adolescent fellowship.

Other Fellowships

In other psychiatric subspecialties, there may be unique opportunities to interact with the legal system. Child and adolescent psychiatrists are often asked to opine on parental fitness; geriatric psychiatrists on guardianship matters; addiction psychiatrists on drug court diversion programs; and consultation–liaison psychiatrists on medical decision-making capacities. These obviously forensic skills are taught in the associated subspecialty fellowship programs and would be well suited to didactic presentations and supervision by the forensic psychiatrist.

Teacher in the Courts/Legal System

The forensic psychiatrist, at his or her best, also functions as an educator to the courts and other segments of the larger sociolegal system, including law enforcement and lawmakers. All of these entities frequently ask for expert psychiatric input into answering questions about defendants, probationers and public policies. There is no question that judicial intervention into patient care has had a variety of effects and, in the second half of the twentieth century, its insistence on the application of due process to involuntary commitment procedures had a major impact on the practice of psychiatry. In sum, the psychiatric expert opinions provided to the courts have helped shape the judicial opinions about the practice of medicine and specifically psychiatry.

Expert Witness Role

The forensic psychiatrist in criminal and civil litigation has an opportunity to function as a teacher, both through the written report and expert witness testimony. Pitfalls for the expert witness are legion: reliance on jargon, self-aggrandizing testimony, pedagogy, and poorly constructed reports, to name a few. Any of these can alienate the fact finder. But if done well the report is the uniquely positioned triumph of the expert witness to provide information so that a member of the jury or the court might make a more reasoned and thoughtful decision.

The expert witness, by reason of education and training, has knowledge not available to the court and as such is given the ability to go beyond testimony of directly witnessed actions and to provide informed opinions. The judge and/or jury then weighs the credibility of the testimony depending on the credentials of the individual expert witness, the clarity of the testimony, what the expert found, and how the expert arrived at his or her conclusions. The testimony of the expert therefore can be conceptualized as a teaching function, explaining with clarity why it was that the information available led the expert to arrive at a particular conclusion. Of course, if not tempered by experience and self-reflection, this teaching function can be an opportunity for arrogance and narcissistic indulgence on the part of the expert; most courts and juries see clearly and, in fact, are appalled by this behavior. Not many people enjoy an arrogant, narcissistic teacher, and testimony of that nature is generally found to have diminished credibility.

Occasionally, the forensic psychiatrist may act as teacher even to the retaining attorney. The forensic psychiatrist must remember that these areas of the law (e.g., competency) that we are frequently asked to consult on are specialized, and not all attorneys have received as much training and experience in these areas of the law as is surgically focused on in a forensic psychiatry training program. The expert also can be of assistance to the attorney in these matters in terms of how to present the medical information. This includes assisting the attorney more than simply as an expert in the specific psychiatric issue, but also as a consultant on other medical aspects of the case, cross-examination, and even jury selection. If the expert witness testifies ethically and credibly, it is conceivable that the community at large will be positively educated by the psychiatric testimony, either through the small number of observers and jurors present for the testimony or through a larger community audience if the trial is adequately and accurately covered by the media. Of course, poor psychiatric testimony can lead to the educational role being perverted into a farce and circus.

Amicus Briefs

In addition to expert witness testimony, the forensic psychiatrist may interact with the courts by participating in the writing of amicus briefs. The American Psychiatric Association Committee on Judicial Action provides amicus briefs at the appellate court levels, including the US Supreme Court of the United States, on matters of concern to psychiatrists and psychiatric patients and other stakeholders. Amicus briefs are informational and, when done well, serve an educational function and may help the court sculpt an informed decision.

Law School

Forensic psychiatrists also have a role to play in the education of attorneys in law schools. Roy LaCoursiere has written about his role in the instruction of lawyers and has provided insights for forensic psychiatrists who may contemplate becoming a faculty member in a law school. "Psychiatrists have considerable knowledge to offer to legal education. This knowledge includes: (1) information from being educated and trained in an analogous profession, (2) knowledge of human relationships, including attorney-client relationships and their distortions and pathology, and (3) more specific knowledge, such as on psychiatric evaluations for competence to stand trial, criminal responsibility, testamentary capacity, civil commitment and guardianship."[13] Psychiatrists may co-teach with law professors courses that focus on mental disability law and relevant landmark cases, for example. Psychiatrists in a law school setting may provide instruction on interview skills and assist young attorneys in working with clients, whether or not the clients are affected by mental illness.

Teacher in the Legislative Process

Another teaching role of the forensic psychiatrist is to help shape legislation, through either direct input to the lawmakers or influential testimony in a case that ultimately may assume landmark status. For example, Perr noted that his involvement with the New Jersey legislature helped defeat a civil commitment bill that was "poorly prepared in wording, scope, and function."[14] The forensic psychiatrist can help lawmakers bridge the gap between legal necessities and psychiatric realities in a fashion that allows for increased feasibility of proposed legislation.

Future Applications of Forensic Psychiatrist as Teacher

We foresee forensic psychiatrists continuing to be teachers in the future, and the role evolving to include new technologies, new audiences, and new applications. Forensic psychiatrists need to be facile with these innovations, and must be prepared to adapt quickly.

New Technologies

New technologies are radically altering how the forensic psychiatrist interacts with the constituents delineated in the preceding. What were "new" technologies a few years ago are becoming standard practice. What were but fanciful technologies in the recent past are now cutting edge technologies. Real-time teleconferencing that allows high-fidelity communication over great distances is becoming standard practice in remote clinical settings, and we foresee the proliferation of distance evaluation and testimony for forensic work expanding, as well. Telepsychiatry is now no longer "cutting edge," but each year brings more options of input devices, signal carriers, and applications for distance communication. Forensic psychiatrists can and do perform evaluations from afar. One author (JJ) has lectured to forensic psychiatry fellows via Skype from across the continent and testified on criminal responsibility internationally via secure teleconference in a combat zone. Obviously, each new technology raises questions about signal fidelity and information security that must be answered before general usage can be recommended for the routine transmission of confidential forensic or clinical data. Each jurisdiction will, of course, determine the admissibility of distance testimony or examinations for itself. However, telecommunications used for transmission of didactic or supervisory teaching between forensic psychiatrist and trainee are used now, and can be expanded. It is conceivable that a forensic training program could be augmented or even fully constituted using distance learning via audiovisual telecommunication and an Internet-hosted virtual classroom.

It is unclear how the advent of social media (e.g., Facebook, Twitter, Instagram) can be used effectively by forensic psychiatrists to teach, and what audiences (if any) these vehicles may effectively reach. There may be a role for these methods of communication in the instruction of the public on psychiatric and forensic matters, much as the already seen "talking heads" of varying degrees of experts have been used for years on television. The credibility of the information disseminated by these means is and will be highly dependent not on the method used to deliver the message, but of course on the quality of the content.

The proliferation of advanced mobile computing devices (e.g., smartphones, tablets) has opened up an entire new market for easily accessed computer programs and applications, commonly known as "apps." There are apps that are marketed for use by the medical profession and psychiatrists in particular. The fidelity, security, and validity of these enticing yet variably quality tools must be evaluated vigorously by the forensic psychiatrist before any should be used. Of course, any use of this technology in a forensic examination also may have to pass the admissibility standards of the Daubert or Frye tests as well. It is unlikely that the makers of cheaply produced apps will have such standards in mind.[15,16]

Forensic psychiatrists already teach courts about the limitations of using psychiatric concepts to answer legal questions, and nowhere has this been more true than in trying to help the criminal justice system weed through the vast amounts of seemingly sound scientific advances in testing of all types. Currently and in the foreseeable future, forensic psychiatrists should stay educated about the advances in medical imaging, especially functional imaging, to help the criminal justice system understand the limitations of these exciting technologies in determining the presence or impact of mental conditions. Similarly, as genetic testing proliferates, the forensic psychiatrist can help the courts decipher whether these new tools can illuminate the psychiatric components of legal questions, but only if the knowledge is current.

New Audiences

The national reimbursement system for clinical psychiatric treatment is changing, like other medical specialties, in response to the Affordable Care Act and associated legislation. Shifting from a fee-for-service model, the focus for payors, including federal and state government payors, is likely to become an outcome-based model. This model is unfamiliar to the average psychiatrist, and generates consternation and apprehension when discussed currently. Change is difficult. The forensic psychiatrist is uniquely positioned within the specialty of psychiatry to teach the discipline how to integrate outcome measures into psychiatric practice. Forensic psychiatrists who perform evaluations of criminal competency and responsibility, and especially those who re-evaluate defendants who have undergone competency restoration or postacquittal treatment after a Not Guilty by Reason of Insanity verdict, are experts in evaluating the results of treatment outcomes. Many forensic psychiatrists are already experts in incorporating standardized tools (e.g., the HCR-20) to measure outcomes. Forensic psychiatrists can take a role in molding how the specialty of psychiatry responds to these outcome-based changes.

Conclusion

The forensic psychiatrist has a number of different roles. The teaching role of the forensic psychiatrist is often overlooked, but is actually a pervasive and valuable part of the subspecialty. The teaching role allows the forensic psychiatrist to effectively share his or her knowledge with the legal system, other physicians, and the public at large. The future will bring change in formats, audiences, and mechanisms, but not in purpose and intent of the forensic psychiatrist as teacher. We must embrace, influence, and harmonize with that change.

References

1. Prosono M. (2003). History of forensic psychiatry. In R Rosner (Ed.), *Principles and practice of forensic psychiatry* (2nd ed., pp. 25–26). London: Arnold.
2. Romano J. (1980). The education of the psychiatrist of tomorrow. *Bull Amer Acad Psychiatry Law, 8*, 356–365.
3. Romano J. (1980). The education of the psychiatrist of tomorrow. *Bull Amer Acad Psychiatry Law, 8*, 361.
4. Accreditation Council for Graduate Medical Education. Program requirements for graduate medical education in psychiatry. www.acgme.org Accessed March 2, 2014.
5. Marrocco M, Uecker J, & Ciccone JR. (1995). Teaching forensic psychiatry to psychiatric residents. *Bull Amer Acad Psychiatry Law, 23*, 83–91.
6. Rotter M, & Prevar D. (2005). Commentary: General residency training. The first forensic stage. *J Amer Acad Psychiatry Law, 33*, 324–327.
7. Barry DJ. (1980). Teaching general psychiatry in a sociolegal clinic: Down from the tower and into the community. *Bull Amer Acad Psychiatry Law, 8*, 366–372.
8. Lamberti JS, & Weisman RL. (2010). Forensic assertive community treatment: Origins, current practice and future directions. In H Dlucacz (Ed.), *Reentry planning for offenders with mental disorders: Policy and practice*. Kingston, NJ: Civic Research Institute.
9. Rosner R. (1982). Accredibility of fellowship programs in the final report of standards. *Bull Amer Acad Psychiatry Law, 10*, 285–292.
10. Joint Committee on Accreditation of Fellowship Programs in Forensic Psychiatry. (1982). Standards for fellowship programs in forensic psychiatry. *Bull Amer Acad Psychiatry Law, 10*, 285–292.
11. Pinals DA. (2005). Forensic psychiatry fellowship training: Developmental stages as an educational framework. *J Amer Acad Psychiatry Law, 33*, 317–323.
12. Scott CL. (2005). Commentary: Developmental stages of forensic psychiatry fellowship training-from a theoretical underpinnings to assessment outcomes. *J Amer Acad Psychiatry Law, 33*, 328–334.
13. Lacoursiere RB. (1980). A fish out of water? A psychiatrist in a law school. *Bull Amer Acad Psychiatry Law, 8*, 387–400.
14. Perr IN. (1980). Legislative acts and psychiatric input: A New Jersey experience. *Bull Amer Acad Psychiatry Law, 8*, 412–425.
15. Frye v. United States. 293 F. 1013 (D.C. Cir. 1923).
16. Daubert v. Merrell Dow. 113 S. Ct. 2786 (1993).

5

The Program in Psychiatry and the Law

A New Direction in Forensic Training and Experience

Thomas G. Gutheil

The Program in Psychiatry and the Law (the "Program") resides in the Department of Psychiatry, Beth Israel Deaconess Medical Center—a teaching hospital of Harvard Medical School. In the context of the book in which this chapter appears, the Program represents a novel and creative manner in which forensic psychiatry can be taught; in which practitioners can expand their knowledge and awareness of developments in the field; and in which attendees can exchange ideas, collaborate on contributions to the professional literature, and counter the isolation that can occur in forensic practice.

Over more than three decades of collaborative work, the Program has evolved from its origins in several ways. To understand this evolution and to appreciate its current form, it may be valuable to place members' contributions into perspective by offering a conceptual biography, as it were, of the Program's defining principles, ideas, and activities. Such a review will also convey some sense of the functioning of the Program itself.

Origins

The Program was founded in 1979 at the Massachusetts Mental Health Center (the "Center") through the efforts of Paul S. Appelbaum, M.D., employing a training grant. From that point the Program in its present form was co-founded by this author, Harold J. Bursztajn, M.D., and Archie Brodsky, B.A. Dr. Appelbaum returned subsequently for a brief interval to lead the group.

The original mandate of the Program was to train young forensic psychiatrists, who would learn through performing supervised medicolegal and ethical consultations with the trainees and staff at the Center. To date the Program has trained 11 chief residents in legal psychiatry, who form an informal nationwide group of Program associates, some of whom still attend its meetings. Additional continuity is achieved by the use of a website pipatl.org, with listings of members, articles, and the like; and two listservs, Programinpsychiatryandthelaw@yahoogroups.com and pipatl@yahoogroups.com, which permit postings of articles, cases, and information about subsequent meetings.

These listservs provide a welcome opportunity for interested scholars and others from all over the world to receive updates and information, to engage in dialogue with interested parties, and to debate controversial issues facing the forensic field. An open forum thus provided keeps listserv participants in touch with novel and interesting developments in law, psychiatry, psychology, social sciences, and ethics, as well as providing stimuli to further explorations in professional meetings and writings.

Early in its development the Program, consisting then of weekly meetings of its three founders, was joined by clinicians concerned about the use of seclusion, especially in the context of political initiatives aimed at superimposing outside regulation on clinical decision making. Other clinicians began to drop in to test out ideas and gain ethical insight into clinical matters.

Conceptual Streams

(Note that the following citations are representative samples only.)

In the early 1980s, the medicolegal training mandate was enlarged by the confluence of several conceptual streams. The first of these streams was the problem in medicine as a whole of making decisions under conditions of uncertainty while minimizing tragic outcomes resulting from either natural or iatrogenic causes. Over the decades, program members have explored a variety of undue influences on clinical decision making that lead to potential iatrogenesis, including implicit cognitive strategies, time-pressured practice contexts, institutional and managed-care constraints, and misleading pharmaceutical marketing. Processes for discovering, questioning, and testing models of clinical and organizational decision making were first outlined in a seminal text, *Medical Choices, Medical Chances*.[1] Since then, the maxim, "Why has no one asked this vital question?" has guided the Program.

A second stream flowed from a demonstrated need for medical decision theory to transcend the limited model offered by the simplifying, certainty-driven mechanistic paradigm of nineteenth-century medicine, and to apply instead the probabilistic paradigm—a model both more realistic and more suited to the inherent uncertainty of modern practice, whereby benefits, risks, alternatives, and uncertainties can and must be shared with patients.

A third stream reflected the unequivocal need in the medicolegal field to ask often unspoken questions via careful empirical study of medicolegal events and the decision making that informed or produced those events. The need for such study is fed in part by public misperceptions of forensic work, such as: "The insanity defense allows huge numbers of felons to escape deserved punishment" or "Psychiatrists are just trying to get criminals 'off.' " We view this need for applied empiricism as so fundamental to our thinking that it has become the Program's motto: "No one has done the study to find out *what actually happens*." Investigations by Program members have included empirical studies of drug refusal,[2,3] involuntary commitment, influences on risk perceptions of psychotropic medication by various populations,[4,5] suicide assessment and liability,[6] the function of the clinical testifying expert,[7–9] pitfalls of attorney–expert relations,[10,11] and the influences on expert witnesses of such factors as professionalism and biases,[12,13] cross-cultural differences in perception of ethical boundaries,[14] and judges' decision making and job satisfaction.[15,16]

A fourth stream responded to the need for new ideas to enrich the dialogue between clinical and legal realms. In particular, although these realms bear in common a process of decision making, there exists no methodology for exploration of the intuitive decision making that all practitioners employ in real life. Such reasoning had been treated by theorists as a "black box," impervious to systematic and reliable empirical analysis. The development by members of the Program of a "gray box" model that "opens up" such intuitive reasoning for scrutiny remains an important contribution to the field.[17] Similarly, the Program addressed clinicians who consciously or unconsciously used subjective data in their decision making but were often uncomfortable with such usage, despite the often pivotal role of such data in the actual decision. The studies in this area addressed not only the valuable role of subjective clinical data (e.g., the clinician's reaction to the patient's facial expression or tone of voice) in making clinical decisions, but also the importance of understanding mental shortcuts called *heuristics* used in making decisions.[18,19]

A fifth stream emanated from issues concerning the therapeutic alliance and the notion of informed consent as a *process* of dialogue rather than as a *pro forma*, legalistically mandated transfer of pure data. These wellsprings have led to the Program's exploration of both the alliance and informed consent as forces directed toward liability prevention through their improvement of the doctor–patient relationship, the central incubator for the emotional substrate of liability.[20]

A sixth stream was developed from the realization that the field of ethics represents a valuable resource for decision making that (1) is older than both medicine and law; and (2) becomes most useful when both of those disciplines have exhausted their possibilities; ethics is not merely a philosophical abstraction or a form of preaching of "right behavior." Program members, beginning with the chief residents in legal psychiatry, would attend teaching rounds in various parts of the hospital and lead discussion of the ethical aspects of challenging cases; these leaders would aid the clinicians in applying ethics reasoning to those cases in "ethics rounds"[21] conducted in the host institution and elsewhere. These principles were also analyzed in Program writings[22–24] and in the occasional functioning of the Program as an "ethics laboratory" in which individuals from outside the Program would present an ethics challenge they faced for discussion by the group.

A seventh stream that has enriched the Program is informed by theories of the stages of moral development and the manner in which these stages influence decision making.[25,26] These theories have enriched a number of Program research projects, making use of a variety of enhanced statistical models.[27,28]

The Program in Action

What does the Program actually look like in action? Its earliest weekly meetings of three founding members (Bursztajn, Gutheil, and Brodsky), styled as workshops to pool ideas and work on drafts of articles, unwittingly served as the embryo of the present "think tank" component of the Program's functioning—with the Program now serving as think tank, consultation service, and clinical research unit. As interested individuals asked or were invited to attend to share ideas, discuss medicolegal points of interest, gain forensic sophistication, study decision analysis, exchange information, and nurture academic interests and concerns, the Program has grown to about 20 active participants meeting weekly. Another dozen individuals—some former "actives"—drop in on occasion.

Attorneys, psychiatrists (including forensic psychiatrists), psychologists, research methodologists, students of various disciplines, and individuals with mixed degree backgrounds (especially clinicolegal) all participate—as a matter of policy, the Program bars no one and invites participation without "admission requirements." The opportunity thus provided—for egalitarian debate, learning, discussion, and mutual peer enrichment around problematic cases, thorny conceptual issues, and empirical investigations—has drawn to our meetings practitioners combating the loneliness of solo practice, investigators seeking guidance on research design, undergraduates considering forensic careers, clinicians eager to sharpen awareness of medicolegal matters, and others.

Remarkably, the Program has operated for 30 years without funding from any source; the driving forces are morale, respect, and credit. Attendance is entirely voluntary, and members contribute as much or as little as they wish. New members regularly join or are added to the Program's listserv; online dialogues provide active discussion and exchanges of ideas, some of which lead to studies and/or publications. Among the cardinal principles of this process are confidentiality, civility, and considerate questioning of one's own cherished convictions and certainties.

One of the Program's most important structural innovations has been to include gifted medical writers as integral members and attendees, to capture ephemeral ideas generated in brainstorming sessions and to edit successive drafts of those materials intended for publication in professional journals and books. As a result, the Program has been a prolific source of "think pieces," empirical studies—some unprecedented in their subject matter and scope—and education on risk management, as well as a stimulus for conceptual advances in the field. Program members have authored or co-authored some 400 publications in the national and international clinical and forensic literature, salient examples of which are cited here,[29-32] and have reached average publication rates of some 10 papers a year. (In one exceptional year the total reached 25.) These contributions include two major amicus briefs filed in significant legal cases that affect psychiatric practice—one addressed liability for recovered memories of child sexual abuse, and another addressed informed consent for release of health information under the Health Insurance Portability and Accountability Act (HIPAA). These briefs are available on the Program's website.

Over the decades, the Program has continued to respond to paradigm shifts in clinical care delivery and other challenging developments at the medical–legal interface.

One of these arose from the revelations of sexual misconduct by psychotherapists that stimulated a professional as well as society-wide examination of ethical boundaries in the clinical professions.[33–35] A second is concerned with the pervasive threats to the integrity of the clinician–patient dyad that are posed by corporate and institutional control of health care, as well as by insufficiently regulated access to electronic medical records.[36,37] More broadly, the Program has been instrumental in developing and setting standards for expert witness practice as well as in providing risk management guidance to the professional community.

Today, the Program continues to lead in empirically questioning the foundations of clinical and forensic mental health and medical decision making, and in identifying distorting factors in the spectrum of evaluations ranging from testamentary capacity to boundary violations. Such collaborative studies have included exploring the extent of potential conflicts of interest in the creation of the American Psychiatric Association's Clinical Practice Guidelines[38] and analyzing the influence of pharmaceutical marketing on clinical decision making.[39] The Program's international stature in the legal, ethical, psychiatric, and medical communities has continued to grow, relative to its collaborations with organizations worldwide through International Academy of Law and Mental Health (IALMH) presentations and UNESCO (The United Nations Educational, Scientific and Cultural Organization) Bioethics Chair publications.[40]

Future Directions

The future evolution of the Program is difficult to predict, but some generalizations can be offered. As the field of forensic mental health expands both in numbers and in subject matter, we can anticipate that our membership, both actual attendees and participants on our listervs, will grow in commensurate fashion. Present technology permits broad and rapid communication of the Program schedule as well as correspondence among members; in addition, use of the Internet, Skype, and similar communication modalities can be expected to increase. The Program has already benefited from distant presenters giving their talks via speakerphone to the attendees; presumably video presence, perhaps even holograms, will make possible even more vivid presentations.

We look forward to the Program's continued leading role in developing resources for enhancing the integrity and reliability of patients' and clinicians' decision making, forensic evaluations, and expert analyses, to the continued provision of risk management guidance to communities of clinicians, and to continuing to ask otherwise unspeakable questions.

Conclusion

In sum, the original think tank model has expanded as noted into a stimulating group discussion that welcomes input, excludes no one from meetings, and allows both attendees and those exposed to the Program's publications and Internet presence to benefit from free discourse in the sometimes restrictive forensic field. Nothing about this model makes it theoretically unavailable for adoption by other institutions, organizations, or group practices; the Program's demonstration of efficacy should encourage such adoption.

Additional information about the Program and its publications is available at:

- The website of the Program in Psychiatry and the Law (www.pipatl.org)
- The website of the Massachusetts Mental Health Center (www.massmentalhealth.org)
- The website of the Harvard Longwood Psychiatry Residency Training Program (www.harvardlongwoodpsychiatry.org)

Acknowledgment

The author acknowledges his gratitude at the invitation of Robert Sadoff, M.D., a founding father in fact of the American Academy of Psychiatry and Law and, by extension, essentially a founding father of American forensic psychiatry in general; gratitude to the Program in Psychiatry and the Law for contributions to and review of this chapter, as well as creating its content; and thanks to Archie Brodsky for his help with the manuscript.

References

1. Bursztajn HJ, Feinbloom RI, Hamm RM, & Brodsky A. (1990). *Medical choices, medical chances: How patients, families, and physicians can cope with uncertainty.* New York: Routledge.
2. Appelbaum PS, & Gutheil TG. (1979). "Rotting with their rights on": Constitutional theory and clinical reality in drug refusal by psychiatric patients. *Bull Am Acad Psychiatry Law, 7,* 308–317.
3. Appelbaum PS, & Gutheil TG. (1980). Drug refusal: A study of psychiatric inpatients. *Am J Psychiatry, 137,* 340–346.
4. Bursztajn HJ, Chanowitz B, Kaplan E, Gutheil TG, Hamm RM, & Alexander V. (1991). Medical and judicial perceptions of the risks associated with use of antipsychotic medication. *Bull Am Acad Psychiatry Law, 19,* 271–275.
5. Bursztajn HJ, Chanowitz B, Gutheil TG, & Hamm RM. (1992). Micro-effects of language on risk perception in drug prescribing behavior. *Bull Am Acad Psychiatry Law, 20,* 59–66.
6. Gutheil TG. (1991). Understanding the psychodynamics of suicide litigation. *Dynamic Psychiatry Lett, 1,* 1–3.
7. Strasburger LH, Gutheil TG, & Brodsky A. (1997). On wearing two hats: Role conflict in serving as both psychotherapist and expert witness. *Am J Psychiatry, 154,* 448–456.
8. Gutheil TG. (2000). The presentation of forensic psychiatric evidence in court. *Isr J Psychiatry Relat Sci, 37,* 137–144.
9. Gutheil TG, & Hilliard JT. (2001). The treating psychiatrist thrust into the expert role. *Psychiatr Serv, 52,* 1526–1527.
10. Gutheil TG, & Simon RI. (1999). Attorneys' pressures on the expert witness: early warning signs of endangered honesty, objectivity and fair compensation. *J Am Acad Psychiatry Law, 27,* 546–553.
11. Gutheil TG. (2001). Adventures in the twilight zone: empirical studies of the attorney-expert relationship. *J Am Acad Psychiatry Law, 29,* 13–17.
12. Commons ML, Miller PM, & Gutheil TG. (2004). Expert witness perceptions of bias in experts. *J Am Acad Psychiatry Law, 32,* 70–75.
13. Gutheil TG, Miller PM, & Commons ML. (2011). Expert professionalism as judged by experts: An empirical pilot study. *J Psychiatry Law, 39,* 411–424.

14. Commons ML, Miller PM, & Gutheil TG. (2006). Clinicians' perceptions of boundaries in Brazil and United States. *J Am Acad Psychiatry Law, 34*, 33–42.
15. Bursztajn HJ, Gutheil TG, Mills MJ, Hamm RM, & Brodsky A. (1986). Process analysis of judges' commitment decisions: A preliminary empirical study. *Am J Psychiatry, 143*, 170–174.
16. Norris DM, Commons ML, Adams KM, Miller PM, & Gutheil TG. (2011). A pilot study of job satisfaction in Massachusetts judges. *J Psychiatry Law, 39*, 321–337.
17. Bursztajn HJ, Hamm RM, & Gutheil TG. (1997). Beyond the black letter of the law: An empirical study of a judge's decision-making process in civil commitment hearings. *Bull Am Acad Psychiatry Law, 25*, 79–94.
18. Gutheil TG, Bursztajn HJ, & Brodsky A. (1983). Subjective data and suicide assessment in the light of recent legal developments. Part I: Malpractice prevention and the use of subjective data. *Int J Psychiatry Law, 6*, 317–329.
19. Bursztajn HJ, & Gutheil TG, Brodsky A. (1983). Subjective data and suicide assessment in the light of recent legal developments. Part II: Clinical uses of legal standards in the interpretation of subjective data. *Int J Psychiatry Law, 6*, 331–350.
20. Gutheil TG, Bursztajn HJ, & Brodsky A. (1984). Malpractice prevention through the sharing of uncertainty: Informed consent and the therapeutic alliance. *N Engl J Med, 311*, 49–51.
21. Appelbaum PS, & Reiser SJ. (1981). Ethics rounds: a model for teaching ethics in the psychiatric setting. *Hosp Community Psychiatry, 32*, 555–560.
22. Gutheil TG. (1985). Medication refusal on religious grounds: Clinical, legal and ethical concerns. *Cura Animarum, 37*, 21–27.
23. Gutheil TG. (1994). Ethical issues in sexual misconduct by clinicians. *Jpn J Psychiatry Neurol, 48*(Suppl), 39–44.
24. Feldman MJ, & Gutheil TG. (1997). Ethical aspects of competence for sexual relationships: A case of adult sibling incest. *J Am Acad Psychiatry Law, 25*, 217–222.
25. Kohlberg L. (1984). Essays on moral development (vol. 2). *The psychology of moral development: The nature and validity of moral stages*. San Francisco: Harper & Row.
26. Commons ML, & Richards FA. (1984). A general model of stage theory. In ML Commons, FA Richards, & C Armon (Eds.), Beyond formal operations (vol. 1). *Late adolescent and adult cognitive development* (pp. 141–197). New York: Praeger.
27. Commons ML, Galaz-Fontes JF, & Morse SJ. (2006). Leadership, cross-cultural contact, socio-economic status and formal operational reasoning about moral dilemmas among Mexican non-literate adults and high school students. *J Moral Educ, 35*, 247–267.
28. Commons ML, Gutheil TG, Rubin E, Lee P, Goldman MJ, & Appelbaum PS. (1995). Moral stage of reasoning and the misperceived "duty" to report past crimes (misprision). *Int J Law Psychiatry, 18*, 415–424.
29. Appelbaum PS, & Gutheil TG. (2007). *Clinical handbook of psychiatry and the law* (4th ed.). Philadelphia: Lippincott Williams & Wilkins.
30. Bursztajn HJ, & Sobel R. (2003). Protecting privacy in the behavioral genetics era. *Ment Phys Disabil Law Rept, 27*, 523–526.
31. Dattilio FM, Commons ML, Adams K, Gutheil TG, & Sadoff RL. (2006). A pilot Rasch study of lawyers' perception of expert bias. *J Am Acad Psychiatry Law, 34*, 482–491.
32. Gutheil TG, Bursztajn HJ, Brodsky A, & Alexander VG (Eds.). (1991). *Decision making in psychiatry and the law*. Baltimore: Williams & Wilkins.
33. Gutheil TG, & Gabbard GO. (1993). The concept of boundaries in clinical practice: Theoretical and risk-management dimensions. *Am J Psychiatry, 150*, 188–196.
34. Gutheil TG, & Simon RI. (2002). Non-sexual boundary crossings and boundary violations: The ethical dimension. *Psychiatr Clin North Am, 25*, 585–592.
35. Gutheil TG, & Brodsky A. (2008). *Preventing boundary violations in clinical practice*. New York: Guilford.
36. Gutheil TG. (2004). Fundamentals of medical record documentation. *Psychiatry, 1*, 26–28.

37. Gutheil TG, & Simon RI. (2011). Empty words in psychiatric records: Where has clinical narrative gone? *Psychiatr Times*, *28*, 16–17.
38. Cosgrove L, Bursztajn HJ, Krimsky S, Anaya M, & Walker J. (2009). Conflicts of interest and disclosure in the American Psychiatric Association's clinical practice guidelines. *Psychother Psychosom*, *78*, 228–232.
39. De Freitas J, Falls BA, Haque OS, & Bursztajn HJ. (2013). Vulnerabilities to misinformation in online pharmaceutical marketing. *J R Soc Med*, 106(5), 184–189.
40. Perlin ML, Bursztajn HJ, Gledhill K, & Szeli E. (2008). *Psychiatric ethics and the rights of persons with mental disabilities in institutions and the community*. Haifa: UNESCO Chair in Bioethics.

6

Reflections of a Forensic Teacher

Phillip J. Resnick

How I Became a Forensic Psychiatrist

In the mid 1960s, all American physicians were required to serve in the military. Physicians had a choice of entering the military upon completion of their freestanding internship and then spending 2 years as a general medical officer, or they could request a deferment and serve their 2 years after completing their specialty training. I chose to take a military internship to support my family because military internships paid more than four times as much as university internships. The army then had a program called OJT (On the Job Training) that allowed some physicians to practice psychiatry because the army did not have enough residency-trained psychiatrists. I was quite fortunate in being allowed to practice psychiatry under supervision for my 2 years in the Army before my psychiatric residency.

I was assigned to Valley Forge General Hospital, an army hospital just outside Philadelphia. I had excellent supervisors who had graduated from top residencies. I was assigned to a women's inpatient ward. Within 1 week I had two women admitted to my ward who had murdered their children. I administered sodium amytal to each to recover memories of what happened at the time of their crimes and treated them intensively for several months. I was encouraged by one of my mentors, Dr. Aaron Lazare, to write an article about child murder.

Although I then had no plans to become a forensic psychiatrist or an academic psychiatrist, I reviewed the world literature on child murder. That was the era before computer searches so I had to review the *Index Medicus* for 50 separate years, searching for articles on filicide (child murder by parents). I reviewed articles in 13 languages. My article, "Child Murder by Parents: A Psychiatric Review of Filicide,"[1] proposed a classification of five types of filicide. I found that mothers who killed their newborns had different motives, diagnoses, and characteristics than those who killed older children. I coined the word *neonaticide* for these cases and wrote a second article about this phenomenon.[2] Writing these articles changed the course of my career. After my articles were published, I was approached by attorneys to evaluate child murderers even while I was a resident in psychiatry. In the last 48 years I have evaluated more than 80 parents who have killed their children. Thus, I was drawn into forensic psychiatry.

How I Learned to Be a Forensic Psychiatrist

In Cleveland, there were no forensic psychiatrists in the early 1970s to mentor me. When I became interested in forensic psychiatry I became an autodidact. As a young assistant professor at Case Western Reserve Medical School in 1975, I decided to take some courses in the Case School of Law. I took criminal law, torts, law and psychiatry, evidence, and domestic relations law.

I went to the Cuyahoga County (Cleveland) Court Psychiatric Clinic and asked for part-time work. I received no instruction so I had to learn on my own the distinction between a sanity report and a competency to stand trial report. Three months went by before I learned the exact standard for insanity in Ohio. In 1976, the psychiatrist director of the Court Psychiatric Clinic retired and I was asked to take over. However, I viewed myself as an academic psychiatrist and I did not want to devote all my time to doing criminal evaluations. I agreed to become director if I could employ several academic psychiatrists to work one-half day each week. The Court Psychiatric Clinic became a teaching setting where we had medical students, law students, psychiatry residents, psychology trainees, and later, fellows in forensic psychiatry.

I started attending every forensic meeting around, especially meetings of the American Academy of Psychiatry and the Law (AAPL), where I absorbed all I could from mentors like Bob Sadoff and Jonas Rappeport. In addition to reading cases for my law courses, I read extensively on law and psychiatry. I was fascinated by forensic psychiatry and did not find it a burden to read about it every night. In Cleveland, I soon became the most knowledgeable psychiatrist about law and psychiatry. I was invited to give lectures to various groups of attorneys and mental health professionals.

How I Became a Teacher of Forensic Psychiatry

I decided to teach an undergraduate course at John Carroll University called Aggression, Psychiatry and the Law. In order to teach this course, I had to become knowledgeable about many aspects of psychiatry and the law. I made a number of videotapes of defendants and victims to illustrate points for my class. My current collection contains 160 videotapes. In 1976, I began co-teaching a course in law and psychiatry with a law professor at Case Law School.

Since I was quite excited about learning new concepts about law and psychiatry, I was eager to teach them to others on a national level. I invited Jonas Rappeport to co-teach a course with me on the psychiatrist as expert witness at the annual meeting of the American Psychiatric Association (APA) in 1981. The course received excellent evaluations and increased my confidence as a teacher. After 3 years, I started teaching the course alone. I have taught that course at APA annual meetings now for 33 years. In 1984, I taught a second APA course on the detection of malingering. I subsequently added APA courses on risk assessment for violence, the insanity defense, child murder by parents, how to give a more effective lecture, and the expert witness in psychiatric malpractice cases. By 2010, I was teaching six half-day courses at the annual meeting of the APA. Since 1981, I have also taught a half-day course at each annual meeting of the AAPL.

As a result of my APA courses and articles, I received invitations to present lectures and workshops in 49 states (all but Wyoming) and in 23 other countries. I believe that my teaching is valued because I always make an effort to include an audience interactive experience such as discussing a videotape, and I provide practical, useful information for participants. Unlike an article, which is final upon publication, teaching is always a work in progress. Every time I give a lecture I tweak it to be better the next time. Although I practice forensic psychiatry, I see myself primarily as an educator.

I am sometimes asked why I do so much teaching. There are several reasons. There is joy in observing learners grasp a new concept. I find pleasure of seeing an audience enjoy my humor when they expected to attend another boring workshop. Many psychiatrists have told me how my teaching changed the way they evaluate patients and write forensic reports. More than one psychiatrist has told me that one of my APA courses has inspired them to become a forensic psychiatrist. Henry Adams observed that "A teacher affects eternity; he can never tell where his influence stops."

Forensic Psychiatry Board Review Course of the American Academy of Psychiatry and the Law

In 1979, Richard Ciccone was asked by the AAPL Executive Council to develop a forensic psychiatry review course to assist psychiatrists preparing to take their examination for the new American Board of Forensic Psychiatry. I was one of the original four faculty along with Dave Barry and attorney Charles Steinberg. The early review courses were given over 2 days. The review course was well received, and participants expressed their appreciation for helping them succeed in their forensic board examinations.

In 1992, I became director of the forensic psychiatry review course. I selected faculty for their ability to present material clearly and to hold the attention of participants. This is not easy when presenting 8 hours per day of dense material. The faculty uses an interactive teaching style, including video clips, audience response clickers, and a report-writing exercise. My long-term faculty included Thomas Gutheil, Charles Scott, and Debra Pinals.

The review course is now given over 3 days with two tracks on 1 day. Thus, 4 days of material are presented. The course includes an 1100-page syllabus and more than 500 self-assessment questions and answers. About 50 fellows in forensic psychiatry take the review course each year. Many psychiatrists take the review course more than once, either to prepare for recertification in forensic psychiatry or to update their knowledge.

The review course is updated each year with new material, new references, and with the landmark cases that are added from the official AAPL list. The peak number of course participants was about 200 when psychiatrists prepared for the final forensic board examination that allowed them to be "grandfathered" without taking a forensic fellowship. Currently, between 100 to 170 participants take the review course each year. The course enjoys a good reputation internationally and has attracted attendees from Scandinavia, Australia, New Zealand, the United Kingdom, South Africa, Switzerland, China, Holland, and Israel.

Case Western Reserve University Fellowship in Forensic Psychiatry

In the 1970s there were only three or four forensic fellowships in the country. One of the earliest was Dr. Seymour Pollack's program at the University of Southern California. In 1979, the National Institute of Justice (NIJ) decided to provide funding to improve the quality of various forensic experts. One concern was the lack of uniform quality of forensic psychiatric evaluations and testimony. The NIJ offered 3-year grants to fund new forensic psychiatry fellowships. Although I had only been practicing forensic psychiatry for 4 years, I submitted a successful proposal for a grant to start a forensic fellowship at Case Western Reserve University. Other fellowships that started with NIJ funding in 1979 are Rochester, Yale, and the Isaac Ray Center in Chicago. From 1979 through 1990 I had one fellowship slot, two in 1991, and three since 1997. In addition to the funded positions, I have had six active duty military fellows who brought their own funding over the years.

In the early years the single forensic fellow shadowed me in all the cases I saw. I sent the fellow to spend 1 week at another fellowship program to get a different perspective of forensic psychiatry. In the first 3 years with external funding, fellows had time to sit in on three law courses. When federal funds were eliminated, some service by fellows in our forensic hospital was required. We have been fortunate in receiving ongoing funds from the Ohio Department of Mental Health so we are able to focus on education with a relatively low proportion of service.

The Case fellowship gained a national reputation through my teaching and presentations at APA and AAPL meetings. The fellowship has been viewed as desirable because of my close personal supervision of each fellow. Rather than delegate supervision to junior faculty, I have continued to provide several hours of personal supervision each week. I try to pour all the hard-won knowledge learned from my mistakes into the fellows each year. I have a personal relationship with each fellow and I feel a responsibility to equip my fellows with the skills to practice forensic psychiatry at the highest level possible.

I view all private forensic cases as teaching cases so fellows sit in on all my evaluations. On only rare occasions, I have had to excuse fellows when a plaintiff objected to their presence. The Case fellowship is accurately known as a demanding fellowship. In addition to their regular work responsibilities, fellows are expected to prepare for didactic seminars and write reports during their evenings.

The Case fellowship focuses particular attention on forensic report writing. Fellow reports are carefully supervised, particularly the opinion section. Each opinion must be logistically supported by evidence drawn from the body of the report. The strongest evidence should be stated first. Because of my longstanding interest in malingering, fellows are taught to always consider possible malingering and how to detect malingered mental illness.

Case fellows learn to give effective court testimony. Although actual testimonial experience is variable, all the fellows go through several mock trials. Their performance is videotaped and specific feedback is given to them on how they might have answered questions better on direct or cross-examination.

When I am referred "paper cases," such as malpractice cases or testamentary capacity cases, one fellow prepares a complete summary and then all the fellows write an opinion. This maximizes the teaching value of each case. Fellows have the opportunity to prepare written opinions on 8 to 12 malpractice cases during their fellowship year. By comparing their opinions to other fellows during supervision, they learn whether they may have a tendency to be plaintiff or defense oriented.

I also teach our fellows how to improve their lecture style. There is a substantial overlap between the ability to give a good lecture and the ability to give effective court testimony. Each fellow is required to present a grand rounds to the Department of Psychiatry. Before the grand rounds I critique the fellow's slides and observe a practice session to give detailed suggestions to improve their presentations.

In addition to presenting lectures, Case fellows have teaching responsibilities throughout their fellowship year. They participate as direct and cross-examiners for a PG4 resident seminar on expert witness testimony. They give seminars to medical students on suicide and violence risk assessment. They also mentor and supervise residents taking electives in forensic psychiatry and teach law students who sit in on their competency and sanity evaluations at the court psychiatric clinic.

Our didactic sessions and landmark case seminar are taught in a Socratic manner. Fellows are expected to know the landmark cases and be prepared to answer questions about them. Fellows take a final examination at the conclusion of their landmark case seminar that helps them to integrate their knowledge of the cases. None of the 81 forensic fellows I have trained has failed to pass the forensic board examinations.

I am usually able to give each fellow an out-of-state travel experience. They fly with me to another city, meet the referring attorney, and participate in the forensic evaluation of a defendant in jail. Fellows have accompanied me to cases throughout the United States, the American Virgin Islands, and to a court martial in Korea. All three of my fellows observed my testimony at the trial of Andrea Yates in Texas. Because I have had an opportunity to evaluate many high profile cases, fellows become aware of the particular pitfalls in this type of case. For example, they learn the importance of absolute confidentiality and how to deal with the media.

I have given preference to fellowship candidates planning an academic career. They are more likely to contribute to the forensic psychiatric literature and share their knowledge with others. More than 10 of my fellow alumni have gone on to become directors of their own fellowships in forensic psychiatry. Mentoring fellows has been one of the highlights of my career.

Current Issues in Forensic Psychiatry

Sometimes forensic psychiatrists offer conclusory opinions without identifying their reasoning or evidence. Although this occurs less frequently today, it still remains a problem. Fortunately, this is rarely done by psychiatrists who have had good fellowship training. The risk that moral judgments may be cloaked in scientific clothing has been a longstanding concern. Halleck noted, "The psychiatrist is the only expert witness who is asked to form opinions as to man's responsibility and man's punishability."[3] When I teach courses on the insanity defense, I emphasize the need for each of us to assess our biases and be humble in offering insanity opinions, especially in close cases.

The public perceives the successful insanity defense as "beating the rap," even though insanity acquittees often lose their freedom for a longer time than if they had been convicted of the crime. Seventy-nine percent of the potential jurors believe that the insanity defense is abused.[4] The public thinks that the insanity defense is raised 40 times more often than it actually is.[5] The public views the following diagnoses as unjustly "getting criminals off": dissociative reaction, the "Twinkie" defense, post-traumatic stress disorder, temporal lobe epilepsy, premenstrual syndrome, and pathological gambling. The closer a defendant is to normality, the more pubic opinion is outraged by insanity acquittals. People are unwilling to excuse conduct that appears to have a rational criminal motive. Evidence of the ability to plan and premeditate a crime flies in the face of the public's perception of mental disease.[6] In reality, a psychotic person is quite capable of rational planning based on a delusional belief.

The public has long been concerned about malingered insanity defenses. After the Hinckley verdict in 1982, columnist Carl Rowan stated, "It is about time we faced the truth that the 'insanity' defense is mostly last gasp legal maneuvering, often hoaxes, in cases where a person obviously has done something terrible."[7] Concern about defendants' successfully faking mental illness to avoid responsibility dates back to at least the tenth century.[8–10] Even though we have more accurate tests for malingering today, the public remains skeptical.

Defendants who raise a legitimate insanity defense have a difficult time succeeding if their case goes to trial. Eighty percent of successful insanity defenses occur when the defense and prosecution experts agree that the defendant was legally insane. If the defense is contested, proving insanity is always an uphill fight. Juror stereotypes of the criminally insane are drooling, raving maniacs or manipulative, malevolent psychopaths.[4] Only 21% of jurors actually listen carefully to the jury instructions and apply the correct test for insanity rather than allowing their own preconceptions to determine their insanity opinion.[4] Most jurors believe that if a defendant has refused psychiatric medication that he is blameworthy rather than insane.[11]

Prosecutors are reluctant to concede an insanity defense in high profile cases even when the evidence is overwhelming. In one Texas filicide case, the prosecution would not agree to an insanity verdict even when his own psychiatric expert, two defense experts, and two court-appointed experts all concurred that the defendant was not guilty by reason of insanity. The prosecutor went to considerable expense in trying the case, although the county did not have sufficient money in their budget to repair the roof of the courthouse. Based on e-mail posts to newspaper articles, the prosecutor was correct in concluding that the public would have been upset with him if he had conceded an insanity verdict.

Future Directions

In the future, more accurate structured instruments will be developed to assess violence risk, suicide risk, and malingering. Some courts have already indicated that mere opinion in the absence of some scientific data has little evidentiary value.[12] Forensic psychologists who routinely use objective testing will have an advantage. The field of forensic psychology is growing faster than forensic psychiatry. More forensic psychologists will be competing for forensic referrals in the future.

More young psychiatrists will be attracted to forensic psychiatry as third-party reimbursement for talking therapy becomes reduced. Some entrepreneurial psychiatrists who previously might have gone into private practice may find themselves attracted to forensic work as the last frontier where third-party reimbursement is not an issue.

The role of computers in forensic psychiatry will expand, which will make it easier to index and manage extensive data. For example, in a recent high-profile criminal case I reviewed more than 70,000 pages of discovery. Courts are beginning to require that all filings be done electronically.

Because of de-institutionalization, the practice of psychiatry will continue to shift to jails and prisons. Although wardens have been reluctant to employ adequate numbers of psychiatrists for mentally ill prisoners, class action lawsuits have mandated that they do so.[13] Some psychiatrists employed by correctional institutions will move into doing other areas of forensic work.

I foresee AAPL remaining the premiere national organization of forensic psychiatrists. The warmth of AAPL's founder, Jonas Rappeport, continues to permeate AAPL meetings. The American College of Forensic Psychiatry was a competing organization on the west coast. However, it did not attract the national leaders of forensic psychiatry and the organization failed in 2011. The AAPL's views have already been presented in some amicus briefs to the United States Supreme Court. I believe that the number of AAPL amicus briefs and practice guidelines will increase in the future.

Forensic psychiatry is now a well-established subspecialty. When I entered the field in the 1970s, some academic departments of psychiatry were wary about employing forensic psychiatrists. Department chairs worried that high-profile trials such as John Hinckley's attempted assassination of President Reagan would cause the public to lose confidence in psychiatry. They feared that the testimony of psychiatrists giving opposite opinions undermined the impression that psychiatry was a true science. For example, after the Hinckley insanity verdict, columnist Andy Rooney, after pointing out that the five psychiatrists paid by the prosecution all testified that Hinckley was sane and the five psychiatrists for the defense all testified Hinckley was insane, put it this way: "The average person... can reach one of two conclusions about psychiatrists: either psychiatrists can be bought, or psychiatry is such an inexact science that it is worthless. I don't want any psychiatrists mad at me, so I'll leave it to them to say which of these two categories they fall into."[14]

In contrast today, many academic departments of psychiatry want to establish a forensic fellowship along with their geriatric and psychosomatic fellowships. Academic department chairs now value consultation with forensic psychiatrists regarding the legal regulation of psychiatry. They appreciate the opportunity to talk about legal aspects of confidentiality, civil commitment, and informed consent. Overall, the future of forensic psychiatry is bright.

References

1. Resnick PJ. (1969). Child murder by parents: A psychiatric review of filicide. *Am J Psychiatry, 126*, 73–83.
2. Resnick PJ. (1970). Murder of the newborn: A psychiatric review of neonaticide. *Am J Psychiatry, 126*, 58–64.
3. Halleck SL. (1966). A critique of current psychiatric roles in the legal process. *Wisc Law Rev, 379*.
4. Skeem JL, & Golding SL. (2001). Describing juror's personal conceptions of insanity and their relationship to case judgments. *Psych Pub Pol L, 7*, 561.
5. Pasewark R, & Seidenzahl D. (1979). Opinions concerning the insanity plea and criminality among patients. *Bull Am Acad Psychiatry Law, 7*, 199–202.
6. Resnick PJ. (1986). perceptions of psychiatric testimony: A historical perspective on the hysterical invective. *Bull Am Acad Psychiatry Law, 14*(3), 203–219.
7. Rowan C. (June 21, 1982). *Cleveland Plain Dealer.*
8. Brittain RP. (1966). The history of legal medicine: The assizes of Jerusalem. *Medicolegal J, 34*, 72–73.
9. Collinson GD. (1812). *A treatise on the law concerning idiots, lunatics, and other persons non compotes mentis*. London: W. Reed.
10. *The New York Times*, December 5, 1881, p. 4.
11. Finkel N. (1995). *Commonsense justice: Jurors' notions of the law.* Cambridge, MA: Harvard University Press.
12. Coble v. State. Texas Ct. of Criminal Appeals, 330 S.W. 3d 253 (2010).
13. Brown, Governor of California et al. v. Plata et al. 131 S.Ct. (1910, 2011).
14. Rooney A. (June 14, 1982). *Columbus Dispatch.*

7

Forensic Psychiatry Fellowship Training

Fundamentals for the Future

Charles L. Scott

My interest in forensic psychiatry, although now passionate, was not immediate. I first became exposed to forensic psychiatric issues during my adult psychiatry residency at Walter Reed Army Medical Center where I was stationed as a United States Army military psychiatrist. Because military psychiatrists are required to conduct forensic evaluations as part of their assigned duties, military psychiatry residency programs mandate training in a range of forensic assessments, including evaluating competency to stand trial and not guilty by reason of insanity claims, conducting psychological autopsies, and determining suicide and homicide risk levels. After completing my adult psychiatry residency requirements, I pursued fellowship training in child and adolescent psychiatry through a combined training program with the University of California, San Francisco and Letterman Army Medical Center. During this 2-year fellowship, I was further exposed to forensic issues that related primarily to child abuse and neglect, juvenile delinquency, and child custody. Although there was a spark of interest related to my exposure to forensic issues in both adult and child/adolescent populations, this interest was really no more than a fleeting flicker.

After completing my child and adolescent psychiatry fellowship, I was stationed in Germany at a military base where I was suddenly responsible for conducting a range of forensic assessments on soldiers, Department of Defense civilian employees, and family members. True, I had some very basic forensic assessment skills; however, because my opinions had significant impact on people's careers and lives, I wanted further forensic training to ensure that my opinions were well founded. My military command provided me the opportunity to attend the American Psychiatric Association's annual meeting where I signed up for a forensic psychiatry course. I remember sitting in the course and realizing that forensic psychiatry emphasized the use of factual evidence to support one's diagnoses and opinions, much like the practice of other medical specialties. That was important to me. At that moment the spark of interest in forensic psychiatry became a fire. The passion was lit.

I subsequently returned to fellowship training where I completed my forensic psychiatry fellowship at Case Western Reserve University under the direction of Phillip Resnick, M.D. After 2 years as an Assistant Professor of Psychiatry with the Forensic Psychiatry Fellowship Program at Tulane University, I joined the University of California, Davis (UC Davis) Division of Psychiatry and the Law in 1998 as the Forensic Psychiatry Fellowship Training Director. In that role, I quickly became immersed in the Accreditation Council for Graduate Medical Education (ACGME) core program requirements and fashioned my program to meet those requirements. At the same time, I wanted the training program to provide more than the minimum. I wanted to train forensic psychiatrists who would have the skills to become leaders in the field through their ability to communicate forensic concepts, to conduct a wide range of civil and criminal evaluations based on current best practices, and to understand forensic research and structured assessment instruments. For the purposes of this chapter, I am highlighting only a few aspects of the UC Davis Forensic Psychiatry Fellowship didactic program designed to accomplish those three goals.

Communicating Forensic Concepts: Teaching How to Teach

Forensic psychiatrists, whether they realize it or not, are teachers. Explaining a complex concept in court, educating a treatment team on a patient's risk factors for suicide, or developing administrative directives governing forensic care that require support from interested parties—all of these activities involve teaching. It is critically important for forensic psychiatry fellowship programs to implement training designed to help their fellows not only "teach," but teach well. Some individuals are naturally gifted educators. Others may have something to say but have great difficulty saying it. Regardless of an individual fellow's baseline communication skill set, every fellow can become a better teacher and as a result, a better forensic psychiatrist.

During my forensic psychiatry fellowship, I was fortunate to have studied with Dr. Phillip Resnick, an incredibly gifted teacher. From that experience, I learned the importance of organizing key message points and delivering those points in a clear and concise manner. At UC Davis, I have concretized that learned lesson by implementing three specific training activities designed to enhance each fellow's teaching skills.

First, fellows are taught how to present an important forensic psychiatry topic at a national conference. During the fellowship application selection process, I inform applicants that those selected for the program are required to present with their co-fellows at a national conference during their training year. Since implementing this requirement in 2005, all fellows have presented at either the American Academy of Psychiatry and the Law

(AAPL) conference or the American Psychiatric Association (APA) conference, and many have presented at both. Because presentation submissions to AAPL are due in March, before the training start date of July 1, I contact incoming fellows in January and request they work as a group to develop a forensic topic of interest that can be submitted for presentation at the October AAPL meeting. I assist them in organizing their abstract and delineating each of their roles and topic areas.

Once the submission is selected, fellows are encouraged to begin a comprehensive literature review of their topic. On the first day of the fellowship, I review the submitted abstract and help fellows organize a time line to ensure they are adequately prepared. Fellows are instructed as to how to create an effective, rather than distracting, PowerPoint presentation. They are specifically taught how to incorporate various audiovisual aids into their presentation, develop interactive exchanges with the audience, utilize live audience response systems, and effectively deliver their verbal content. Fellows present their presentations in multiple public formats before the national meeting, and faculty members provide extensive feedback on how to improve their teaching.

Second, fellows are evaluated on their ability to provide education to other providers as a forensic consultant. In particular, fellows provide forensic consultation on complex cases at Napa State Hospital, an 1100-bed forensic inpatient psychiatric hospital. Fellows present their diagnostic findings and recommendations to the patient's team and forensic staff. Attendees provide written feedback on how effectively the fellows communicated and supported his or her opinions.

Third, fellows are instructed how to educate a judge or jury in a courtroom setting through a series of practice mock testimony exercises and two videotaped mock trials. At the mock trial, a local district attorney cross-examines each fellow with the general psychiatry residents and forensic faculty in attendance. At the conclusion of the testimony, fellows are given immediate feedback in regard to their effectiveness as a forensic teacher in addition to extensive written feedback provided on an evaluation form that is completed during their testimony. The evaluation form provides a Likert rating for each of the following communication skills: avoiding the use of psychiatric jargon; communicating in a clear manner; waiting for the attorney to finish his or her question; answering questions directly; requesting clarification of a question when appropriate; identifying compound cross-examination questions; responding to cross-examination challenges without appearing defensive; presenting as fair and objective rather than as an advocate; demonstrating knowledge of the case; knowing the relevant legal standard; and supporting the opinion with specific evidence.

Mastering Forensic Psychiatric Evaluations

I direct a psychiatry case seminar that focuses on the practical aspects of conducting civil and criminal forensic psychiatric evaluations. Forensic ethics, forensic report writing, deposition and courtroom testimony, and attorney consultation are heavily emphasized. This seminar meets for 3 hours weekly during the 12-month fellowship. During the first week of training, fellows are trained on forensic report writing. I give them numerous sample forensic reports to help them quickly master basic report writing skills.

This seminar revolves around cases that are assigned to fellows and/or faculty (when appropriate). In addition, a library of hypothetical case materials covering key forensic referral topics has been developed to ensure that all fellows are guaranteed training on the most common types of civil and criminal forensic psychiatric referrals. My goal is for fellows to leave the program with a wide range of reports they have written that they can use in their subsequent practice. Forensic referral issues in criminal cases include competency to stand trial, competency to represent oneself, not guilty by reason of insanity, violence risk assessments, and sexual offender risk assessments. Fellows must write their own report on civil forensic issues listed in Box 7.1. In addition, each fellow must be deemed competent to independently evaluate these civil cases based on their performance in this seminar.

To assist fellows in obtaining competency in the range of criminal and civil forensic issues described in this chapter, they are assigned actual or example cases, complete with the relevant history and record summary. Each fellow writes a parallel report that includes a diagnosis and opinion on the forensic referral question. In this group seminar, every report is reviewed line by line with "on the spot" cross-examination to train fellows on the importance of providing evidence to support statements they make.

In addition to the cross-examination of their written reports, this seminar provides skill-based testimony training in a sequential format. First, fellows undergo a mock *voir dire* that challenges their forensic expertise and credentials. Second, each fellow learns how to effectively provide testimony during direct examination with an emphasis on testifying in a jargon-free manner using specific examples from the evidence to support their opinion.

BOX 7.1 Required Adult Civil Case Competencies

- Americans with Disability Act
- Competency to manage financial affairs
- Deliberate indifference
- Disability
- Fitness for duty
- Impaired professionals
- Malpractice
    - Suicide risk assessment
    - Violence risk assessment
    - Medication management
- Psychic harm
- Psychological autopsy
- Sexual harassment
- Testamentary capacity

Responding to cross-examination is especially highlighted and numerous techniques commonly used by attorneys are demonstrated with appropriate responses to such techniques modeled. The fellows' testimony skills are also evaluated through two separate mock trials described in the preceding.

Finally, in this seminar, I provide detailed training on the practical mechanics of practicing forensic psychiatry. Specific skills that are taught include how to draft a forensic fee agreement, estimate retainer and evaluation costs, write a forensic resume, produce a court declaration, respond to a subpoena, and prepare for a deposition and/or trial.

Because I am also a child and adolescent forensic psychiatrist, I have developed a list of child and adolescent criminal and civil forensic issues that are preferentially assigned to child and adolescent psychiatrists in the program. For further details about the child and adolescent forensic psychiatry track, please see "The Child and Adolescent Track in the Forensic Fellowship."[1]

Understanding Structured Assessments and Forensic Research

University of California Davis is fortunate to have an outstanding forensic research psychologist, Dr. Barbara McDermott, who directs the forensic research and structured testing seminar.

This seminar meets weekly for the academic year and has three primary goals.

Goal 1: Provide fellows with in-depth education on the role of structured assessments in forensic evaluations and training on how to administer and/or interpret these assessments.

The UC Davis program recognizes that it is critical for forensic psychiatrists to become informed on the ethical use and administration of a number of important assessment tools for several reasons. First, the scientific evidence indicates that forensic risk assessments are often improved with more structured approaches when the selected assessment is appropriately matched to the evaluee. Second, statutes and regulations are increasingly requiring specialized assessments to distinguish "high-risk" individuals for detention and "low-risk" individuals for release. Structured instruments are commonly utilized, and in some states required, to accomplish this goal. Third, forensic psychiatrists who collaborate with a testing psychologist, either in a treatment setting or as part of a forensic evaluation, should have a practical working knowledge of the assessment instrument to understand, or potentially challenge, the test results.

Fourth, the structured assessment instruments are standard components of forensic research. In the past, forensic psychology has been at the forefront in the development and research of risk assessment instruments. Over the last several years, forensic psychiatrists have begun to incorporate many of the structured assessment approaches in their research and related publications. For forensic psychiatrists to become leaders in forensic research, to include risk assessment and prevention research, they must have an in-depth knowledge in this area. Fifth, forensic psychiatrists should play vital leadership roles as administrators overseeing the delivery of care in forensic settings. In this role, the psychiatric administrator must have an understanding of these assessment tools, to include both their strengths and weaknesses and appropriate populations for their use. Without such knowledge, the administrator must either proceed blindly or delegate their responsibility to an informed surrogate. Sixth, the forensic psychiatrist is likely to encounter other experts who have utilized structured instruments in their case analysis. The forensic psychiatrist must be trained in this subject area in order to understand the methodology and appropriateness of the assessment instrument used by other evaluators in this area.

This seminar focuses on the following four general categories of structured assessments used to enhance the forensic psychiatric clinical assessment: violence risk assessment; sex offender risk assessment; malingering assessment, and competence to stand trial. Specific instruments in each of these categories are summarized in Box 7.2.

The UC Davis position that forensic psychiatry fellows should achieve competency in administering a limited number of assessment tools does not suggest that forensic psychiatrists can or should administer all forms of psychological assessments and should not be taken out of this context to suggest otherwise. Rather, it is important to acknowledge that there are several instruments appropriate for psychiatrists to administer consistent with each instrument manual's guidelines and commensurate with the knowledge and skills of a forensic psychiatrist.

In addition, the UC Davis program provides specific training on the following areas for each assessment instrument reviewed in the program: ethical and appropriate use; limitations; population norms; research application and utility; reliability and validity, governing statistical principles, and administration procedures; relevant legal issues and restrictions; and the instrument's role in a comprehensive forensic evaluation process. Training on these instruments is rigorous and comprehensive with established standards to determine and document competency.

Goal 2: Provide fellows with skills in understanding research methodology and research applications relevant to forensic psychiatry.

The scope of this goal is broad, ranging from research design issues to the admissibility of research findings and psychological testing cited by expert witnesses. Fellows are required to complete a tutorial on the Institutional Review Board (IRB) process to better understand issues related to research with human subjects. In addition, fellows learn federal regulations and guidelines for research (especially to vulnerable populations), research design methods, and basic statistical techniques to assist them in reading and understanding data in relevant articles. Finally, fellows are required to develop a research idea based on their interest in ongoing research within the UC Davis Psychiatry and Law Program.

BOX 7.2 Structured Assessment Instruments for Forensic Psychiatric Use

Violence Risk Assessment

Hare Psychopathy Check List-Revised (PCL-R)
Historical Clinical Risk-20 (HCR-20)
Psychopathy Check List: Youth Version (PCL:YV)
Structured Assessment of Violence Risk in Youth (SAVRY)
Violence Risk Appraisal Guide (VRAG)

Sex Offender Risk Assessment

Abel Assessment of Sexual Interest (AASI)
Rapid Risk Assessment for Sexual Offense Recidivism (RRASOR)
Sex Offender Risk Appraisal Guide (SORAG)
Sexual Violence Risk-20 (SVR-20)
Static-99 and Static 99-Revised

Malingering

Atypical Scale of the Georgia Court Competency Test
b Test
Inventory of Legal Knowledge (ILK)
Medical Symptom Validity Test (MSVT)
Morel Emotional Numbing Test (MENT)
Miller Forensic Assessment of Symptoms Test (M-FAST)
Structured Interview of Reported Symptoms-Second Edition (SIRS-2)
Structured Inventory of Malingered Symptomatology (SIMS)

Competency to Stand Trial

Competency Assessment Instrument-Revised (CAI-R)
Georgia Court Competency Test
MacArthur Competency Assessment Tool-Criminal Adjudication (MacCAT-CA)
The Competency Assessment for Standing Trial for Defendants with Mental Retardation (Cast-MR)

Goal 3: Teach fellows how to prepare an academic paper for journal submission.

The forensic psychiatry fellow is required to write a paper of a quality to be submitted to a peer-reviewed journal. The paper must focus on a topic in forensic psychiatry. Fellows can choose to write a paper summarizing their forensic research or write an overview of a specific area in the field of forensic psychiatry.

Future Directions

The American Board of Psychiatry and Neurology (ABPN) first formally recognized forensic psychiatry as an area of subspecialization in 1992. Although forensic psychiatry may be considered a relatively new field, our specialty should nevertheless strive to meet recognized standards for the field of forensic science in general. In 2005, Congress enacted a statute authorizing the National Academy of Sciences (NAS) to conduct a study on the state of forensic science in the United States.[2] The NAS committee issued a report titled, "Strengthening Forensic Science in the United States. A Path Forward."[3] The committee commented that the term *forensic science* encompasses a broad range of forensic disciplines, and forensic psychiatry was specifically mentioned as a forensic discipline.[3] A review of the NAS committee findings and their applicability to forensic psychiatry is relevant and important to review when planning future training needs. In particular, the committee emphasized that research is desperately needed, particularly in forensic disciplines that rely more on subjective assessments. The committee outlined two factors that should govern the admissibility of forensic evidence in court:

1. "The extent to which a particular forensic discipline is founded on a reliable scientific methodology that gives it the capacity to accurately analyze evidence and report findings;
2. The extent to which practitioners in a particular forensic discipline rely on human interpretation that could be tainted by error, the threat of bias, or the absence of sound operational procedures and robust performance standards." (p. 9)[3]

In accordance with the NAS's strong recommendations, forensic psychiatry must utilize the most current and objective approaches when conducting forensic evaluations. In many cases, structured assessments and psychological testing provide valuable additional data and enhance objectivity. In my opinion, forensic psychiatry training programs should dedicate the necessary resources to train forensic psychiatry fellows on the appropriate and ethical use, administration, and interpretation of standard assessments methods in order to enhance their ability to conduct research and to conduct forensic evaluations.

It is also my opinion that only psychiatrists who are well trained in the administration, scoring, and interpretation of recommended assessments should give them. An unqualified psychiatrist can and should inform the court that they cannot perform relevant structured assessments or psychological testing. Some may argue that the default position can always be for the psychiatrist to consult with a psychologist on these specific assessment tools. This approach is certainly acceptable. However, should forensic psychiatric educators not even attempt to render future psychiatrists knowledgeable or qualified in this area? If so, why should this be the default approach?

The National Academy of Sciences has sounded the alarm that all forensic sciences, including forensic psychiatry, should rely on evidence-based procedures with sound methodology and robust performance standards. Giving forensic psychiatrists the fundamental skills to ethically and competently answer this call to arms is crucial for our field to lead and light the way forward.

References

1. Scott CL. (2011). The child and adolescent track in the forensic fellowship. *Child Adolesc Psychiatric Clin North Am*, *20*, 565–575.
2. H. R. Rep. No. 109–272, at 121 (2005) (Conf. Rep.).
3. Committee on Identifying the Needs of the Forensic Science Community, Committee on Science, Technology, and Law Policy and Global Affairs, Committee on Applied and Theoretical Statistics, Division on Engineering and Physical Sciences. (2009). *Strengthening forensic science in the United States: A path forward*. Washington, DC: The National Academies Press.

8

The Development of a Fully Integrated Forensic Psychiatry Residency Within a General Department of Psychiatry

Stephen Bates Billick

From the earliest times, learning to be a physician has utilized the preceptorship model. The student would shadow the learned physician and observe the evaluation, diagnosis, and treatment for patients. In my PGY-2 year of general psychiatry residency at the Hospital of the University of Pennsylvania, Dr. Robert L. Sadoff, Director of the Center for Studies in Social-Legal Psychiatry, gave a series of lectures "Introduction to Forensic Psychiatry and Its Relevance to the Clinician." They were incredibly fascinating in content. Dr. Sadoff presented the material with enthusiasm and plenty of clinical examples, encouraging questions and class discussion. After one of the lectures, I asked him further questions and he invited me to come with him on Tuesdays when he would drive around the Pennsylvania and New Jersey countryside examining defendants in jails, testifying in courts, and browsing rare book stores. I explained to him that I could not take up the invitation as I was doing inpatient psychiatry and needed to cover my patients. To my great surprise, my three fellow residents were listening to our conversation and interrupted to say that they would take turns covering my patients on Tuesdays so that I could accept Dr. Sadoff's offer of a personal preceptorship. For the remainder of that year and throughout the entire PGY-3 year, I had a weekly tutorial in forensic psychiatry. Dr. Sadoff would give me literature to read and in the car we would discuss the material. Thankfully, this was before the era of cell phones, so my professor of forensic psychiatry was a captive educator and I was the singular captive audience. During that time, he suggested taking an elective in forensic psychiatry in the PGY-4 of final general psychiatry training.

Establishing a Forensic Training Program and Clinic

I asked my training director about this proposal, and he outlined the core requirements for the upcoming year. With some careful scheduling, he helped me arrange for 50% of the time devoted to forensic training. Dr. Sadoff then labeled this last year of residency training a "forensic fellowship." Under his tutelage, I organized a weekly "forensic psychiatry case conference," a continuing weekly didactic forensic psychiatry lecture, and most important I helped to develop a forensic psychiatry evaluation clinic. We would receive referrals from the municipal and family courts. The cases would be child custody cases, abuse and neglect evaluations, and juvenile delinquency and competency cases. My three colleagues eagerly accepted cases for evaluation, wrote up the relevant forensic psychiatric reports, and presented them at the case conferences. They also attended the didactic schedule. A PGY-3 resident asked to join us and Dr. Sadoff accepted his participation. With the training director's approval, Dr. Sadoff appointed each of the residents as "forensic psychiatry fellows" and named me the "chief fellow in forensic psychiatry." Dr. Sadoff and I continued our Tuesday preceptorship, but Dr. Sadoff added clinical forensic exposure by inviting me to first observe some of his own private referrals, and then to participate in the evaluation and formulation of the cases. In this year, Dr. Sadoff was not only teaching me forensic psychiatry, but was also teaching me how to be a teacher myself, as well as how to design and administer a program.

Identifying Child and Adolescent Forensic Psychiatry

In one of the private cases that Dr. Sadoff had done previously in a delinquency proceeding, the judge felt that the original evaluation didn't fully explain why the adolescent had committed the offense. Dr. Sadoff is a true physician. He is sure of his expertise and performs the evaluations with incredible care and attention to detail. His true physician-hood is also apparent insofar as he is always willing to entertain the possibility that he has made an error. He was quite willing to accept the judge's request to re-evaluate this adolescent, even though the very act of requesting re-evaluation implied the judge felt Dr. Sadoff's evaluation was either not complete or perhaps simply wrong. Dr. Sadoff asked me to participate and I accepted. Dr. Sadoff asked the adolescent many questions in his warm, empathic professional manner and he obtained much factual information. I could tell that Dr. Sadoff's original assessment of what we would now label Antisocial Behavior was also his continuing assessment after commencing this re-evaluation. The youth had had a rather stoic demeanor and was not willing to form even a modest therapeutic relationship during the interview. Dr. Sadoff invited me to ask some questions. I asked the adolescent offender about his childhood. Just prior to the offense, his family had moved from an upper middle class neighborhood in a large urban setting in the South. Both his school and his neighborhood were integrated. His friends were both white and black.

His father, who worked in a high position for a large corporation, had received a promotion and was reassigned to the company's New Jersey facility. The adolescent's new southern New Jersey neighborhood was virtually 100% white and his was the only black family. He was the only black person in the school. The offense involved a white female. As we were discussing his move and the emotional toll on him, the adolescent began sobbing. He talked of his despair, loneliness, and social isolation. He was at the core quite gregarious and loved to be around people. Having been well taught by Dr. Sadoff, I asked about the instant offense in detail and in careful chronological order. As the adolescent related the events, it became clear to Dr. Sadoff and me, that the offense was most likely actually committed by the female friend, the adolescent's one and only friend. It was apparent that the adolescent male had taken the rap to protect her from getting into trouble. After we finished and the adolescent had left, Dr. Sadoff made two important proclamations. First he said that the adolescent was innocent and that he and his family should relocate back to an integrated urban upper middle class neighborhood and would be recommending this to the judge. Dr. Sadoff later told me that the judge, after reading the follow-up report, had profusely thanked Dr. Sadoff and told him that this finally made sense, and that the judge planned on following Dr. Sadoff's recommendations.

From Preceptor to Mentor

His second proclamation was directed to me. He told me that I had to do a child and adolescent psychiatry residency and join the perhaps five living child and adolescent forensic psychiatrists in the United States. In every interaction, Dr. Sadoff has always tried to use it for maximum assessment accuracy and for teaching. Now my preceptor educator was transforming into my mentor. I found a wonderful clinical child and adolescent residency at St. Vincent's Hospital/NY Medical College. It had close faculty/resident contact and interactions. It had outstanding therapy patients, and it had a real rotation for half time, 3 months doing evaluations in NY County (Manhattan) Family Court. This was the beginning of my career in child and adolescent forensic psychiatry.

Forensic Opportunities in General Psychiatry

Within 3 years, my career had taken an unusual and unexpected twist and turn. I was appointed the Chief of Inpatient Psychiatric Service. Three units reported to me directly: a geriatric/private patient unit, a unit for the most severely mentally ill, and an adolescent unit. I also coordinated with the alcohol and substance abuse unit. Within a few years, we established a child psychiatry unit, which I also coordinated. We had a total of 100 beds, which ran an annual occupancy rate of more than 95%. I began teaching courses on forensic psychiatry to the general psychiatry residents. For the PGY-1 and -2 classes, I taught basic inpatient forensic issues, competency, right to refuse treatment, and so on, with an introduction to forensic outpatient clinical issues. For the PGY-4 residents, the course was titled, "How to Stay out of the Courtroom as the Defendant." It was very well attended. These courses and my own preceptorial approach to onsite clinical inpatient psychiatry made it possible for me to interest some residents in choosing a career in forensic psychiatry.

I would invite the residents to design a research project with me, on competency to consent to hospitalization and treatment, as an example. We would write the protocol, submit to the hospital research committee for approval, and then submit to the IRB for review. Once approved, we would perform the research and collect data, which we then analyzed statistically with a review by a statistician. Once the findings were established, the research would be submitted to the American Academy of Psychiatry and the Law (AAPL) or the American Psychiatric Association (APA) for presentation at the annual scientific meeting. The research would be written up and submitted for publication. Most residents used these forensic experiences to enhance their future clinical treatment practices. Some used it as an inspiration to pursue research, and others to pursue a career in forensic psychiatry.

Outreach Teaching and Recruitment

We would also sometimes present research at the annual meeting of the American Academy of Child and Adolescent Psychiatry (AACAP). At these presentations at AAPL, APA, and AACAP, I would meet medical students and residents from other institutions and states. I would offer to mentor them in a research project or in academic writing. Some accepted and we had excellent results, with some of them going on to train in forensic psychiatry. Additionally, I would form panels, symposia, and workshops with other senior forensic psychiatrists from around the country and include at least one resident as a member of the group. Dr. Sadoff would often accept my invitation to speak at one of these events. He enjoyed them and offered mentorship to many new psychiatrists.

As a child and adolescent forensic psychiatrist, with only a handful of colleagues in the United States, I established the Child/Adolescent Forensic Psychiatry Committee of AAPL. Although the AAPL committees were limited to the number of official members, I invited all child/adolescent psychiatrists to attend. For 10 years I was the chair and we always presented one or several submissions of diverse topics for panels, symposia, and workshops at the annual scientific meeting for AAPL. This group also functioned as a support group for the growing number of child/adolescent forensic psychiatrists in the United States.

The Accreditation Council for Graduate Medical Education and American Board of Psychiatry and Neurology Recognition of Forensic Psychiatry

Because of the careful, steady and hard work of the AAPL, forensic psychiatry was recognized as a distinct subspecialty of psychiatry. The Accreditation Council on Graduate Medical Education (ACGME) established standards for forensic psychiatry residency training. Through the residency review committee (RRC) these newly formed residency programs were reviewed and accredited. The American Board of Psychiatry and Neurology

(ABPN) created certifying exams and later recertification exams. The open-ended "fellowships" of the past were replaced with recognized academic residency programs. Dr. Sadoff created a residency program at the Hospital of the University of Pennsylvania—and continued to incorporate a large preceptorship experience within it.

St. Vincent's Hospital Model for Forensic Training

I was asked to set up a residency program at St. Vincent's Hospital/NY Medical College (SVCMC). St. Vincent's was one of two academic medical centers for the medical school. I had integrated forensic teaching within the general residency and I didn't want to create a forensic residency in its own forensic world. Most programs in the United States were accredited through their medical schools, but the training and education took place in somewhat isolation from the greater departments of psychiatry. I wanted them to facilitate knowledge in both directions. The main clinical experience for the new forensic psychiatry residents would be to evaluate patients for competency, involuntary hospitalization, right to refuse treatment, and other pertinent forensic questions. They would present their findings to me, the unit attending and full clinical staff at all levels, residents, medical students, nurses, social workers, and occupational therapists. This was to create an enhanced educational experience for all in attendance along with the forensic psychiatry resident. Additionally, this provided a direct opportunity for the forensic psychiatry resident to testify under supervision in an actual courtroom with a real judge. For their criminal experience, they rotated through the Criminal Court Clinic run by New York University (NYU). In exchange for giving our residents this experience, the NYU residents each had a 3-month preceptorial child/adolescent forensic psychiatry experience under my direction participation. This was the model that Dr. Sadoff has used to educate me. All of the New York City–based programs participated in the AAPL Tri-state Chapter Wednesday lecture series, which covered virtually every topic in forensic psychiatry. This reduced duplication of efforts.

The SVCMC forensic psychiatry residents participated in giving the forensic lectures to the general psychiatry residents. Their mailboxes were in the general psychiatry lounge. They were fully integrated into the department. This was not the norm for most subspecialty residency programs. When I had been a resident in child/adolescent psychiatry at SVCMC, we had mailboxes in our separate clinic area. I never really got to know any of the general psychiatry residents or faculty during that period. When the general psychiatry resident would be on call for consultation/liaison to the medical/surgical part of the hospital, the forensic psychiatry resident would provide counsel on relevant forensic issues.

As part of the ACGME requirements, the residents were required to have a correctional psychiatry experience. In collaboration with the Community Medicine Department of SVCMC, the residents rotated through the Manhattan Borough jail. There they would evaluate prisoners, diagnose them for any existing psychiatric disorders, and begin treatment.

This provided a wonderful opportunity to educate primary care providers on forensic psychiatric issues.

The residents would meet with me for 1 to 1½ hours weekly and review their rotations, experiences, the faculty, and the lectures. They were also encouraged to bring up any relevant topic. These were particularly lively meetings, and quite educational to all, myself very much included. Of my first three SVCMC forensic psychiatry residents, one went on to create a forensic psychiatry residency as a combined Columbia/Cornell program. I was pleased to provide continuing mentorship and give advice to this graduate of my program. Another has become the director of forensic psychiatry for the New Jersey correctional system and has also gone on to create a forensic psychiatry residency at the University of Medicine and Dentistry of New Jersey in Newark. The third resident went into academic child psychiatry and is on a tenured track at UCLA, using his forensic knowledge to enhance his teaching and clinical supervision of child/adolescent psychiatry residents and faculty.

Evaluation of Forensic Knowledge of General Psychiatry Residents

At an APA meeting in San Francisco, a PGY-3 psychiatry resident came up to me to inquire about opportunities for training in forensic psychiatry. He told me that there was virtually no education for his residency in forensic psychiatry. We devised a questionnaire/forensic psychiatry exam that could be given to the general psychiatry residents at Stanford, SVCMC, NYU, and Columbia. He contacted the chief resident in each program and asked if they would participate by coordinating efforts to fill out the questionnaire. Each chief resident received permission from his or her training director to participate in this survey. The questionnaire was a simple set of expected forensic information taken in part from *Kaplan & Sadock's Study Guide and Self-Examination Review in Psychiatry.*[1] Along with being the chief of inpatient psychiatry, and the new director of the forensic psychiatry residency at SVCMC, I also ran the medical student teaching program for NY Medical College (NYMC) at SVCMC. We had the first-year medical students in their behavioral science course, the third-year students on their clinical clerkship rotations for 6 weeks, and also multiple fourth-year electives. Weekly, with the third-year students, I assigned reading in the Synopsis and then gave them practice exams on Friday using the self-examination questions. On Monday, before receiving the next reading assignment, we would review the previous Friday's exam—providing the correct answers and the reference in the Synopsis. Although I corrected and scored each exam, I didn't tell the students that I did not actually keep their results. Their clerkships were graded in two parts: clinical skills demonstrated on the clerkship with patients and a standardized psychiatry board exam. The "exams" I gave them were to alert each student how he or she was learning the material and to provide some practice at taking an exam in psychiatry. These "exams" were simply a learning tool, not an assessment.

The Stanford resident received the data and analyzed it. The residency with the best knowledge base in forensic psychiatry for general psychiatry residents was SVCMC. The worst, abysmal knowledge base was Stanford, where there was no forensic psychiatry program. New York University and Columbia scored in between. To optimize the general psychiatry resident education, as required by the RRC and assessed by the ABPN for the general psychiatry boards, we found that having an integrated forensic psychiatry fellowship as part of the greater department of psychiatry clearly produced the best results for achieving this required education and knowledge base. Not having a forensic psychiatry fellowship at all produced the least education and produced a deficiency. The SVCMC model was optimal. This survey was accepted for presentation as a poster at the next AAPL annual scientific meeting.[2]

This long distance mentoring had a further impact on the participating resident, as I encouraged him to apply for a Rappeport Fellowship from AAPL. This is an honorary fellowship that is for PGY-4 general psychiatry residents who have evidenced a serious interest in forensic psychiatry. It carried a stipend and paid travel/registration expenses to the annual scientific meeting of AAPL. According to the chair of the selection committee, his training director had written quite a short letter containing little substance. However, I had written a multi-paged letter detailing his interest and his accomplishments. Based on my clear enumerations the Stanford resident was designated a Rappeport Fellow. During his PGY-4 general psychiatry residency, he applied to and was accepted at a very competitive forensic psychiatry fellowship, which he completed. Many years later, he is currently practicing forensic psychiatry and teaching the general psychiatry residents at Stanford using lectures and mentoring.

Child/Adolescent Forensic Psychiatrists

Not only has the integration of forensic psychiatry been achieved with general psychiatry, but perhaps more important, there has been a steady increase in the number of child/adolescent psychiatrists pursuing fellowship training in forensic psychiatry. Since the ACGME established forensic psychiatry fellowships, I have been training both SVCMC/NYMC and NYU forensic psychiatry fellows. Additionally, with the creation on the Columbia/Cornell forensic psychiatry fellowship program, I have been teaching and mentoring in that program as well. Some of the child/adolescent forensic psychiatrists whom I have helped to train are now on faculties around the country training the next generation. Several have told me that they utilize the mentoring model that I learned from Dr. Sadoff and have employed for more than 30 years of teaching. From our early modest research projects, some are now receiving their own research grants from the National Institute of Mental Health (NIMH) that will further enhance our knowledge base as we continue to strive for evidence-based practice in medicine.

Keeping Abreast of Scientific Progress

There has also been a dramatic increase in the neuroscience basis for brain function and dysfunction. The faculties of the residency programs need to keep abreast of this new knowledge so that they can teach residents how to apply it appropriately in the forensic context, establishing the generally accepted criteria of the forensic scientific psychiatric community for each new area of scientific discovery. I was the third author on the first published research study of the use of single photon emission tomography in differential psychiatric diagnosis, and I have helped to show where this knowledge could be used in forensic psychiatric testimony. Perhaps more important, I have written on how it can be misused and misleading in the courtroom. All of my research projects and academic writing projects have followed my career-long path of including and encouraging medical students, residents, and junior faculty. Evaluating and applying new neuroscience discoveries have also included mentoring.

The Future

The future of forensic psychiatry lies well within general psychiatry as an important subspecialty that will also greatly help the clinical general psychiatrist. As psychiatry takes on a new, more consultative, and leadership role of a multidisciplinary mental health treatment team in the US medicine of the future, it should be ready to impart important forensic principles to the primary care providers. It is likely that the primary care coordinator of the medical treatment (including psychiatric treatment) for the seriously chronically mental ill may very well be the psychiatrist. Knowing and understanding forensic principles will be essential to good health care.

References

1. Kaplan, & Sadock BJ. (August 8, 2011). *Kaplan & Sadock's study guide and self-examination review in psychiatry.* Lippincott Williams and Wilkins, Philadelphia, PA.
2. Greene JM, Billick SB, Sullivan SP, et al. (October 20, 2000). *General psychiatry residents and forensic psychiatry.* Research poster presentation at the 31st Annual Meeting of the American Academy of Psychiatry and the Law, Vancouver, BC.

SECTION THREE

Child and Adolescent Forensic Psychiatry

9

"The Child Is Father of the Man"*

Mutual Influences of Child and Adult Forensic Psychiatry

Annie Steinberg and Laurentine Fromm

Child psychiatrists who subspecialize in child forensic psychiatry have trained in adult psychiatry and adult forensic psychiatry, as well as child psychiatry and child forensic psychiatry. These training and practice experiences enrich the forensic evaluation and forensically based treatment of child and adult evaluees and detainees in multiple ways. Because the evaluative, report writing, and treatment recommendation principles of adult forensic work guide the practice of child forensic psychiatry, the neurodevelopmental and experiential perspectives emphasized in child training and practice inform the understanding and practice of adult forensic psychiatry. In 2002, Thomas Gutheil referred to child forensic psychiatry as "a shadowed and undiscovered country."[1] In the last decade, exploration of this country has proceeded apace. The child psychiatrist explorer traverses the terrain using landmarks established by pioneers in adult forensic psychiatry, but encounters situations unique to the child forensic domain. At the same time, recognition of the complex interplay of developmental and environmental factors that contribute to a child's vulnerabilities (and resilience) convinces the explorer that the path of adult adjustment is embarked upon in childhood.

This chapter reviews the application of the principles of adult forensic practice to child forensic work, and illustrates through examples the ways in which the biopsychosocial and developmental perspectives of child psychiatry inform the understanding of adult behavior

*William Wordsworth.

which may come before the legal system. In this chapter, for simplicity's sake, the term *parent* is used to refer to the child's legal guardian.

The Emergence of Child Forensic Psychiatry as a Subspecialty of Forensic Psychiatry

The subspecialty of child forensic psychiatry came into existence only within the past 30 years; the first text on the subject was not published until 1980. As a field it has emerged slowly, along with the gradual acknowledgment that children have legal rights. Psychiatrists, psychologists, and other mental health professionals are frequently called as expert witnesses in court proceedings related to children and adolescents for their unique skills in communicating the child's needs and behaviors to the courts. Despite the acknowledgment that specialized information and clinical expertise is needed, there remains no formal fellowship to train individuals in the subspecialty of child forensic psychiatry, and most child psychiatrists who serve as experts in the court have not been trained formally in forensic psychiatry. As such, their training has been limited to a handful of lectures in adult psychiatry training on topics such as civil commitment, duty to warn, confidentiality, malpractice, right to treatment, and right to refuse treatment; some programs in adult psychiatry residencies and most in child psychiatry include single lectures on child abuse/neglect, civil competence/guardianship, competence to stand trial, and child custody. However, it has been noted that most training directors rated topics in child forensic psychiatry toward the lower end of the spectrum when asked to rank the importance of the topics.[2]

Custody evaluations have been noted to be particularly complex and best, if not only, handled by psychiatrists subspecializing in child forensic psychiatry.[3] A curriculum in child forensic psychiatry for child psychiatry residents has been described as including child custody, competency to consent to treatment, right to treatment when in conflict with parents' wishes, child abuse and neglect, and termination of parental rights.[3] Training for the practice of forensic psychiatry should incorporate continuous exposure to these aspects of forensic psychiatry throughout general and child psychiatry residencies, with clear differentiation of the role the forensic adult and child psychiatrist plays in legal matters; the distinction between psychiatric treatment and the provision of expert testimony in court.[3] Within the latter capacity, it is critical to learn how to follow legal standards in each case (and when to refer questions to a third-party evaluator).

The concept of forensic specialization in training was proposed by Dietz in 1987; he suggested that the field of forensic psychiatry should narrow its fellowship training focus to four tracks: criminal behavior, mental disability, forensic child psychiatry, and legal aspects of psychiatric practice.[4] Child abuse and juvenile delinquency, according to Dietz, fall into both the forensic child psychiatry and criminal behavior branches of forensic psychiatry. He outlined the three goals of a 2-year forensic psychiatry program: to attain in-depth knowledge of one of the branches; competence in the other three branches; and investigatory commitment to a set of intellectual problems. His premise was that instead of developing a broad knowledge base in all fellows, we should create centers of excellence in each of the four branches.

Although most forensic programs have not developed specialized tracks in criminal behavior, mental disability, or the legal aspects of practice, a few adult forensic psychiatry programs have developed a track or specific focus on child and adolescent issues.[5] Despite the challenge of recruiting child and adolescent fellows to complete yet an additional training year (after two residencies in adult and child psychiatry), highly motivated applicants now seek programs that have developed these specialized tracks in child forensic psychiatry.

Training that meets the Accreditation Council for Graduate Medical Education (ACGME) program requirements in forensic child psychiatry must incorporate both knowledge of child and adolescent emotional development and psychiatric disorders as well as the evaluative, report writing, and treatment recommendation approaches particular to adult forensic work.[6] The training requires child-focused as well as adult learning sites and relevant (additional) didactic curricular instruction and supervision. Clinical work supervised at correctional facilities for adults and juveniles, outpatient community mental health centers, and forensic units serving both populations, and court-based or public legal aid clinics, now form the core of these child tracks. These clinical experiences are augmented by seminars and case conferences, participation in child advocacy, juvenile or family law clinics at affiliated law schools, and observation of and practice in parallel report writing, depositions and trial testimony (including mock trials). Supervision by child forensic psychiatrists in practice enables trainees to seek additional experience in areas of particular interest, and facilitates the development of a collegial network for future consultation in complex forensic matters.

Unique Aspects of Child Forensic Psychiatry: Implications of the Child's Dependent Status

To understand the experience of the child who encounters the legal system, it is helpful for the trainee to appreciate some implications of the "child" (as opposed to "adult") status in psychiatry and forensic psychiatry. In the wider societal context, children are acknowledged to need a higher degree of protection than adults, and to be less responsible for their actions. In child psychiatric treatment and in child forensic psychiatric evaluation, this need for a higher degree of protection results in the requirements of what might be called the "four Cs" of child psychiatry: custody, consent, confidentiality, and clinical care. Each of these factors has features that differentiate child psychiatry from adult practice.

Custody recognizes that the child is dependent on an adult or agency ("parent") for care. The parent is legally responsible for the care of the child, and consents to the child's evaluation and treatment. The child's custody has several implications in child forensic psychiatry. The identity of the child's legal custodian must be confirmed before an evaluation is done or treatment given. This may require some investigation, as an adult with physical custody may assume that he or she is the legal custodian. Attorneys may not inquire about the child's custody status. In ambiguous cases, the evaluator may need to require that the retaining attorney produce court documentation of the child's legal custodian. If only one parent is involved, documentation that the parental rights of the other parent have been terminated may be requested.

Determination of the child's legal custodian may be the issue before the court, and the forensic evaluator asked for recommendations about the child's legal custody and/or visitation schedule. In this situation, the evaluator recognizes that an adversarial legal process is not usually salutary to the child, and conducts the evaluation in as impartial a manner as possible. It is recommended that one evaluator be court appointed or agreed to by both parties, and evaluate all parties.[7]

Consent to evaluation or treatment is given not by the child, but by the legal custodian. In forensic evaluation, just as in treatment, the identity of the legal custodian must be confirmed to assure that the consent is valid. State laws regarding legal consent to forensic evaluation for children should be reviewed by the evaluator. When the biological parents are not married to each other, and both parents retain parental rights, the forensic evaluator should request the retaining attorney to attempt to obtain the informed consent of both parents. If one parent refuses consent, the forensic evaluator may need to confer with the retaining attorney about the obstacle to the evaluation posed by that lack of consent.

Older children and adolescents, who are able to understand the purpose of the evaluation, may assent, or agree to, the evaluation, although the parent's consent is required. The evaluator should explain to children and youth in developmentally appropriate language the purpose of the evaluation (including the limits of confidentiality), so that the child my give informed assent. If the older child or adolescent refuses, the evaluator may explore the reasons with the family, and should consider deferring the evaluation until such assent is given. If the parents decline to allow an evaluator to explain the nature, purpose, and limits of confidentiality of a forensic evaluation to an older child or adolescent, the evaluator should again consider deferring the evaluation until the parents are willing to tell the child the purpose of the evaluation. Attorneys may need to be educated by the evaluator about this necessary step in the process. In this way, the evaluator accords the child the dignity of participating knowingly in the evaluation to the extent developmentally possible.

Confidentiality in the case of children differs from confidentiality in adult evaluations. First, the parent is interposed in the information flow between the evaluator and the child. Some parents may decline to allow the child to be seen by the evaluator out of their presence (especially if the evaluator is retained by the attorney for the "other side"). Child forensic psychiatrists must decide how they will proceed with the evaluation given in this circumstance. The evaluator may request that the attorney explicate the need for a period of individual assessment of the child before the evaluation, and if necessary, request the court to order the individual assessment, educating the court as to its purpose and advisability, particularly in cases in which the child may have been coached. If the evaluator opts to allow the parents (and child) to decide whether part of the evaluation will be done out of the parents' presence, and the parents or child refuse, it should be documented that the individual interview was requested, refused, and be considered in the evaluation as part of the family dynamics. If the parents are present, communications (verbal and nonverbal) between the parents and the child during the individual evaluation convey information about the influence of the parents on the child's account.

The custody evaluation is a special case in which it is important to have an opportunity to interview the child out of the presence of either parent, so that the child has a chance to tell the evaluator preferences about where to live and how much to visit without fear of offending either parent/caregiver. The evaluator may tell the child, and be sensitive in verbal and written communications to the court, that although the report will reflect the child's wishes, the evaluator need not quote the child directly. This approach preserves confidentiality to the extent possible (in an effort to preserve the child's relationship with both parents) while conveying to the court the basis of recommendations that incorporate the child's experiences of both parents. The evaluator needs to bear in mind that the parent is likely to learn or surmise what the child has told the evaluator sooner or later, and that the child will live with the consequences, if any. Therefore, confidentiality, in the case of children, begins with the question of how much confidentiality is allowed by the parent.

Clinical care of children requires a higher standard of protection than for adults. Societal standards recognize that children are dependent, and require a mature person (adult) to be responsible for their care and make decisions on their behalf. In medicine, this attitude is reflected in the recognition that the child's dependent status requires a higher level of vigilance on the part of clinician about the child's safety. This is why physicians are required in every state to report suspected abuse or neglect to relevant authorities. The child forensic evaluator remains a mandated reporter of suspected abuse or neglect, despite not being a treating physician. If the safety of the child requires the forensic child psychiatrist to step out of the neutral role, this change in role should be discussed with the retaining attorney.

Principles of Adult Forensic Psychiatry Applied to Child Forensic Psychiatry

The American Academy of Child and Adolescent Psychiatry (AACAP) develops practice parameters based on empirical evidence when available, and on clinical consensus, to provide clinicians with principles on which to base practice skills. The AACAP's "Practice Parameter on Child and Adolescent Forensic Evaluations" acknowledges principles of adult forensic psychiatry that differentiate forensic evaluation from clinical assessment, in recognizing the lack of a therapeutic relationship, and acknowledging limits to confidentiality, two critical aspects of the child forensic evaluation.[8] As we have seen, however, application of these principles is complicated in the child evaluation by the child's dependent status. Despite the reality that children do not function autonomously, medical ethics accords them the dignity of recognizing their independent personhood and allows them a developmentally appropriate degree of self-determination. This recognition and respect is not only ethically required, but also increases the likelihood that the results of the evaluation are meaningful and valid.

The AACAP Practice Parameter comprises the following 16 principles, all of which have origins in adult forensic psychiatric practice. Please see the Parameter in its entirety for explication of these principles. The following comments and examples illustrate their application in child forensic practice:

Principle 1. Clinicians who provide mental health treatment for children and adolescents should clarify their role if those children are involved in legal proceedings.

"Except in unusual circumstances... clinicians in a treatment role should not serve in a forensic role for the same child or adolescent." This principle is articulated in the article "On Wearing Two Hats."[9] The roles of treating physician and forensic evaluator are conceptualized to have fundamental differences in goals, confidentiality, and duty of the clinician. Clinicians who provide treatment or make treatment recommendations for children in the juvenile justice setting need to clarify their roles to youth and families.

In another common child psychiatric dilemma, a treating child psychiatrist may be requested by an attorney to give an opinion related to a legal determination of, for example, damages resulting from an injury, or to custody or visitation decisions. In this situation, the clinician wearing the treatment "hat" should avoid assuming the role of forensic expert, because of fundamental differences in role, perspective, and confidentiality expectations.

Principle 2. The role of the forensic evaluator is distinct from that of treatment provider and all involved with the child must understand and respect the distinction between these functions.

This extension of Principle 1 originates in the AAPL ethical guideline that the forensic evaluator should strive for objectivity.[10] The striving for objectivity in the gathering, evaluating, synthesizing, and reporting tasks of the forensic evaluator is conceived as fundamentally different from the healing, advocating, and treating goals of the therapeutic clinician. Nevertheless, the higher level of clinical care due to a child requires that the physician retain a primary concern for the safety of the child. If a child is at risk, the physician has to step out of the objective role, and take on the advocacy role of notifying appropriate authorities. This change in role must be conveyed to the retaining attorney or the court. Aside from preserving the child's safety, a clinician doing a child forensic evaluation must be alert to the tendency to slide from an objective stance into, for example, to an attitude of rescuing a child from a stressful family conflict, or healing a child who has suffered trauma. The child psychiatrist, familiar with the enduring effect of adverse childhood experiences, may find it difficult to determine the line between appropriately educating the court and advocacy for the child in the legal setting.

The roles of treatment and evaluation are easily blurred in child forensic work. An evaluator may get a referral from a parent or an attorney for a child who has been injured and needs treatment. The expectation that may or may not be expressed is that the clinician will, at some later point, provide a report as part of legal proceedings. Similarly, a child who is already in treatment may become involved in a legal proceeding and the treating clinician is asked to provide documentation or testimony because he or she knows the child best. The forensic evaluator may become aware that the legal proceedings themselves are unfolding in an emotionally destructive manner, and form the opinion that this needs to be discussed with the attorney(s), guardian *ad litem*, and/or the court. In situations in which it is not possible to observe a strict boundary between evaluation and treatment, the clinician should strive to recognize the blurring of boundaries, and clarify the distinction in any report or testimony.

> *Principle 3. The forensic evaluator should have adequate education, training, or experience.*

The American Board of Psychiatry and Neurology does not at this time offer separate certification in child and adolescent forensic psychiatry. Issues particular to child and adolescent forensic psychiatry comprise part of the knowledge base required for certification in forensic psychiatry. Because of the complex legal issues and potential role conflicts of child forensic practice, forensic child psychiatrists should readily consult with peers about these issues.

> *Principle 4. The forensic evaluator should have an understanding of the pertinent legal system and system of care.*

The standard of protection required in child work requires that the forensic child psychiatrist be aware of the suitability of, for example, a likely disposition of a juvenile who is adjudicated delinquent.

> *Principle 5. The forensic evaluator should clarify the question being asked by the person or agency making the referral.*

In child evaluations there are often multiple parties with roles in the legal process, and each of them (e.g., judge, child welfare agency, attorney, guardian *ad litem*, parent) may have distinct questions that pertain to the legal action. The evaluator of a child or adolescent should clarify who is requesting the evaluation and who will frame the questions that shape the evaluation, as well as who has legal custody of the child, and who will (therefore) be consenting to the evaluation. If the biological parents are not married, or are not together presenting the child for the evaluation, the evaluator should ask whether both parents consent to the evaluation. It should be clarified that the evaluator's fee is payable by the retaining attorney or agency, to avoid possible conflicts arising if a parent providing the fee feels a sense of "owning" the evaluation. The child should have, if possible, a developmentally appropriate understanding of the purpose of the evaluation, and the limits to its confidentiality. The evaluator should confirm that the attorney and/or parents have appropriately prepared the child or adolescent for the evaluation, so that the evaluation is not conducted under false pretences (i.e., that the child is not in some way tricked into agreeing to the evaluation—consistent with a fundamental respect for the dignity of the child).

Principle 6. The forensic evaluator should know and understand the applicable legal test and standard of proof for the question being evaluated and focus the evaluation on those issues pertinent to that test.

In child evaluations, the evaluator should clarify the legal question that the evaluation is asked to address, the child's legal custodian, the court in which the proceeding will take place (adult vs. juvenile), and the level of proof to which the evaluator will be asked to testify.

Principle 7. The forensic evaluator should determine the amount of time, collateral information, and resources that are necessary to complete the evaluation.

Collateral information, although always important, is critical in child forensic evaluations because the child may be preverbal or communicate largely through behavior and play. In civil matters such as alleged damages resulting from an injury, behavior at home and school may corroborate or refute a claim. The diverse perspectives of, for example, each parent, teacher, guidance counselor, pediatrician, and therapist gives a fuller picture of the child's functioning in various settings. The retaining attorney should confirm that the parents are willing to allow the evaluator access to themselves, as well as to the child's school, counseling, and medical records. It may be necessary to obtain permission from the child/adolescent, as well as the child's parents, in order to access the child's electronic communications. Such materials should be obtained by the retaining attorney and made available to the evaluator. Reviewing and synthesizing these multiple sources of information may require extensive time.

Additional time may be needed to observe the child's interaction with significant adults (particularly in custody evaluations). In child work, actions speak louder than words if the child lacks the developmental maturity to put thoughts into words, or feels inner or outer pressures to give a "correct" (as opposed to a genuine) answer to an evaluator's questions. Observations of interactions and play give information that confirms (or belies) verbal communication. The child's preparation for the evaluation by an adult may influence communications. If, for example, the child has been coached, it may influence the manner in which the child answers questions. A child's behavior may also be inhibited if he or she feels that certain ideas or experiences are unacceptable.

Attorneys, parents, and occasionally the court, may need to be educated by the evaluator as to the time required to review these multiple sources of collateral information and to make the required behavioral observations.

Principle 8. The forensic evaluator should carefully consider the impact of the presence of parents or of the youth's attorney during the interview.

As the parameter states: "Clarification of who will be attending the assessment is important. If others will be present, the evaluator should recommend guidelines for their conduct and confidentiality. Any conflicts will be addressed by the court."

This principle has particular importance in the interview of a youngster, because the child/adolescent is dependent on the parents for basic necessities of life, as well as for emotional needs. Therefore, information that the child imparts may be influenced by what the child perceives as the expectations or emotional needs of the caregiver (see Confidentiality).

Several adults may be involved in the child's care, and on behalf of the child, in the legal case. This can result at times in an unwieldy number of adults requesting to be present at the child's evaluation: both parents, attorneys for both sides, the child's treating therapist, for example. In this situation, it is better for the evaluation to be conducted in a one-way mirror setting, or monitored remotely by video camera, rather than have the child at the center of a large group of adults during the evaluation.

Principle 9. The forensic evaluator should be competent in conducting evaluations in a culturally sensitive manner.

This principle has added importance in the child evaluation because of the greater role of culturally specific nonverbal communications and styles of family interaction. The family may have expectations regarding behavior and communication with themselves and the child that differ from those of the evaluator's culture. The use of professional forensically competent consultants and interpreters is necessary when the evaluator is not familiar with the child's family's culture or when the family and evaluator do not share a language. For obvious reasons, neither the child nor a family member should interpret for each other. Attorneys may need to be educated as to the necessity of involving this additional professional. Child-rearing practices and family styles of living reflect their cultural context, and the evaluator may need to seek information about whether a certain family style is culturally normative. At the same time, it is important to identify abusive behaviors, even if culturally common.

Principle 10. The forensic evaluator should consider whether to record the forensic evaluation by audio or video recording.

Consider that if the child is recorded, the recording is likely to last a long time, and that control of the recording may be uncertain. Although the parents may consent to the recording, most children are not likely to understand the implications of being recorded. Recording should be reserved for those situations in which the potential benefit (e.g., avoidance of multiple interviews of a traumatized child) outweigh the risks (the potential loss of confidentiality).

Principle 11. The forensic evaluator should have an understanding of psychological testing and make use of it as appropriate.

The need for, and scope of, any psychological testing is determined on a case-by-case basis; based on the referral questions posed, or guided by history or record review.

For example, intelligence testing of the child is typically only considered when questions are raised regarding cognitive capacity, or when a child's special needs might be critical to answering a referral question. Psychological testing is most helpful if it precedes any interviews, as test data may suggest areas of inquiry that might otherwise be overlooked. In addition, examiner bias is minimized when psychological testing occurs before interviews.

In addition to "traditional" child psychological testing instruments, risk assessment instruments, such as the J-SOAP II (Juvenile Sex Offender Assessment Protocol II) and the SAVRY (Structured Assessment of Violence Risk in Youth) are now available.[11,12] Use of these risk-assessment instruments parallels the use of risk-assessment tools such as the Hare PCL-R in the adult forensic setting, although most have fewer years of use and more limited validation.[13] Similar to adult self-administered instruments, the literacy level and processing of written material by children and adolescents should be considered before administering these tools, and from the most pragmatic perspective, some will require an additional 30 minutes for completion.

These instruments should be used by those with the appropriate training. They are not a substitute for a clinical evaluation including synthesis of the relevant history, interviews, and collateral information with the psychiatric examination of the youth. In adult risk assessment, the structured professional judgment (SPJ) model incorporates risk factors in a structured fashion, allowing for flexibility by the clinician in the weighting and relevance of factors.[14] Further research will elucidate the use and value of these instruments for children and adolescents.

Principle 12. The forensic evaluator should be aware of the types of and level of clinical services available and different indications when making treatment or placement recommendations.

In some cases, the court will specifically request placement and treatment recommendations. Other evaluations, such as personal injury or child custody, may not explicitly request recommendations, and while bearing the evaluation role in mind, the clinician's professional judgment may be that the evaluation has revealed information that mandates treatment recommendations. The evaluator has a professional responsibility to record and communicate those treatment recommendations felt to be necessary for the child's health and safety.

For many children and adolescents, the forensic evaluation will provide the most time and consideration given to their social situation and emotional needs. In most cases, the evaluator should not assume treatment of the child, but if indicated, may provide appropriate referrals to community resources.

Principle 13. The forensic evaluator should be prepared to document the findings of the evaluation and the opinions reached in a report.

The report of a child forensic evaluation synthesizes information from multiple sources into a coherent narrative that represents the evaluator's best understanding of the factors contributing to the opinion recorded.[15] This narrative should serve to humanize the child's experience to the court and to explain interpersonal relationships related to the legal matter. The reasoning in the report should be sound and recorded in the report. The writer should strive for objectivity of language as well as viewpoint. Emotionally charged expressions such as "this unfortunate child suffered" should be avoided in favor of more neutral language such as "this child underwent." Sensitive family and personal information should be included only if relevant to the legal question under consideration. Since the report becomes part of the legal record, the evaluator should respect shielding of the child's identity by the use of initials or a pseudonym (e.g., "child Doe"). The writer should bear in mind that this document may form part of the child's legal history for many years and statements about prognosis should be circumspect; children can change dramatically over the course of maturation, and educating the court about the capacity for growth is a specific and important component of many child forensic evaluations, particularly those involving the juvenile court or children waived to adult court.

Principle 14. The forensic evaluator should be prepared to testify in depositions and in court.

In the adversarial setting of the deposition or courtroom, attorneys actively advocate for their side. In this setting, they may intentionally use faulty logic and emotionalized language to try to sway a judge or jury's opinion. The testifying expert is well served by a soundly reasoned and neutrally expressed opinion that has been recorded in writing. Such an opinion redirects the attention of the court to genuinely relevant issues. If the expert becomes temporarily flustered under aggressive questioning, briefly referring to the written report will help to remind the expert of reasoning carefully thought through in calmer moments.

Principal 15. The forensic evaluator should consider the pros and cons of whether a child should testify.

The expert should be prepared to educate attorneys and the court about issues related to developmental and family dynamics. Regarding cognitive level, for example, the child's understanding of time (how long, how many times) differs with age; a "hundred times" has different meanings for toddlers and adolescents. Regarding truthfulness, despite having recognized to the court's satisfaction the nature of a lie, and acknowledged that to lie is wrong, a child may be motivated to lie out of fear of alienating an important attachment figure or a person on whom one is dependent. Regarding accuracy of memory, in addition to the complex issue of suggestive questioning, the expert may need to distinguish for the court the difference between historical and emotional truth[16]; a child may report an incident as true because it is an emotionally accurate record of the child's experience, although not an historic fact. The complex arena of evaluating the accuracy of children's statements requires a foundation in child development and knowledge of the scientific evidence that has emerged; accuracy is optimal in the first report of a child, presuming appropriate and nonleading questions; inaccuracy can be related to perception, poor recall, cognitive limitations, and other factors.

Principle 16. The forensic evaluator should adhere to the ethical guidelines of his or her respective professional organizations.

The Parameter acknowledges that, "ethical principles for forensic psychiatric evaluations of minors have not been fully developed." Therefore, in complex evaluative and testimony situations, it is helpful for the child forensic psychiatrist to consult with a colleague to explore the issues and decisions involved, as well as to benefit from supportive exploration of what can be emotionally trying professional experiences.

Principles of Child Forensic Psychiatry Applied to Adult Forensic Psychiatry

Example 1. Developmental Maturation: Criminal Culpability and Mitigation in the Sentencing of Juveniles

In the juvenile justice arena, the child forensic psychiatrist is asked to assist the court in determining a juvenile's psychiatric diagnosis, amenability to treatment, and risk of future dangerousness. There also may be the question of competency to waive Miranda rights, competency to participate in delinquency proceedings, competence to stand trial as an adult (including eligibility for being tried in adult court, or waiver to adult court, and competency to stand trial if insanity is raised as a defense). In recent years, the testimony of developmentally informed child forensic experts has had a significant impact on decisions, including important Supreme Court decisions such as *Roper v. Simmons* and *Graham v. Florida*, establishing that children are constitutionally different from adults for sentencing purposes, citing differences in maturity, sense of responsibility, impulsivity, risk-taking behaviors, and vulnerability to peer influence.[17,18] The impermanence of the adolescent phase of development and the likelihood of change was also cited. Both *Roper* and *Graham* explained why it was wrong for juvenile offenders, even when they commit terrible crimes, to be given the harshest of sentences. *Roper v. Simmons* held that the Eighth Amendment bars capital punishment for children, and *Graham v. Florida* concluded that the Amendment prohibits a sentence of life without the possibility of parole for a juvenile convicted of a nonhomicide offense.

In a more recent decision, two 14 year olds were charged with murder in the course of arson (while intoxicated and using drugs) and sentenced to statutorily mandated life without parole. The Supreme Court held that the Eighth Amendment forbids a sentencing scheme that mandates life in prison without possibility of parole for juvenile homicide offenders in *Miller v. Alabama*.[19] As a result, juvenile homicide offenders now have the opportunity to be re-evaluated as part of the judicial process in order to determine whether or not they should have the possibility of parole.

Familiarity with the adolescent brain (and its difference from the adult brain with respect to impulse control, risk aversion, and cognitive skills, such as problem solving and assessment of consequences), psychosocial and socioeconomic variables affecting the juvenile at the time of the crime, and the history of complex trauma that so often results in adolescent criminal behavior are but a few of the critical aspects of the retrospective examination of the crime and the individual's developmental trajectory (including character and moral capacity) since the time of the crime and while incarcerated.

The developmental construct of child and adolescent forensic psychiatry informs the adult forensic expert to retrospectively examine adolescent risk-taking and thrill-seeking behaviors, inability to conceptualize the future, egocentrism and sense of invincibility, and peer influences as a basis for distinguishing identity, familial influences and values, and social skills, as well as the gradual nature of cognitive developmental changes, identity consolidation, morality, and capacity for reasoning. The Miller cases revisited also present an opportunity to assess the impact of incarceration, the atypical environment of the prison, and the peer group of inmates, often adult, on the moral development and general life trajectory of the adolescent.

Example 2. Adult Presentation of Childhood and Developmental Disorders: Autistic Spectrum Disorders, Intellectual Disability, and Crime

In *Atkins v. Virginia*, the US Supreme Court found that the execution of offenders with intellectual disabilities was unconstitutional, as it violated the Eighth Amendment prohibition on cruel and unusual punishment.[20] However, states were left to determine the criteria for defining intellectual disability. In *Hall v. Florida*, Hall was sentenced to death because he scored one point above the cutoff for intellectual disability on a recent IQ test.[21] In hearing this matter, the Supreme Court found the state's threshold in deciding this matter to be unconstitutional, as it does not reflect medical practice, in which intellectual disability is defined by the presence of deficits in both intellectual and adaptive functioning, in evidence in the developmental period. This decision acknowledged the reliance on medical professionals, their diagnostic framework and informed assessments, as well as the imprecise nature of IQ testing, noting that a fixed numerical cutoff by the states would fail to honor the Eighth Amendment's protection of human dignity. The decision will determine how the Atkins mandate will be implemented in future cases involving serious offenders with intellectual disabilities, setting a national standard for how intellectual disability should be defined in the legal arena, where cutoff IQ scores have been used until now despite much broader definitions in the clinical arena. The child forensic context can help inform expert testimony by educating the court as to the limited utility of categorical cutoff scores in matters such as developmental age, levels of functioning, and the numerous other factors that influence the developmental capacity of an individual with a lifelong developmental disorder.

Autism is another example of a domain in which the child forensic perspective can inform the adult forensic expert and the court. A pervasive and lifelong developmental disorder that results in intensely focused and stereotypic interests, autism profoundly affects almost every aspect of an individual's functioning in the community at large. These conditions have their onset in the first years of life, disrupt diverse developmental processes, and can be associated with cognitive impairment. The history obtained by the forensic expert must examine the entire developmental trajectory from birth forward to ensure that it is consistent with this diagnosis and to assist the court in understanding the profound impact of autism spectrum disorder on past behaviors, the capacity to understand social encounters, to make decisions independently, and to understand the full consequence of the choices in the social situation. The autistic brain works in fundamentally different ways than the brains of same-age peers; delayed and dysfunctional neural development can undermine every decision, in particular, social judgment, developmental maturity, most evident in the areas of not only judgment, but also rational thinking, organization of sequential behaviors, abstraction, mental flexibility, social cognition, and perceptions of social interaction.

The court needs to understand the organic nature of autism, and what is known neuropathologically as well as neurochemically and genetically. As a severe developmental disorder of the brain that many researchers believe to be both heritable and the result of an antenatal event occurring quite early in pregnancy, there is still wide phenotypic variation that must be explained to the court. The forensic expert may also need to address misperceptions and negative stigma about the incidence of violence among individuals with developmental disorders such as autism; the number of reports of violence or offense by people with autism or Asperger's syndrome is actually very small and indeed, because of the very rigid way in which many tend to keep to rules and regulations, they may well be more law-abiding than the general population. Aside from largely anecdotal reports of inappropriate social response, especially to strangers that may result in police involvement and crimes related to obsessional interests, there is little evidence in support of the prevalence of individuals with autism committing criminal acts.

In the forensic context, the role of the expert is, in large part, to help others understand the developmental nature and severity of neurobiological disorders that result in social maladjustment, isolation, conspicuous eccentricity with an obsessive quality, as well as features that may increase risk of criminal involvement necessitating psychiatric input, for example, a desire for intimate partners but lack of skills, impaired social interactions, interpersonal naïvete, and the likelihood of immediate confession. For individuals with pervasive developmental disorders, the biological impairment of the expression of remorse and empathy must be explained to police and others who evaluate the individual's ability to appreciate the nature of the crime and capacity to conform to typical behaviors.

Expert assessment may avoid the case coming to court or help to mitigate punitive action. Incarceration of adults with developmental disorders such as autism in the general population will likely result in control, exploitation, and abuse by other inmates because of their social inexperience. Therefore, the separation from other offenders is critical in ensuring safety. Uneducated staff may misinterpret the rigid or obsessive autistic individual as rude or incorrigible and react punitively. When it is necessary to incarcerate an individual with autism or other developmental disorders, the forensic expert may need to guide placement, because severe social and language disabilities have a profound impact on the ability to function and respond appropriately in confinement with other adults. These individuals require programs that recognize and address their unique characteristics and needs, and the developmental perspective of child forensic psychiatrist can inform the correctional system so that undue harm can be avoided.

Example 3. Sensitive Periods in Brain Development: Adoption/Family Law and Trauma

Trauma is another area in which the child developmental context informs the forensic expert. In civil litigation, there are assessments of trauma and evaluations of posttraumatic stress disorders in childhood (and adulthood), including implications of the event for the developmental life of the child; assessment of psychiatric damages resulting from personal injury or loss. There are evaluations assessing allegations of neglect, emotional, physical, and sexual abuse, and in dependency matters and family law pertaining to children who may have experienced trauma, there are determinations of child custody, evaluations of parental capacity, termination of parental rights, and complex cases that must assess what is in the best interests of the child (least detrimental alternative).

Brain development research links early adverse life events with alterations in neural circuitry with long-lasting negative consequences, not only on mental health, but also on social and health-related behaviors. Early caregiving environments are also increasingly shown to correlate with the development of neural circuits that regulate emotional reactivity; critical windows during which one may provide appropriate environmental and emotional stimulation and avert neural changes, language delays, and cortisol fear/stress responses also have been outlined; this translational research evidence is information that must be shared with the court to facilitate decision making relevant to both child and adult matters.

In civil litigation involving physical injury to the child (e.g., a motor vehicle accident), the impact of the injury often is alleged to include psychological distress beyond the acute stress reaction to include persistent posttraumatic symptoms that impede full recovery. The child forensic perspective addresses the manner in which child stress responses are both similar and different from adult manifestations. The malleability of childhood is such that the caregiver and family factors (e.g., parental response and level of distress) impact treatment and outcome significantly, predicting both resilience and maladaptive responses, often regardless of the severity of the trauma. Intrinsic preinjury traits such as anxiety, the nature and context of the injury and its meaning to the child and family, as well as the familial and social support network in place after the injury are also key factors in the assessment of trauma and its etiologies, and play particularly strategic roles in recovery, regardless of the injury or trauma. Furthermore, because of the unique developmental trajectory of early childhood (including limited language and emotional control, critical nature of the primary caregivers, and attachment relationship in supporting self-regulation, as well as neurobiological and neurochemical changes secondary to trauma), all of these factors are inextricably intertwined in childhood and adolescence, rendering determinations of direct causation challenging for the forensic expert charged with this task.

With the recent changes in diagnostic criteria for posttraumatic disorders, it will be even more incumbent on the child forensic expert to understand the developmental context, obtain collateral information that confirms or refutes the child's and parents' reports, explore impact on social, occupational, and school functioning as well as home behaviors, ponder the potential legal import of subthreshold presentations, and ensure the coherence of the assessment so as to sustain a potential Daubert challenge.

In all family matters, the child developmental context can also be seen; direct or indirect exposure to intrafamilial violence impacts the child's capacity to learn, think, and develop, and may result in anxiety and depression, as well as aggression and other behavior problems, including acts of delinquency and substance abuse. The child forensic perspective informs forensic experts involved in mitigation of sentencing juveniles and explains to the court how exposure to violence is a destructive lesson about the use of physical power and domination to relieve stress and exert control. In cases of complex trauma or exposure to multiple traumatic events, including abuse or neglect, the cumulative impact extends far beyond childhood and adolescence into adulthood, with resultant disability, dysfunction, and societal cost. Informing the court about how the developmental trajectory that has gone astray can help guide difficult legal decisions and place into proper perspective the value, or even necessity, of ensuring safety and protection for children and adolescents.

Conclusion

Child forensic psychiatry has developed as a subspecialty relatively recently. It is based on principles established in forensic psychiatry, but the application of these principles is complicated by the child's dependent status and higher need for protection. The child psychiatrist's understanding of the complex neurodevelopmental, experiential, and social factors contributing to behavior assists judges and juries to understand the behavior of children and adolescents, as well as adults with histories of trauma, developmental atypicalities, and other disorders beginning in childhood.

Child and adolescent forensic psychiatrists have unique training and are needed to evaluate and consult regarding youths involved in the child welfare and juvenile justice systems as well as civil litigation and family matters such as custody. As models of sustainable training initiatives emerge to address this underserved area of forensic psychiatry, the relevance of the child and adolescent forensic psychiatrist's specialized expertise is amplified not only for children and adolescents involved in the court, but also in providing the necessary developmental contextual framework to inform and enrich the assessment of adults who come before the court.

References

1. Gutheil TG. (2002). A voyage of discovery. In D Schetky, & E. Benedek (Eds.). *Principles and practice of child and adolescent forensic psychiatry* (p. xii). Washington, DC: American Psychiatric Publishing.
2. Marrocco MK, Uecker JC, & Ciccone JR. (1995). Teaching forensic psychiatry to psychiatric residents. *Bull Am Acad Psychiatry Law, 23*(1), 83–91.
3. Lewis CF. (2004). Teaching forensic psychiatry to general psychiatry residents. *Am Psychiatry, 28*(1), 40–46. doi: 10.1176/appi.ap.28.1.40
4. Dietz PE. (1987). Forensic psychiatrist of the future. *Bull Am Acad Psychiatry Law, 15*(3), 217–227.

5. Scott C. (2011). The child and adolescent track in the forensic fellowship. *Child Adolesc Psychiatr Clin North Am*, 20, 565–575.
6. ACGME program requirements for graduate medical education in forensic psychiatry. Available at http://www.acgme.org/acgmeweb/Portals/0/PFAssets/ProgramRequirements/406_forensic_psych_2016_1-YR.pdf. Accessed November 16, 2014.
7. Practice parameters for child custody evaluation. (1997). *J Am Acad Child Adolesc Psychiatry, 36*(10 Suppl), 57S–68S.
8. Practice parameters for child custody evaluation. (2011). *J Am Acad Child Adolesc Psychiatry, 50*(12), 1299–1312.
9. Strasburger LH, Gutheil TG, & Brodsky A. (1997). On wearing two hats: Role conflict in serving as both psychotherapist and expert witness. *Am J Psychiatry, 154*, 448–456.
10. American Academy of Psychiatry and the Law. (2005). *Ethics guidelines for the practice of forensic psychiatry.* Available at http://www.aapl.org/pdf/ethicsgdlns.pdf. Accessed March 11, 2014.
11. Prentky R, & Righthand S. (2003). *Juvenile sex offender assessment protocol-II (J-SOAP-II): Manual.* Available at http://www.psicologiagiuridica.eu/files/didattica/jsoap2.pdf. Accessed March 30, 2014.
12. Borum R, Bartel P, & Forth A. (2005). Structured Assessment of Violence Risk in Youth (SAVRY). In T Grisso, G Vincent, & D Seagrave (Eds.), *Mental health screening and assessment in juvenile justice* (pp. 311–323). New York: Guilford.
13. Hempel I, Buck N, Maalke C, & van Marle H. (2013). Review of risk assessment instruments for juvenile sex offenders: What is next? *Int J Offender Ther Comp Criminol, 57*(2), 208–228.
14. Guy LS, Packer IK, & Warnken W. (2012). Assessing risk of violence using structured professional judgment guidelines. *J Forensic Psychol Pract, 12*(3), 270–283.
15. Steinberg A, & Fromm L. (2012). The uses of narrative and persuasion in the child forensic psychiatric report and testimony. *J Psychiatry Law, 40*(1), 23–42.
16. Fonagy, P. (1999). Memory and therapeutic action. *Int J Psychoanalysis, 80*, 215–223.
17. Roper v. Simmons, 543 U.S. 551 (2005).
18. Graham v. Florida. 130 S. Ct. (2011).
19. Miller v. Alabama. 132 S. Ct. 2455 (2012).
20. Atkins v. Virginia. 536 U.S. 304 (2002).
21. Hall v. Florida. 572 U.S. (2014).

10

Childhood Maltreatment and Chronic Unmediated Stress

A New View for Forensic Psychiatry

Steven Berkowitz

The author is a child and adolescent psychiatrist with expertise in childhood trauma and maltreatment. He was interviewed on the local National Public Radio radio station on the topic of violence in the community and an attorney, who heard the show, invited him to present on the relationship between child maltreatment and criminality.

Subsequently, he was asked to be an expert in a capital case for purposes of mitigation during the sentencing phase in which the death penalty was considered a highly probable outcome. A PowerPoint presentation was shown to the jury on the Adverse Childhood Experiences (ACE) study and many of the neurodevelopmental findings that result from childhood maltreatment and toxic stress (chronic unmediated stress in childhood). The defendant's history and ACE score of 8 were presented and described. Because of the arrangement of the courtroom, the presentation was done across the courtroom from the jury, as the stand was next to the jury stand. As the author returned to the stand he overheard jury members discussing the number of ACEs they had. The defendant received a life term.

An all too common misconception for both mental health professionals and the lay public is that disorders and symptoms caused by traumatic experiences are simply some version of PTSD/ASD. The DSM-5 has made some attempt to rectify this by creating a chapter of trauma and stress related disorders that includes posttraumatic stress disorder (PTSD), acute stress disorder, reactive attachment disorder, and adjustment disorders.[1] Although a step in the right and scientifically supported direction, our psychiatric nosology still doesn't encompass the wide range of psychiatric and behavioral symptoms and disorders that are often etiologically related to chronic adversity, stress, and trauma experienced in childhood.[2–7] For instance, most mental health professionals are aware that many individuals displaying antisocial and criminal behavior have been maltreated, yet when providing this diagnosis no etiological explanation is required. However, there is increasing research and information that provides support for forensic evaluations to assess and provide these findings in a scientific and compelling manner that abrogates the necessity of making diagnoses that do not capture the complexity of the defendant's history and behaviors.

Perhaps the most cutting edge issue now facing forensic psychiatry is neuroforensics (see chapters 28–31). The validity of the various types of imaging and their specific findings in those accused of crimes is in its infancy and their acceptance varies by jurisdiction. However, there is a great deal of convergence in a range of research involving the effects of stress during childhood and adolescence. Neuroimaging studies, epidemiology, and clinical phenomenology of childhood maltreatment all support the large impact that trauma and adversity have on neurodevelopment, neurophysiology, and epigenetics, and subsequently on psychiatric and physical health as well as functional and behavioral capacities. By integrating the epidemiology of maltreatment with the neuroscience of childhood trauma and stress, the forensic psychiatrist adds significant weight and validity to the argument regarding mitigating circumstances.

The importance of the convergence of these studies' findings for the forensic psychiatrist cannot be understated. Although perhaps not as useful when evaluating an individual regarding criminal guilt or innocence, they are relevant to issues of intent and so may influence whether a defendant is convicted on a more or less severe charge. Almost certainly the most salient and compelling use of the findings around maltreatment and later outcomes for the forensic psychiatrist is during the penalty phase. Last, the findings regarding the effects of childhood maltreatment and trauma on the brain and genome have tremendous potential to change policies in the criminal and juvenile justice system.

Epidemiology

Perhaps the most compelling group of findings regarding the effects of childhood trauma, chronic unmediated stress (toxic stress), and maltreatment come from the Adverse Childhood Experiences (ACE) Study, which grew out of research conducted at Kaiser-Permanente-San Diego.[2] Importantly, the participants, by virtue of their enrollment at Kaiser-Permanente were a solidly middle class population and so may be considered to represent a statistically normal subsample of the US population. The initial phase of the study occurred between 1995 and 1997 and included 17,000 participants. Each participant had a physical exam and completed a survey regarding his or her experiences before the age of 18 of maltreatment and family dysfunction and current health status and behavior.* All results were integrated to develop the baseline data set for the ACE study. Although no new subjects are being enrolled for the study, longitudinal follow up is continuing to assess the relationship between childhood maltreatment as measured by the ACE survey and a range of behavioral, psychiatric,

*The ACE Health Survey is available at www.acestudy.org.

health, and social outcomes.[3] Also, several states and municipalities have adopted the ACE survey and in 2010 five states collected ACE information for the Behavioral Risk Factor Surveillance Survey (BRFSS). Data from these new studies are beginning to be published. Although there are some findings specifically related to juvenile and adult crime, more studies of this population subset are underway.

Vincent Felitti and Robert Duda developed the ACE Questionnaire and the Health and Behavior Survey (see the Questionnaire and links to the survey in the following). The survey inquires about childhood abuse, neglect, and exposure to other traumatic stressors, which the developers named Adverse Childhood Experiences (ACE). The study found that ACEs are common with approximately 66% of respondents reporting at least one ACE. Perhaps more remarkable is that 17% reported experiencing four or more ACEs before the age of 18 and only 33% reported none. The ACE survey is simply summed to arrive at the ACE score, so the ACE score is simply the addition of each of the 10 items. No item is weighted, for instance; being sexually abused is scored as a 1, as is parental divorce, loss, or separation. The score is used to assess the total amount of stress during childhood and as such functions as a measure of chronic unmediated or unbuffered stress experienced by the individual during childhood and adolescence. Remarkably, the study has demonstrated that as the score increases, the risk for a range of health, mental health, social, and behavioral issues increases in a graded fashion. However, it appears that an ACE score of 4 or higher increases the risk for a range of detrimental outcomes to a much higher degree.[4]

Adverse Childhood Events Survey

Prior to your 18th birthday:

1. Did a parent or other adult in the household often or very often... Swear at you, insult you, put you down, or humiliate you? or Act in a way that made you afraid that you might be physically hurt?
   No _____ If Yes, enter 1 _____

2. Did a parent or other adult in the household often or very often... Push, grab, slap, or throw something at you? or Ever hit you so hard that you had marks or were injured?
   No _____ If Yes, enter 1 _____

3. Did an adult or person at least 5 years older than you ever... Touch or fondle you or have you touch their body in a sexual way? or Attempt or actually have oral, anal, or vaginal intercourse with you?
   No _____ If Yes, enter 1 _____

4. Did you often or very often feel that... No one in your family loved you or thought you were important or special? or Your family didn't look out for each other, feel close to each other, or support each other?
   No _____ If Yes, enter 1 _____

5. Did you often or very often feel that... You didn't have enough to eat, had to wear dirty clothes, and had no one to protect you? or Your parents were too drunk or high to take care of you or take you to the doctor if you needed it?
   No _____ If Yes, enter 1 _____

6. Was a biological parent ever lost to you through divorce, abandonment, or other reason?
   No _____ If Yes, enter 1 _____

7. Was your mother or stepmother: Often or very often pushed, grabbed, slapped, or had something thrown at her? or Sometimes, often, or very often kicked, bitten, hit with a fist, or hit with something hard? or Ever repeatedly hit over at least a few minutes or threatened with a gun or knife?
   No _____ If Yes, enter 1 _____

8. Did you live with anyone who was a problem drinker or alcoholic, or who used street drugs?
   No _____ If Yes, enter 1 _____

9. Was a household member depressed or mentally ill, or did a household member attempt suicide?
   No _____ If Yes, enter 1 _____

10. Did a household member go to prison?
    No _____ If Yes, enter 1 _____

Now add up your Yes answers. This is your ACE score.

At present there have been two waves of health data collection that correlated ACE scores with a range of outcomes in which the risk increases in a graded fashions. These include: (1) alcoholism and alcohol abuse, (2) chronic obstructive pulmonary disease (COPD), (3) depression, (4) fetal death, (5) health-related quality of life, (6) illicit drug use, (7) ischemic heart disease (IHD), (8) liver disease, (9) intimate partner violence, (10) having greater than 50 sexual partners, (11) sexually transmitted diseases (STDs), (12) smoking and its early initiation, (13) suicide attempts, (14) unintended pregnancies, (15) early initiation of sexual activity, and (16) adolescent pregnancy.[4]

A more recent analysis evaluated the population attributable risk (the proportion of a disease in a population related to an exposure) to a number of negative health outcomes and behaviors. Some of these findings are truly remarkable. Adverse Childhood Experiences scores of 4 or greater correlated with a *78%* risk of intravenous drug abuse, *65%* of alcoholism, *58%* of suicide attempts, *54%* of depression, *50%* of drug abuse, *48%* of having more than 50 sexual partners, and 39% of ever smoking.[4]

As previously mentioned, there are few studies evaluating the relationship between ACE scores and criminality. The most direct US study of criminality and the ACE score[7] evaluated 151 men referred to outpatient treatment after being convicted for child physical abuse, domestic violence, stalking, or sexual offending of adults. Their ACE scores were compared to men drawn from the ACE study database. Nearly half of the offender group (48%) had an ACE score of 4+, compared with only 13% of men in the general ACE study. All 10

ACEs were found in higher proportions in the offender group than in the Kaiser-Permanente group. Only 10% of the offenders reported no ACEs, compared with 38% of the male control sample. A recent study of 141 incarcerated women in Norway evaluated ACE scores with primary outcomes of attempted suicide and substance abuse. Seventeen percent reported having experienced no ACEs, whereas 34% reported having experienced more than five ACEs, which is almost three times the findings in the Kaiser-Permanente population.[8] After controlling for age, immigrant background, and marital status, the number of ACEs significantly increased the risk of attempted suicide and current drug abuse.[8] In another examination of ACEs and delinquency, the Tacoma Urban Network and Pierce County Juvenile Court measured ACE prevalence among juvenile offenders. They found that juvenile offenders have approximately three times the number of ACEs documented in the original ACE study, and those with the highest ACE scores had higher rates of school failure, multiple suspensions, substance abuse, and suicidal behaviors.[9] In the now-often-cited studies by Widom and colleagues in which the term *cycle of violence* was coined, childhood maltreatment—including abuse and neglect—was a significant risk factor, not only for juvenile delinquency, but also for adult criminal behavior.[10] Although these studies did not use the ACE methodology, the primary outcomes were of delinquent and criminal behavior. They studied 900 individuals with substantiated childhood abuse and neglect and compared them with 667 individuals without a history of childhood maltreatment. The groups were matched for age, sex, race, and family socioeconomic status. Arrest records were examined when the cohort averaged 26 years of age and again when the cohort averaged 32.5 years. Those persons who suffered childhood maltreatment were more likely to have been arrested as juveniles (27%) than those without a history of childhood abuse (17%). A greater proportion of the abused cohort were arrested as adults (42% vs. 33%) and for violent crime (18% vs. 14%). The maltreated group offended at nearly twice the rate, was arrested more frequently, and was younger at first arrest. Gender analyses demonstrated that maltreated females increased rates of both general criminal and violent behavior. In males abuse and neglect did not increase the risk for violent behavior, but increased the rate of arrest violent crime compared with the controls. Importantly, childhood neglect was found to be more pernicious than had traditionally been thought, as it was also a significant risk factor for juvenile and adult criminal behavior.

The ACE study, the Cycle of Violence studies, and the more recent studies using the ACE survey with the delinquent and criminal populations highlight the need for forensic psychiatrists to think beyond the practice of evaluating under the rubric of DSM psychiatric diagnoses or cognitive deficits alone and recognize that chronic stress and adversity during childhood is a primary factor predisposing individuals toward criminal and delinquent behavior. Thus, childhood histories of maltreatment and chronic stress must be thoroughly assessed to demonstrate these key mitigating factors. Importantly, it is also essential that the psychiatrist demonstrate that chronic and severe childhood stress changes both neurophysiology and brain structure and understand the biological bases for these alterations. Although most people intuitively recognize that "violence begets violence," demonstrating that actual brain injury results from the psychological stress caused by maltreatment and trauma that correlates with a range of difficulties and poor behavior seems to make the phenomena resulting from maltreatment and trauma more "scientific and real" to those unfamiliar with the issues. Again, the convergence of the increasingly sophisticated research in genetics (primarily epigenetics) and neuroimaging of the effects of chronic unmediated stress and maltreatment are powerful evidence that environmental stress has deleterious effects on brain development and the related deficits in psychiatric and behavioral functioning.

Neurophysiology of Stress

The dysregulations of the hypothalamic pituitary axis (HPA), especially in posttraumatic stress disorder (PTSD), have been well described and replicated (although not without continuing controversy), and although the knowledge base regarding HPA dysregulation is not as well defined for maltreated children and adults without PTSD, there is increasing expert agreement regarding HPA axis dysregulation in individuals with childhood adversity.[11,12] Many HPA axis neurotransmitters and hormones are dysregulated in this population, with norepinephrine and cortisol having been the most studied with the most replicated findings.[11,12] Many studies have concluded that cortisol appears to be a primary cause of damage to the developing brain. Importantly, the concept that a hormone that is especially released as a response to stress could cause damage in excess is readily understandable by the lay public.

Hypothalamic pituitary axis dysregulation results in multiple problematic effects on neurogenesis, dendritic branching, synaptic pruning, and myelination.[11,12] Depending on stage of brain development and age, the structural consequences can be as profound as whole brain shrinkage in very young children and shrinkage in specific brain areas such the hippocampus, the medial and dorsal later prefrontal cortex, the corpus callosum, insula, visual cortex, and so on.[12] Shrinkage in these areas of the brain correlate with a number of psychiatric and behavioral issues that are commonly found in individuals involved in the justice system, as seen in the studies cited. Specifically, some of the correlated phenomenological findings include difficulties with memory, especially for childhood events, emotional regulation, impulsive and aggressive behavior, and issues with planning, judgment, decision making, and social interaction.[13]

Undoubtedly this convergence of increasingly sophisticated research in genetics (primarily epigenetics and neuroimaging around the effects of chronic unmediated stress and maltreatment) are powerful evidence for the effects of environmental stress on brain development and deficits and related psychiatric and behavioral issues.

Mechanisms

For the purpose of illustration, the focus of this section is on how cortisol becomes dysregulated in the face of trauma and maltreatment. These mechanisms have been elucidated in the last 10 years, and it appears that the explanation for neurotransmitter dysregulation and the subsequent impairment of brain development has its basis in epigenetics. Epigenetics is the study of changes in organisms caused by modification of gene expression rather than alteration of the genetic code itself. The most well-studied of these epigenetic changes involves methylation of the promoter region of various genes. The first studies of early stress' impact on brain development were done in animal models, which demonstrated that rat pups raised by stressed rat mothers regardless of the biological mother had fewer glucocorticoid receptors (GR) in their hippocampus and increased methylation in the promoter region of the GR gene.[14] Similar findings have been found for a number of gene products involved in neurodevelopment and maintenance,[15,16] and these same findings in rat models have now been replicated in humans.[17,18]

Additional epigenetic studies have demonstrated a number of differences in methylation between adults maltreated as children and controls.[19]

Conclusion

The burgeoning knowledge base regarding the long-term effects of child maltreatment on adult physical and mental health and behavior as demonstrated by the ACE study and other research is powerful mitigating information for many criminal defendants. When integrated with the neuroimaging findings of the impact of child maltreatment on brain development and the now-understood underlying epigenetic mechanisms that explain how maltreatment and chronic stress impact the brain and behavior, we can offer a scientific and replicated explanation of how many defendants do not have the capacity for intellectualized intent, despite appearances. Their childhood experiences have changed their biology, and it has often been repeated that they live in instinctual survival mode and their behavior is truly instinctual.

References

1. American Psychiatric Association. (2013). *DSM 5*. Washington, DC: American Psychiatric Association.
2. Felitti VJ, Anda RF, Nordenberg D, et al. (1998). Relationship of childhood abuse and household dysfunction to many of the leading causes of death in adults. The adverse childhood experiences (ACE) study. *Am J Prev Med, 14*, 245–258.
3. Accessed on March 22, 2014 from WWW.ACEstudy.org.
4. Accessed on March 22, 2014 from WWW.CDC.gov/ACE.
5. Brown DW, Anda RF, Henning T, et al. (2009). Adverse childhood experiences and the risk of premature mortality. *Am J Prev Med, 37*, 389–396.
6. Anda RF, Felitti VJ, Bremner JD, et al. (2006). The enduring effects of abuse and related experiences in childhood: A convergence of evidence from neurobiology and epidemiology. *Eur Arch Psychiatry Clin Neurosci, 256*, 174–186.
7. Dong M, Anda RF, Felitti VJ, et al. (2004). The interrelatedness of multiple forms of childhood abuse, neglect, and household dysfunction. *Child Abuse Negl, 28*, 771–784.
8. Green JG, McLaughlin KA, Berglund PA, et al. (2010). Childhood adversities and adult psychiatric disorders in the National Comorbidity Survey Replication 1: associations with first onset of DSM-IV disorders. *Arch Gen Psychiatry, 67*, 113–123.
9. Reavis JA, Looman J, Franco KA, & Rojas B. (2013). Adverse childhood experiences and adult criminality: How long must we live before we possess our own lives? *Perm J. 17*(2), 44–48.
10. Friestad C1, Åse-Bente R, & Kjelsberg E. (2014). Adverse childhood experiences among women prisoners: relationships to suicide attempts and drug abuse. *Int J Soc Psychiatry, 60*(1), 40–46.

11. Grevstad JA. (2010). *Adverse childhood experiences and juvenile justice.* PowerPoint presentation delivered to the Washington State Family Policy Council, June 8, 2010.
12. Widom CS, & Maxfield MG. (2001). *An update on the "cycle of violence."* Washington, DC: US Department of Justice, Office of Justice Programs, National Institute of Justice.
13. McCrory E, De Brito SA, & Viding E. (2010). Research review: The neurobiology and genetics of maltreatment and adversity. *J Child Psychol Psychiatry, 51*(10), 1079–1095.
14. Cameron NM, Soehngen E, & Meaney MJ. (2011). Variation in maternal care influences ventromedial hypothalamus activation in the rat. *J Neuroendocrinol, 23*(5), 393–400.
15. Teicher MH, Andersen SL, Polcari A, Anderson CM, & Navalta CP. (2002). Developmental neurobiology of childhood stress and trauma. *Psychiatr Clin North Am, 25*(2), 397–426, vii–viii.
16. Beers SR, & De Bellis MD. (2002). Neuropsychological function in children with maltreatment-related posttraumatic stress disorder. *Am J Psychiatry, 159*(3), 483–486.
17. Murgatroyd C, & Spengler D. (2011). Epigenetics of early child development. *Front Psychiatry, 2*, 16.
18. Naumova OY, Lee M, Koposov R, Szyf M, Dozier M, & Grigorenko EL. (2012). Differential patterns of whole-genome DNA methylation in institutionalized children and children raised by their biological parents. *Dev Psychopathol, 24*(1), 143–155.
19. McGowan PO, Sasaki A, D'Alessio AC, et al. (2009). Epigenetic regulation of the glucocorticoid receptor in human brain associates with childhood abuse. *Nat Neurosci, 12*(3), 342–348.

11

Social Policy, Child Abuse and Neglect, and Forensic Psychiatry

Richard J. Gelles and
Debra Schilling Wolfe

The case was unremarkable as reports of child abuse and neglect go. A mother and father were riding a public bus with their 3-month-old baby. At some point in the ride, the mother stood up and began walking up and down the aisle asking riders if they wanted to buy her baby. One rider called 911 and after about 10 minutes a police officer boarded the bus and took the mother, father, and child into custody. The officer called the county Department of Children's Services and a caseworker traveled to the police station, took down the basic facts about the incident, and received permission from her supervisor to take the baby into custody. The mother's family lived in a different state, but the father's brother and sister-in-law lived nearby. A quick check of the child abuse registry, criminal history of the brother and sister-in-law, and a home visit confirmed that the brother and sister-in-law would be an appropriate kin placement. A subsequent court hearing approved the placement. After a check of hospital records for the baby, a home visit, and interviews with the mother and the father, the county agency substantiated the report for child neglect. Nearly 8 out of 10 (78.3%) of substantiated reports of child maltreatment in 2012 were child neglect.[1]

Sixteen months after the child was substantiated as a victim of child neglect, the county department referred the case to the University of Pennsylvania Field Center for Children's Policy, Practice and Research. The staff of the Field Center was asked to conduct a complete forensic evaluation of the mother, father, child, and kin placement and make subsequent recommendations to the county department as to the appropriate permanency plan for the child.

The genesis of what would become the Field Center began in 1999 when faculty from the University of Pennsylvania's School of Law, School of Medicine, School of Nursing, and then School of Social Work (now called the School of Social Policy & Practice), came together to discuss how to pool their efforts and expertise to improve the quality of child welfare policy and practice. Each faculty member possessed decades of experience in his or her own specialization; and yet, each felt frustrated that his or her knowledge and expertise was not making a sufficient impact on behalf of victims of abuse and neglect. Richard Gelles, from the School of Social Work, had more than 30 years of research experience and had recently helped draft the Adoption and Safe Families Act of 1997 (PL 105-89). Yet he felt frustrated that he was not able to translate his research findings into better practice. Another faculty member, a pediatrician from the School of Medicine and Children's Hospital of Philadelphia, directed a child abuse clinic at Children's Hospital and wanted to know more about state-of-the-art research on child maltreatment. Faculty from the School of Law also wanted to know how to differentiate solid and applicable research from claims-making that at first glance appeared to be based on research but also seemed more anecdotal than empirical. What we all knew intuitively, and from experience, was that child maltreatment was a multidisciplinary phenomenon. Moreover, each of us had some forensic experience—expert witness work and some case evaluations, and realized that our own disciplinary expertise was often insufficient to address the totality of the forensic questions and issues we were asked to address. The nascent multidisciplinary center was started with some seed money from the Dean of the School of Social Work, which would be augmented by an initial gift from interested alumni of the university. In 2003, Marie and Joseph Field endowed what is now the Field Center for Children's Policy, Practice and Research. Faculty Directors representing each of the four partner schools and the Children's Hospital of Philadelphia now lend their academic and disciplinary expertise to the center.

When we received the "baby selling" case, the staff of the Field Center, led by Executive Director Debra Schilling Wolfe, initiated our normal forensic assessment. Debra obtained the full case file from the county department—with redactions to protected noninvolved children and adults. The team's clinical psychologist consultant scheduled time to interview the mother, father, and kin caregivers. The interviews were conducted in the Field Center clinic that has a two-way mirror, viewing room, and audio and visual taping capacity. The viewers signed standard confidentiality agreements and the interview subjects also signed standard informed consent procedures.

The details of the case were that mother had, indeed, tried to sell her baby on the bus, but she claimed it was merely a joke between her and her husband. The mother worked, had no ongoing substance abuse issues, but presented as someone who was more interested in winning her case and getting her baby back than actually caring for her child. The father had suffered a traumatic brain injury during a deployment in Iraq with his National Guard unit. He was receiving physical and psychological treatment at the local Veteran's Administration hospital and was receiving disability payments from the Veteran's Administration. The kin caregivers were appropriate and were providing excellent care to the now nearly 2-year-old child. One of the troubling aspects of the placement was that the father had unfettered access to his child, including being allowed to have overnight visits and being allowed to drive a car while transporting his child. Our psychologist was quite concerned that the father's physical and psychological issues resulting from the traumatic brain injury could put the child at risk while in the father's care. The mother, who had no prior child protective service involvement or criminal justice history, engaged the department in a running battle in which she denied she had a problem and demanded the return of her child. The mother was sporadically compliant with demands that she attend parenting classes and accept social services. During her interview with the psychologist the mother spent all her time complaining about her caseworkers and how she was going to win her battle with the department. The clinician was unable to direct the mother's attention to focusing on how she planned to care for her child if and when the child was returned to her custody. The mother and father's relationship had ended, so the father would not be living with the mother if and when the child was returned home. The mother worked full-time during the day, but the psychologist could not seem to get the mother to explain who would provide child care if the child returned home.

After our case record review and the interviews were complete, the full Field Center team, including the clinical psychologist, met with the county department caseworker and supervisor. Our first question was, "What is your current case plan and goal for the child?"

The supervisor's response was a bit surprising. The department's plan was to change the case goal from reunification to adoption and seek a termination of the mother and father's parental rights. The father had already agreed to voluntarily terminating his parental rights and the department expected to file for termination of the mother's rights. The goal change and case plan elicited two comments from the Field Center staff. The faculty co-director from the School of Law asked what would be the basis of terminating the mother's parental rights. The supervisor explained that the termination would be based on the fact that the child had been in out-of-home care for 15 months and according to the provisions of the federal Adoption and Safe Families Act (ASFA), when a child had been in out-of-home placement for 15 of the previous 22 months, the state or county is obligated to seek a termination of parental rights. Richard Gelles quickly jumped in and pointed out that the "15/22 month rule" does not apply when a placement is with kin and the child in question was in kin care for the full 15 months. "Oh no," the supervisor replied, "that is not the case in Pennsylvania—we have to seek termination after 15 months, no matter where the child is placed." Gelles responded that that simply was not the case and if an attorney with the department thought that was the law, the attorney was most assuredly incorrect. The School of Law faculty co-director pointed out that in the Commonwealth of Pennsylvania the standard for terminating parental rights was clear and convincing evidence of parental unfitness. Termination was not simply the result of poor parenting or failure to comply with the case plan; the department had to prove that the parent was inadequate. The sum total of our multidisciplinary evaluation was that there was not clear and convincing evidence of the mother's inadequacy as a parent, the 15/22 rule from ASFA did not apply, and if the department went to court seeking a termination they would most surely fail. The case plan and the goal change would not work. On the other hand, the mother was not prepared to accept responsibility for caring for the child and the father did not want to assume sole responsibility for child care. The father was more than happy to terminate his own parental rights provided the mother did so as well. Last, the department had not thought through its permanency plan. Assuming the child was freed for adoption, who would adopt the child? Presumably, the likely candidates would be the paternal uncle and aunt. However, would and could the aunt and uncle assure the safety and well-being of the child vis-à-vis the physical and psychological limitations of the father? Pennsylvania is a closed-adoption state, which means the biological father would have no legal right to know where his child is or have any access to the child once parental rights were terminated. Yet it would be naïve to assume that the father would not visit and want to have time with his child, given the child was with his brother and sister-in-law. Then there was the issue of the mother. The Field Center team continued to stress that the department could not succeed in obtaining an involuntary termination from the court. Perhaps the mother could be counseled to voluntarily terminate her parental rights. But in a closed-adoption state, she would then lose the right to know where her child was or have access to her child. The mother would not be happy to know the father could continue to see the child but she could not. Federal and state policy creates significant constraints to finding the most appropriate outcome for this case. The Field Center team also stressed that the most appropriate outcome was not simply complying with policy, but also making a decision that assured the safety, permanency, and well-being of the child.

Child Welfare Work Is Not Brain Surgery

Protecting children from abuse and neglect is not brain surgery—it is much more difficult. Brain surgeons have the advantage of a decade of specialized training and the use of the latest and most advanced technology. Front-line child protective service caseworkers often have only a bachelor's degree in the liberal arts and job tenure of 3 to 5 years. The latest technology in child protective service work is a cell phone and, if budgets allow, a laptop computer.

Brain surgeons never have to choose between fixing the brain and losing the patient or saving the patient and letting the brain stop functioning. Child protective service work involves choices among three often incompatible goals—preserving the family, assuring the safety and well-being of the child-victim, or assuring that the child has permanent caregiving from a loving parent. Prioritizing safety can lead to removing children from parents who might have responded to help. Preserving often leads to re-abuse and even fatality. Permanency by placement with birth parents runs the same risks as preservation. To achieve permanency through adoption requires the early termination of parental rights.

Applying Federal Law to Evaluations and Recommendations

Khalil Wimes was 6 years old when he was starved and beaten to death by his mother and father. The Wimes case made headlines in Philadelphia for weeks, but was not a case referred to the Field Center for an evaluation. Nonetheless, we discussed this case at weekly Field Center meetings because of its implications for better system response to child abuse and neglect. The key facts are a matter of public record. Khalil was the 10th of his parents' 11 children. At least five of Khalil's older siblings had previously been removed from their parents' care by the city Department of Human Services.

Khalil's case was initially reported to the Department of Human Services shortly after his birth. Relatives were concerned that Khalil and the six other siblings in the home were living in deplorable conditions of neglect. Khalil initially was placed with a relative after the Department of Human Services substantiated the case for neglect. Three years later, Khalil was returned to his parents. Khalil was home schooled and often hidden in the basement for the next 3 years. At the time of his death, he weighed 29 pounds.

Why was Khalil returned to his parents, even over the objection of his social worker? Why would he be returned when his siblings were in out-of-home placement? One answer is that federal law mandates the case plan of "reunification." The Adoption Assistance and Child Welfare Act of 1980 (PL 96-292) mandates that states make reasonable efforts to keep children in the home or assist parents whose children have been removed before moving for a termination of parental rights. It was exactly the "reasonable efforts" provision that Congress addressed in 1997 with the Adoption and Safe Families Act (PL 105-89). A provision in ASFA (as the law is referred to) stated that there were certain conditions or "aggravating circumstances" that allowed states to "bypass reasonable efforts." The aggravating circumstances included inflicting grievous injury to a child or having one's parental rights previously terminated by a court. In the Wimes household, before Khalil's murder, there had been no grievous injury inflicted on any of the children prior to their removals. But the parental rights of some of the children had been terminated, so why had the Department of Human Services not bypassed the reasonable efforts mandate and sought a termination of parental rights for Khalil when he was first removed? The answer is that the parents had voluntarily terminated their rights to their other children—therefore the bypass condition was not applicable in Khalil's case.

It often seems humane and efficient to obtain voluntary terminations of parental rights from parents who harm their children or are inadequate. This was the case in the *Book of David: How Preserving Families Can Cost Children's Lives.*[2] In *The Book of David,* as with Khalil Wimes, the local child agency obtained a voluntary termination of older children only to have a younger child murdered by the parents.

A close understanding and application of the "aggravating circumstances" bypass provided by ASFA is essential to any forensic assessment of abused and neglected children.

Constraints of State Law

An early case the Field Center assessed illustrated the constraints imposed by unique state laws. We were asked to assess the case of a mother and her child. The mother had a recurring substance abuse problem and had been reported and substantiated for child neglect on a number of occasions. Numerous attempts to resolve the substance abuse problems through in-patient and outpatient services failed to yield long-term sobriety. The child had been in foster care for 14 months and, because a non-relative provided the care, the case was coming up on the 15-month AFSA deadline. Our lead clinician found that the mother was closely attached to her child, deeply desired to be a caring and adequate parent, but was immersed in a drug culture. Our clinician wrote a 20-page report that provided a detailed history and accounting of the mother's strengths and weaknesses. But the bottom line was that the mother was still not able to be an adequate caregiver and the prospects for her achieving adequacy in the near future were minimal. Our clinician was clearly torn about her recommendation and so she reluctantly concluded that mother's parental rights should be terminated. But, in order to support the mother and enhance her psychological health, our clinician recommended that the mother be able to visit and have time with her child on a regular basis.

Although there has been considerable advocacy and change on the matter over open adoption records, the Commonwealth of Pennsylvania remains a "closed adoption" state. In other words, once a parent's rights are terminated, the parent has no legal rights with regard to his or her former child. Our clinician's compassionate recommendation was at odds with state law. Worse, we said, the recommendation of continued parental contact might undermine the most important finding of the report, that the mother was not, nor would be, adequate as a caregiver.

Our clinical insights and compassionate instincts cannot determine our forensic assessments. One must apply a full knowledge of state law to all forensic work in the field of child maltreatment.

Disproportionality: When the Law Provides No Guidance

One of the more difficult cases the Field Center evaluated was that of a 9-year-old girl. The girl's mother was single, homeless, unemployed, and had a persistent substance abuse problem. After multiple substantiated neglect reports and failed attempts to help the mother accept services, the local child welfare department removed the child and placed her in non-kin foster care. The maternal grandparents expressed an interest and willingness to care for the granddaughter, but the department opted for non-kin placement. The prevailing opinion among the caseworkers and supervisors was that the grandparents might be too old to be able to take on the task of raising their granddaughter. Another concern was that the caseworkers and supervisors doubted the grandparents' ability to prevent their daughter from seeing her child and possibly removing the child from the grandparents' care. The non-relative foster parents expressed an interest in adopting the child. After the girl was in foster care for 15 months, the department successfully petitioned to terminate the mother's rights. The case plan changed from reunification to adoption.

At the point we were asked to assess the case, the grandparents were mounting a challenge to the adoption. The foster parents had permitted the grandparents to maintain regular visitations and overnight visitations. But now, the foster parents wanted to move away from the city to elsewhere in the state. Two demographic facts created the dilemma. The child and her family were black, whereas the foster parents were white. The city was multiracial and -ethnic, with nearly half the population being black. The foster parents planned to move to a region of the state that is 97% white.

The issue of racial disproportionality has hung over the child welfare system for decades. One of the first battlegrounds was trans-racial adoption. In the late 1970s, the National Association of Black Social Workers declared trans-racial adoption "cultural genocide."[3] For decades child welfare agencies would race-match foster placements and adoptions. The Multiethnic Placement Act of 1994 (MEPA; PL 93-382) was supposed to end the practice of race matching. However, critics of the child welfare system pointed out that minority children were disproportionately swept into the child welfare system and minority families were disproportionately likely to have their parental rights terminated.[4] Our case was one in which a perfectly acceptable placement was available that would not have involved a trans-racial adoption.

On one side of the argument, our team knew that the child had developed a bonded and nurturing relationship with her foster parents. But we worried what might take place in 5 or more years when the child became a teenager and was the only girl of color in her community and school. One the other hand, all the research in trans-racial adoption exploded the myth that minority children fared badly in trans-racial adoptions.[5,6] The fact that the child had achieved a permanent relationship with her foster parents and was doing well ultimately trumped our legitimate concerns over the trans-racial adoption. More importantly, we could use high-quality evidence on trans-racial adoption to inform our evaluation and recommendation. The multidisciplinary composition of the Field Center was critical in generating a deep and thoughtful evaluation of the case.

A Case for the Multidisciplinary Approach

Traditional evaluations in the child welfare arena typically focus on one issue or purpose, and are conducted through only one lens. The court may request a "bonding evaluation," as was requested on the "baby selling case." This sort of evaluation asks if the child is bonded with the biological parent, and is often used to assist the judge in determining what is in the best interest of the child. In the "baby selling case" we wondered, what would a bonding evaluation actually contribute? If a parent's sole contact with his or her child since infancy has been in weekly supervised visits, is the child truly able to view that parent as anything other than someone who plays with him or her and perhaps brings gifts? A bonding evaluation often reveals little to address the crux of the issue: the parent's capacity to care for the child.

Many evaluations are based solely on clinical interviews or psychological testing, without the benefit of an in-depth case history or record review. Child welfare cases are highly complex, involving a multitude of issues and often, lengthy agency involvement. A longitudinal perspective, rather than a snapshot in time, can provide critical insight into determining parental fitness and addressing the best interest standard. By conducting an evaluation that includes a comprehensive record review across multiple agencies and systems, a more robust examination will result.

The multidisciplinary team is truly one in which the whole is greater than the sum of its parts. The interplay of a team comprised of a variety of disciplinary lenses—in our case, clinical psychology, law, pediatric medicine, social policy, child and family therapy, forensic psychiatry, and nursing—provides rigorous analysis and leads to a far more comprehensive and productive evaluation. Had only one team member conducted an evaluation of the "baby selling case," the end result would have been far different. A recommendation may have been made, based solely on psychological testing and/or clinical interviews, that the mother would never be capable of parenting the child and that her rights should be terminated. Without input from the legal or policy perspectives, action would likely have been taken to attempt to terminate the mother's rights, a case that surely would not have prevailed in court. The end result would have been returning the child to her mother's care and the system yet again placing a child in harm's way.

Multidisciplinary versus Interdisciplinary

When the Field Center's team of experts first began to meet and discuss cases, each offered his or her own perspective and viewpoint. Team members benefited greatly from hearing the thoughts and ideas of colleagues with different academic training and professional experience. This multidisciplinary team construct was an important first step. However, it was merely "parallel play." In moving from *multi*disciplinary to *inter*disciplinary, team members actually began seeing cases through each different lens and subsequently integrated the ideas of others. As a fully integrated interdisciplinary team, evaluations take on a multisystemic perspective, with all team members contributing to reports and recommendations. No one discipline directs the work. Because children do not live in the systemic silos that we create for them, evaluations determining their future should reflect their reality and be truly interdisciplinary. The complexity of these cases precludes a simple and singular approach.

Implications for Forensic Psychiatry and the Child Welfare System

Forensic psychiatry traditionally involves one psychiatrist evaluating one patient. In our model, forensic evaluations take a broader approach. The forensic clinician serves as the lead of a multidisciplinary team, conducting clinical interviews, offering his or her expertise to the group, and receiving input from the various disciplines sitting around the table. This alternative model not only expands the role of the forensic psychiatrist, it provides far more material for the evaluative process. The forensic psychiatrist becomes a member of a team, rather than the sole evaluator, a significant shift in practice from the traditional medical model. It represents a change in culture, requiring a comfort in collaboration and a willingness to not be the sole voice on a case.

Assessing cases of child abuse and neglect and formulating recommendations for case management, goal setting, and court action is an inherently multidisciplinary process that involves psychiatric assessment, application of research evidence, and an understanding of federal and state law, as well as agency practice. This interdisciplinary approach to forensic evaluation defies the traditional silos of services and program funding. The clinical hour takes on new meaning when a team is evaluating or treating a patient. Not only does this have implications for forensic psychiatry, it also points out a major flaw in the child welfare system. Services and funding streams must transcend traditional systemic silos to reflect the multisystem needs of children. It is the interaction of the various disciplines that touch the lives of victims of child maltreatment that can best inform these highly complex and troubling cases.

References

1. U.S. Department of Health and Human Services, Administration for Children and Families, Administration on Children, Youth and Families, Children's Bureau. (2013). *Child maltreatment 2012.* Available from http://www.acf.hhs.gov/programs/cb/research-data-technology/statistics-research/child-maltreatment
2. Gelles RJ. (1996). *The book of David: How preserving families can cost children's lives.* New York: Basic Books.
3. Gelles RJ, & Spigner CW. (2008) Child welfare policy. In IC Colby, KM Sowers, & CN Dulmus (Eds.), *Comprehensive handbook of social work and social welfare* (vol 4). New York: Wiley.
4. Roberts D. (2002). *Shattered bonds: The color of child welfare.* New York: Civitas Books.
5. Simon R, Allstein H, & Melli M. (1994). *The case for transracial adoption.* Washington, DC: American University Press.
6. Simon R, & Allstein H. (2002). *Adoption, race and identity: From infancy to young Adulthood* (2nd ed.). New Brunswick, NJ: Transaction Publishers.

12

Juvenile Sentencing and the Possibility of Parole Following *Miller v. Alabama*

Catherine Mao and Susan Rushing

Edel Gonzalez was involved in gang activity by the age of 11.[1] He was a victim of childhood abuse and had never met his father; older gang members were his adult role models.[2] In 1991, an intoxicated,16-year-old Gonzalez and a number of adult gang members participated in a carjacking; during the robbery, one of Gonzelez's peers shot the car owner Janet Bicknell, a Huntington Beach school employee.[3] Gonzalez neither pulled the trigger nor carried a weapon but was charged with felony murder because of his participation in the robbery.[4] An Orange County Superior Court jury found him guilty, and in November of 1993 he was sentenced to life without parole.[5] For the next two decades, Gonzalez took advantage of educational opportunities and maintained a "pristine" behavioral record in prison.[6,7]

In January 2013, California enacted Senate Bill 9 (S.B. 9), the "Fair Sentencing for Youth Act," which allows California inmates who have served 15 to 25 years of a life sentence that they received for crimes committed as a juvenile to apply for a resentencing hearing.[8] As a result, Gonzalez, once the youngest individual in Orange County sentenced to life without parole, has now become the first inmate to be resentenced under the Act.[9] Charles Manson has been eligible for parole 12 times,[10] but, until now, Gonzalez would never have been eligible for parole.

S.B. 9 comes on the heels of *Miller v. Alabama*, a landmark Supreme Court Case ruling that mandatory juvenile life without parole sentences violate the Eighth Amendment of the Constitution.[11] Criminal law recognizes the core principle of penal proportionality, and, increasingly, trends in juvenile sentencing mitigation recognize the significance of adolescent immaturity in assessing culpability.[12]

Mandatory Juvenile Life Without Parole: A Legal History

The first American juvenile court was created in Illinois in 1899 with the intention of providing a social welfare alternative to criminal courts.[13] At its inception, juvenile court—in purpose and practice—echoed emerging trends in juvenile punishment primarily centered on reform and rehabilitation.[14] In the 1960s, however, a series of United States Supreme Court rulings set forth a transformation in juvenile justice that ultimately resulted in a substantive and procedural convergence between juvenile and adult criminal courts.[15]

Most notably, the 1967 case *In re Gault* granted juveniles certain constitutional rights such as the Sixth Amendment right to confront witnesses and receive legal counsel and the Fifth Amendment right against self-incrimination.[16] In 1970, the Court ruled in *In re Winship* that a determination of guilt in juvenile proceedings was subject to the same standard of reasonable doubt as in adult criminal trials.[17] Five years later, *Breed v. Jones* determined that the double jeopardy clause applied to juvenile courts.[18] Providing due process protections previously only afforded to adult criminal defendants would inevitably alter the nature and purpose of juvenile justice. Indeed, in his dissent, Justice Stewart noted that *Gault* "serve[d] to convert a juvenile proceeding into a criminal prosecution."[19] By the end of the century, the difference between the two would diminish dramatically.

"Get Tough Laws" and Juvenile Punishment

In time, juvenile courts evolved from a purely rehabilitative system to one heavily influenced by retributive and deterrent philosophies. For example, the State of Washington implemented a Juvenile Justice Act in 1977 to ensure that juvenile offenders were "held accountable for their offenses" and to "provide for punishment commensurate with the age, crime, and criminal history of the juvenile offender."[20]

In the 1980s and 1990s, the surge of violent juvenile crime led to a series of legislative decisions that advocated for more punitive measures, particularly with recidivist offenders.[21] As a result, several states enacted statutes that permitted harsher maximum sentences and imposed mandatory minimum sentences for specific crimes—including mandatory life without parole.[22] Known as "Get Tough Laws," many of these statutes also allowed for juveniles to be tried in adult criminal courts, and therefore receive the same sentences as adults.[23] Many states lowered the age of transfer, allowing and sometimes requiring for adolescents younger than 14 to be tried in adult criminal courts. Other states mandated offenders of a certain age and crime be tried as adults—Virginia, for example, required any child 14 or older charged with murder to be tried as an adult.[24]

In all, Get Tough Laws resulted in an estimated 250,000 youth being transferred into the adult criminal system per year.[25] Proponents of these laws asserted that reform toward retribution and deterrence was all too necessary; clearly, the rehabilitative model had failed society. Conversely, critics argued that the progressive influence of retributive intent dangerously blurred the fine line between treatment and punishment.[26] It would take another 20 years before contemporary juvenile justice would begin to choose a side.

Juvenile Justice Sentencing Reform: *Thompson, Roper,* and *Graham*

It is commonly believed that the judicial system began to point juvenile punishment back toward its rehabilitative beginnings with a series of landmark cases starting in 2010: *Roper,*[27] *Graham,*[28] and *Miller.*[29] In fact, the process first began in 1988, when the Supreme Court ruled in *Thompson v. Oklahoma* to restrict the death penalty to offenders over the age of 16.[30] Twelve years later, *Roper v. Simmons* precluded any court from imposing the death penalty on any juvenile on the grounds that doing so constitutes cruel and unusual punishment in violation of the Eight Amendment.[31] In its analysis, the Court compared capital punishment for juveniles to capital punishment for the mentally retarded, noting that "[r]etribution is not proportional if the law's most severe penalty is imposed on one whose culpability or blameworthiness is diminished, to a substantial degree, by reason of youth and immaturity."[32] Furthermore, the Court recognized the difficulty "even for expert psychologists to differentiate between the juvenile offender whose crime reflects unfortunate yet transient immaturity, and the rare juvenile offender whose crime reflects irreparable corruption."[33]

The Court applied the same reasoning in 2010 when it categorically prohibited juvenile life without parole for non-homicide charges in *Graham v. Florida.*[34] In its decision, the Court noted both a domestic and international consensus against life without the possibility of parole sentences for juveniles. At the time, no other country allowed for life without parole sentences for juvenile non-homicide offenders, and within the United States, only 11 jurisdictions chose to impose such punishments.[35] In particular, Florida imposed life without parole sentence on juvenile non-homicide offenders at 19 times the rate expected given an analysis of comparable states.[36] Furthermore, the Court once again pointed to the limited culpability of adolescent offenders, citing their 1991 decision in *Harmelin v. Michigan* that "age and the nature of the crime each bear on the analysis."[37] Citing *Roper,* the Court noted that like the death penalty, "the differences between juvenile and adult offenders are too marked and well understood to risk allowing a youthful person to receive a sentence of life without parole for a nonhomicde crime despite insufficient culpability."[38]

Eliminating Mandatory Juvenile Life Without Parole

Most recently, in 2012, the US Supreme Court addressed mandatory juvenile life without parole for homicide in *Miller v. Alabama.*[39] Like *Graham,* the *Miller* decision likened juvenile life without parole sentences to the death penalty. Writing for the majority, Justice Kagan reiterated the foundational principle that imposition of a State's most severe penalties on juvenile offenders cannot proceed without considering the youth of the offenders. To give the lengthiest possible incarceration is an "especially harsh punishment for a juvenile," because he will almost inevitably serve "more years and a greater percentage of his life in prison than an adult offender."[40] The penalty of life in prison without the possibility of parole when imposed on a teenager, as compared with an older person, is therefore "the same... in name only."[41]

With this equivalence in mind, the Court not only relied on the precedent set by *Roper* and *Graham,* but also the 1976 case *Woodson v. North Carolina,* in which a 5-4 decision ruled unconstitutional legislation that mandated the death penalty for all first-degree murders.[42]

In *Woodson*, the Court held that the compulsory nature of the statute failed to "allow the particularized consideration of relevant aspects of the character and record of each convicted defendant before the imposition upon him of a sentence of death."[43] Similarly, the *Miller* Court—also a 5-4 decision—found that "the mandatory penalty schemes at issue... prevent the sentencer from considering youth and from assessing whether the law's harshest term of imprisonment proportionately punishes a juvenile offender."[44]

Miller obligated 29 jurisdictions, including the federal government, to discontinue issuing mandatory juvenile life without parole sentences.[45] It is important to note that *Miller* does not categorically ban juvenile life without parole sentences—courts remain free to impose these sentences so long as they consider all mitigating factors. However, although "a state is not required to guarantee eventual freedom" to juvenile offenders, it must provide them with "a meaningful opportunity to obtain release based on demonstrated maturity and rehabilitation."[46] Furthermore, the Court recognized that although its ruling in *Miller* was limited to mandatory sentences, discretionary life without parole for juveniles should be uncommon.[47]

The Role of Neuroscience in Juvenile Justice

The Supreme Court has long recognized youth to be a relevant mitigating circumstance.[48] In fact, starting with *Roper*, three integral differences between juveniles and adults have permeated nearly every judicial analysis of juvenile punishment.[49] First, juveniles are comparably immature and irresponsible. Second, juveniles are more vulnerable to negative external influences, including but not limited to peer pressure. Last, the character of a juvenile is simply not as well formed as that of an adult, and therefore more transient.

Much of this analysis is backed by substantial research in psychosocial immaturity, which delineates four dimensions of distinction between adolescent and adult judgment: (1) susceptibility to peer influence; (2) perception of risk; (3) future orientation; (4) capacity for self-management.[50] It is important to remember that regardless of cognitive development, psychosocial immaturity independently contributes to deficiencies in adolescent decision making.

From a neurobiological standpoint, however, technological advances in modern brain research now allow for "unprecedented access to the developing human brain."[51] In particular, developments in neuroimaging techniques have been monumental in "relating the dramatic maturation of cognitive, emotional, and social functions with the brain structures that ultimately underlie them."[52] Trends in juvenile justice, backed by scientific insight, show an increasing deference to the importance of accounting for adolescent immaturity, vulnerability, and amenability to reform when sentencing juveniles.

Biological Bases for Adolescent Immaturity

Adolescent deficiencies in decision making and reasoning capabilities are well established, both to scientists and laypeople. The *Roper* Court noted that a "lack of maturity and an underdeveloped sense of responsibility are found in youth more often than in adults... often result in impetuous and ill-considered actions and decisions."[53] Indeed, studies show that the cognitive control system not only develops later than the motivational system, but that it also does so at a slower rate—particularly in adolescents.[54]

As a result, adolescents are more influenced by potential rewards and less inhibited by risk. Specifically, their brains are both less capable of cognitive control than their adult counterparts and more active in regions associated with risky, impulsive, and sensation-seeking behavior.[55,56,57]

Cognitive Control over Behavior

The frontal lobes and the prefrontal cortex—a crucial part of the brain responsible for "response inhibition, emotional regulation, planning and organization"[58] are markedly underdeveloped in adolescents in two distinct ways affecting cognitive control.[59]

The human brain is composed of approximately 85 billion nerve cells called *neurons*. Neurons connect adjacent and distant brain structures to one another to assure integration of information across brain regions. The gray matter of the brain, where neurons reside, thins with maturity through processes called "synaptic pruning." Pruning leads to greater efficiency and strengthens the complex information processing, which support consistent exercise of good judgment."[60] Before the development of magnetic resonance imaging technology, it was commonly believed that pruning was a gradual, lifelong process and that gray matter volume peaked shortly after birth. Research has revealed that gray matter volume—particularly in the prefrontal cortex—actually increases before adolescence, and continues to thin well beyond adolescence. The implication is significant: the greater amount of adolescent gray matter is directly correlated to an impeded "ability to process complex information" and to make "executive plans supporting voluntary control of behavior."[61]

Brain connectivity is also enhanced though a developmental process that insulates neurons with a fatty sheath called *myelin*. The presence of myelination makes "communication between different parts of the brain faster and more reliable" and myelin continues to accumulate well into adulthood.[62] "[T]he development of improved self-regulatory abilities during and after adolescence is positively correlated with white matter maturation."[63] Thus, myelination is essential to improving cognitive abilities such as impulse control and decision making.

Developmentally, the brain is also organized from deep, internal, primitive brain structures to the distant outer cortical areas, which are uniquely and highly developed in adult human brains. The deep, primitive structures of the brain include: the limbic system (the amygdala, the cingulate, the thalamus, and the hippocampus), the basal ganglia (including the nucleus accumbens), the hypothalamus, the pituitary gland, and the brainstem. These primitive brain structures develop early in life and are fully developed during adolescence. The prefrontal cortex, the center of executive function, is one of the last brain structures to mature. For most humans, the development of the prefrontal cortex remains incomplete in the early twenties. The prefrontal cortex is responsible for complex decision making, including the ability to integrate information, plan, reason about choices, and to predict outcomes. The prefrontal cortex is the area of the brain governing judgment and behavioral control.

Reward-Seeking and the Hyperactive Motivational System

The relative latency of cognitive control system development is particularly meaningful in light of the adolescent motivational system, which, as a result, becomes less regulated than in adults. In other words, this temporal gap "creates a period of heightened vulnerability to risk taking during middle adolescence."[64] The dominance of the adolescent motivational system can be observed through the comparably rapid development of impulsive and reward-seeking areas, as well as through specific neurochemical imbalances in the adolescent brain.[65]

Neuroimaging studies show that the nucleus accumbens, located in the ventral striatum, is activated in reward-related processing, and hyperactivated in adolescent decision making.[66] This suggests that adolescents tend to "overvalue rewards in risk-reward assessment."[67] Additionally, the prefrontal cortex—underdeveloped in adolescents—is responsible for modulating function of the amygdala, the "neural system that evolved to detect danger and produce rapid protective responses without conscious participation."[68] Together, the nucleus accumbens and the amygdala create a portrait of the adolescent brain that is hypersensitive to rewards and ill-equipped for avoiding harm.[69]

Another neurobiological basis for juvenile susceptibility to rewards is the comparably lower level of seratonin in adolescents, a neurotransmitter known to support inhibitory control.[70] Similarly, research with rodents has also revealed indications that dopamine receptor density in the striatum and prefrontal cortex decreases in preadolescence—resulting in a significant *increase* in dopamine.[71] "Because dopamine plays a critical role in the brain's reward circuitry," this surge of dopaminergic activity in the prefrontal cortex "is likely to increase reward-seeking behavior and, accordingly, sensation seeking."[72]

Vulnerability and Susceptibility as Mitigating Factors

Extenuating external pressures are a common source of mitigation in criminal sentencing. More so than their adult counterparts, adolescent offenders are subject to environmental factors that they cannot control or alter. "Difficult family and neighborhood conditions are major risk factors for juvenile crime."[73] By virtue of their status "as legal minors, they lack the freedom that adults have to extricate themselves from a criminogenic setting."[74] Yet this lack of freedom is not merely a physical one. Significant research, both psychosocial and neurobiological, corroborates the comparative vulnerability of adolescents.[75]

Several cognitive factors contribute to adolescent susceptibility to external pressure. The deficiencies in myelination account for one: "[r]ecent research on the neural underpinnings of resistance to peer influence in adolescence indicates that improvements in this capacity may be linked to the development of greater connectivity between brain regions, and likely facilitates the better coordination of affect and cognition."[76] Recent studies have also shown that adolescents "show heightened activation within incentive processing regions in response to a variety of social stimuli."[77] Similarly, peer presence alters brain activity in impulse regulating regions as well.[78] The disparity in adolescent brains between reward-sensitivity and impulse control is only heightened in social contexts, rendering adolescents much more vulnerable to peer pressure than children or adults. It is unsurprising, then, that "[m]ost adolescent decisions to break the law take place on a stage where the immediate pressure of peers is the real motive."[79]

Implications for Adolescent Behavioral Reform

In *Roper, Graham*, and *Miller* the Court acknowledged that "because a child's character is not as well formed as an adult's, his traits are less fixed and his actions are less likely to be evidence of irretrievable depravity."[80] The comparative neurobiological deficiencies in adolescent brain development have serious implications for the rehabilitative aspects of the juvenile justice system as well. In addition to the fact that adolescent character is relatively unformed, dopamine plays a crucial role in reinforcement learning.[81] Thus, the adolescent capacity for learning may translate to "enhanced amenability for rehabilitation."[82] As the *Graham* court noted: "[i]ncorrigibility is inconsistent with youth."[83]

In 2011, the Office of Juvenile Justice and Delinquency Prevention of the United States Department of Justice published what is thus far the most comprehensive data set available on serious juvenile offenders after running a 7-year study following 1354 juvenile offenders postconviction.[84] Approximately 50% of the youth were under some form of supervision postconviction; approximately 20% were receiving community-based services. The study found that, regardless of intervention or punishment, approximately 91.5% of the studied adolescents "decreased or limited illegal activity during the first three years following court involvement"—suggesting that age has a tangible effect on teenage rehabilitation. Furthermore, only a "small proportion of offenders studied continued to offend at a higher level." This is consistent with prevailing psychosocial beliefs about adolescent character: "until late adolescence, individuals' values, attitudes, beliefs, and plans are likely to be tentative and exploratory expressions rather than enduring representations of personhood."[85] Just as courts consider "out-of-character" behavior as a mitigating factor for adult defendants, so too must they account for the transitory character of juveniles. Because adolescent character is not yet formed, a determination of bad, unchanging character must be a rare exception.

The Future of Juvenile Life Without Parole

The response to *Miller* was both swift and muddled: Within a year of its ruling, states such as Delaware, Wyoming, and California passed legislation effectively abolishing all juvenile life without parole sentences.[86] Washington abolished life imprisonment without parole for all juveniles under the age of 16 at the time of their crime.[87] Yet several salient questions remained unanswered as states scrambled to comply with *Miller*.[88] Naturally, judicial and legislative attempts at resolving these questions have thus far varied from state to state. One of the greatest challenges to efficiently implementing *Miller* is the lack of guiding principles for re-sentencing juveniles whose sentences have been vacated. Florida, which in 2009 had 266 juveniles serving life without parole,[89] has faced monumental difficulty responding to *Graham* and *Miller*. Florida courts looked to the lawmakers for guidance on resentencing and the legislature took 3 years and proposed legislation four times before settling on a sentencing range of 40 years to life for juveniles who commit or attempt capital murder with the opportunity for a sentence review after 25 years if the teen had not previously engaged in a violent felony.[90] Florida's law also allowed for sentence review after 15 years if the victim did not die.[91] Although *Miller* established that "developmental and neurological differences matter when meting out long sentences to juveniles," it fails to "provide nuanced answers for *how* they matter."[92]

Post-*Miller* Standards for Resentencing Evaluation

Although the Supreme Court declined to explicitly outline the requirements of a post-*Miller* resentencing hearing, it did prescribe several considerations fundamental to mitigation.[93] First, resentencing hearings must consider "hallmark features" of "chronological age" such as "immaturity, impetuosity, and failure to appreciate risks and consequences." Second, they must take into account the family and home environment of the offender, from which juveniles "cannot usually extricate" themselves. Third, hearings cannot "neglect the circumstances of the homicide offense, including the extent of participation in the conduct and the [effect of] familial and peer pressures." Fourth, they must assess whether youth-related incompetence resulted in undue legal disadvantage during the criminal proceedings. Last, resentencing hearings must consider the possibility of rehabilitation.

The Alabama Supreme Court proffered a long list of factors considered in determining whether a juvenile life sentence should be imposed with or without parole: the juvenile's chronological age at the time of the offense and the "hallmark features of youth;" the juvenile's diminished capability; the circumstances of the offense; the extent of the juvenile's participation in the crime; the juvenile's family, home, and neighborhood environment; the juvenile's emotional maturity and development; the presence of familial and/or peer pressure on the juvenile; the juvenile's past exposure to violence; the juvenile's drug and alcohol history; the juvenile's ability to deal with the policy; the juvenile's capacity to assist his or her attorney; the juvenile's mental health history; and the juvenile's potential for rehabilitation.[94]

In June 2013, Delaware Governor Markell signed Senate Bill 9, which eliminated juvenile life without parole by providing for sentence review for all those under 18 years of age who were sentenced to more than 20 years in prison in Delaware.[95] The new law replaced automatic life-without-parole for first-degree murder with a sentencing range of 25 years to life in prison. Juveniles previously sentenced to life in prison without parole may petition for a reduction in their sentence after serving 30 years and will be sentenced using the new range of 25 years to life.[96]

Similarly, West Virginia passed bill H.B. 4210 in March 2014, providing that individuals convicted and sentenced for a crime that occurred before they were 18 years old are eligible for parole after serving 15 years.[97] The bill outlines 15 mitigating factors for the parole board to consider, including age at the time of the offense; impetuosity; family and community environment; ability to appreciate the risks and consequences of conduct; intellectual capacity; peer or familial pressure; level of participation in the offense; ability to participate meaningfully in his or her defense; capacity for rehabilitation; school records and evaluations; trauma history; faith and community involvement; and involvement in the child welfare system.[98] A comprehensive mental health evaluation also may be considered.[99] Although the legislation is clear that no such evaluation is compelled, it does require any evaluation under consideration to include family interviews, prenatal history, developmental history, medical history, history of treatment for substance abuse, social history, and a psychological evaluation.[100]

Retroactivity: *Miller* and *Teague*

Miller is also conspicuously silent on the issue of retroactivity—whether a new ruling can be applied to cases with a final legal disposition. Retroactivity is especially relevant in cases in which a form of due process was denied. The 1989 Supreme Court ruling in *Teague v. Lane*, which prohibits the retroactive application of constitutional criminal procedure rules on final convictions, provides an exception only where *substantive* constitutional rules are concerned.[101] As expected, courts have been divided in reconciling *Teague* and *Miller*. As of May 2014, Delaware, Illinois, Florida, Mississippi, Iowa, Massachusetts, Texas, Wyoming, and Nebraska—as well as the federal courts, have definitively determined *Miller* to be retroactive. On March 6, 2014, the Michigan Supreme Court heard oral arguments on the issue of *Miller* retroactivity.

Federal courts are similarly inconsistent. In 2012, the Eastern District of Pennsylvania granted a petition for a writ of *habeas corpus* in light of *Miller*.[102] The Eastern District of Michigan ruled that "if ever there was a legal rule that should—as a matter of law and morality—be given retroactive effect, it is the rule announced in *Miller*. To hold otherwise would allow the state to impose unconstitutional punishment on some persons but not others, an intolerable miscarriage of justice."[103] At the appellate level, the Court of Appeals for the Fourth Circuit granted a motion for re-file a petition for a writ of *habeas corpus*, noting that "a new rule of constitutional law" was "made retroactive to cases on collateral review by the Supreme Court."[104] Yet contrarily, the Courts of Appeal for the Fifth and Eleventh Circuits both concluded that *Miller* represented a procedural rule that did not apply retroactively.[105]

Changes in Juvenile Justice

Despite its deficiencies in clarity, *Miller* has prompted nationwide reform of juvenile life without parole. In 2012, both Pennsylvania and North Carolina passed laws restricting juvenile life without parole to only convictions of first-degree murder.[106] Wyoming and Delaware, states that previously mandated juvenile life without parole, enacted legislation eliminating *all* juvenile life without parole.[107] Similarly, Connecticut introduced H.B. 5221 in February 2014 (previously H.B. 6581, which in 2013 advanced to the Senate but was not voted on), applying retroactively to offenders after 1990 and also abolishing juvenile life without parole.[108] Currently, juveniles may receive life without parole sentences in seven states.[109]

The Court in *Miller* devoted significant attention to adolescent development and its implications under the law. Several states have advanced legislation in recognition of fundamental differences between juveniles and adults.[110] For example, the text of Connecticut H.B. 5221 requires a court to consider "any scientific and psychological evidence including, but not limited to, evidence showing, as compared to an adult: a child's lack of maturity and underdeveloped sense of responsibility; a child's vulnerability to negative influences and outside pressures from peers or family members, or both; a child's increased capacity for change and rehabilitation; a child's reduced competency in appreciating the risks and consequences of his or her own actions, negotiating the complexities of the criminal justice system, and assisting in his or her own defense."

Although California did not previously have a mandatory life without parole scheme,[111] the recently enacted S.B. 9 is similarly cognizant of these considerations. S.B.9 delineates eight factors to be considered in determination of whether a hearing is granted, including: whether the offender had "insufficient adult support or supervision" and "suffered from psychological or physical trauma" before the offense; whether the offender suffered from "cognitive limitations" influencing his or her involvement in the offense; whether the defendant has performed acts indicating rehabilitation; whether the defendant maintained family ties; whether the defendant eliminated contact with individuals outside of prison involved in crimes; and whether the defendant initiated violence while incarcerated, resulting in disciplinary actions. In addition, it excludes offenders who were convicted without an adult co-defendant and offenders of crimes in which the victim was tortured or a public safety official. In Connecticut and California, individuals who have already served a significant portion of their sentence are not eligible for resentencing; whereas in Delaware an offender is eligible for resentencing after serving 30 years in prison. Clearly, there has not been a consistent re-structuring of juvenile sentences across the United States following the Court's decision in *Miller* and likewise there will not be an equal opportunity for all juvenile offenders to demonstrate rehabilitation.

Conclusion

This is a landmark time for juvenile justice. Advancements in neuroimaging have allowed scientists to gain a more comprehensive understanding of adolescent brain development. This understanding is not confined to the field of neuroscience. Popular culture has taken an interest in developmental neuroscience—advertisements and parenting books frequently make allusions to the comparable deficiencies in adolescent brains.[112] More important, American jurisprudence has grown increasingly cognizant of fundamental neurobiological and psychosocial differences between juveniles and adults.

Currently, more than 2,500 juveniles have been sentenced to life without parole in the United States and many more have been sentenced to die in jail because of virtual life sentences.[112] Although *Miller* has already prescribed and inspired a considerable reform in juvenile justice, its practical implications—and its corresponding impact on those sentenced to life without parole as juveniles—remain unclear. Inmates such as Edel Gonzalez now have the possibility, for the first time since childhood, of pleading for parole before a board. Countless others wait for their states to fully determine the reach of *Miller*, which, although explicit on the issue of resentencing, provides little guidance as to its implementation. Courts and legislatures are already slowly and inconsistently unraveling the complicated issues that *Miller* presents. Although it is unlikely that a nationwide resolution will arise in the near future, the next few years will likely bear witness to substantial changes in juvenile sentencing. We hope that the possibility of eventual release of offenders back into the community will incentivize states to enhance rehabilitation efforts aimed at juvenile offenders.

References

1. Elizabeth Calvin. (January 13, 1993). Growing up behind bars. *L.A. Times.*
2. Ibid.
3. Matt Lait. (April 9, 1993). Youth guilty of murder in woman's death. *L.A. Times*; see also Calvin, supra note 1.
4. (December 18, 2013). Sentenced to life as a teen, convicted killer now sees chance of becoming free man. *CBS Los Angeles.*
5. Ibid.
6. S. Parker Yesko. (December 19, 2013). First youth offender resentenced under SF lawmaker's bill. *S.F. Examiner*
7. Claudia Koerner. (December 18, 2013). O.C. man receives parole eligibility for teenage crime. *Orange County Register.*
8. S.B. 9, 2011-2012 Reg. Sess. (Calif. 2012).
9. Greg Risling. (December 18, 2013). Man convicted as teen resentenced under new law. *U.T. San Diego.*
10. Michael Martinez. (April 12, 2012). Charles Manson denied parole. *CNN.*
11. *Miller v. Alabama*, 132 S. Ct. 2455 (2012).
12. Steinberg & Scott. (2003). Less guilty by reason of adolescence: developmental immaturity, diminished responsibility, and the juvenile death penalty, *Am. Psychol*, 58, 1009, 1016 (hereinafter Steinberg & Scott).
13. See, e.g., Barry C. Feld. (1991). *The transformation of the juvenile court*, 75 Minn. L. Rev. 691.
14. See, e.g, Julianne P. Sheffer. (1995). *Serious and habitual juvenile offender statutes: Reconciling punishment and rehabilitation within the juvenile justice system*, 48 V and L. Rev. 479, 491.
15. See Feld, *supra* n.i.
16. *Application of Gault*, 387 U.S. 1 (1967).
17. *In re Winship*, 397 U.S. 358, 368 (1970)
18. *Breed v. Jones*, 421 U.S. 519, 541 (1975).
19. *Gault* at 79.
20. Wash. Rev. Code Ann. § 13.40.010(2) (West 1977 & Supp. 1988).
21. Elizabeth S. Scott, Laurence Steinberg. (2008). Adolescent development and the regulation of youth crime. *The future of children.* 18:2. Juvenile Justice Princeton-Brookings.
22. Danielle R. Oddo. (1998). *Removing confidentiality protections and the "get tough" rhetoric: What has gone wrong with the juvenile justice system?* 18 B.C. Third World L.J. 105, 114.
23. See, e.g, Julianne P. Sheffer. (1995). *Serious and habitual juvenile offender statutes: Reconciling punishment and rehabilitation within the juvenile justice system*, 48 V and. L. Rev. 479, 491.
24. Fox Butterfield. (May 12, 1996). States revamping laws on juveniles as felonies soar. *N.Y. Times.*
25. See Scott, supra n.21.
26. See, e.g., Barry C. Feld. (1991). *The transformation of the juvenile court.* 75 Minn. L. Rev. 691.
27. *Roper v. Simmons*, 543 U.S. 551 (2005).
28. *Graham v. Florida*, 560 U.S. 48 (2010).
29. *Miller v. Alabama*, 132 S. Ct. 2455 (2012).
30. *Thompson v. Oklahoma*, 487 U.S. 815 (1988).
31. *Roper.*
32. *Id.* at 572.
33. *Id.* at 573 (citing Steinberg & Scott. (2003). Less guilty by reason of adolescence: Developmental immaturity, diminished responsibility, and the juvenile death penalty. *Am. Psychol, 58*, 1009, 1014).
34. *Graham.*
35. Annino PG, Rasmussen DW, & Rice CB. *Juvenile life without parole for non-homicide offenses: Florida compared to nation.* Florida State University: Public Interest Law Center.
36. Ibid.
37. *Graham* at 50 (quoting *Harmelin v. Michigan*, 501 U.S. 957, 1001). Ironically, *Harmelin* actually upheld the Eighth Amendment constitutionality of a juvenile life without parole conviction for cocaine possession.

38. *Graham* at 78 (citing *Roper* at 572-573) (internal quotations omitted).
39. *Miller.*
40. *Graham* at 50 citing *Roper* at 272.
41. *Id.* at 2466 (citing in part *Graham v. Florida*, 560 U.S. 48, 70 (2010)) (internal quotations omitted).
42. *Woodson v. North Carolina*, 428 U.S. 280 (1976).
43. *Id.* at 303.
44. *Miller* at 2458.
45. *Id.* at 2471.
46. *Miller* at 2469.
47. *Id.* at 2481 ("Even when a life without parole sentence is not mandatory... appropriate occasions for sentencing juveniles to this harshest possible penalty will be uncommon.").
48. *See, e.g., Roper; Graham; Miller; Eddings v. Oklahoma*, 455 U.S. 104, 115-116 (1982). ("Even the normal 16-year-old customarily lacks the maturity of an adult.")
49. *Roper* at 569-70.
50. Steinberg & Scott at 1014.
51. Sarah Durston et al. (2001). Anatomical MRI of the developing human brain: What have we learned? *J Am Acad Child Adolesc Psychiatry, 40*, 1012.
52. Elizabeth R. Sowell et al. (1999). Mapping cortical change across the human life span. *Nat Neurosci*, 6, 859.
53. *Roper* at 569 (citing *Johnson v. Texas*, 509 U.S. 350, 367 (1993)).
54. Laurence Steinberg. (2009). Adolescent development and juvenile justice. *Ann Rev Clin Psychol, 16*(3), 47, 57 (hereinafter L. Steinberg).
55. L. Steinberg at 54.
56. L. Steinberg at 54.
57. L. Steinberg at 54.
58. Eveline Crone et al. (2009). Neurocognitive development of relational reasoning. *Dev Sci, 12*(1), 55, 56.
59. See Brief for the American Medical Association and the American Academy of Child and Adolescent Psychiatry as Amici Curiae In Support of Neither Party, *Miller v. Alabama*, 132 S. Ct. 2455 (2012) (hereinafter AMA Amici Curiae).
60. AMA Amici Curiae at 21 (citing Robert F. McGivern et al.. (2002). Cognitive efficiency on a match to sample task decreases at the onset of puberty in children. *Brain Cogn, 50*, 73.
61. AMA Amici Curiae at 22.
62. Ekhonon Goldberg. (2001). *The executive brain: Frontal lobes & the civilized mind* (p. 144). New York: Oxford University Press.
63. AMA Amici Curiae at 26.
64. L. Steinberg at 54.
65. AMA Amici Curiae at 30.
66. Ariana Galvan et al. (2006). Earlier development of the accumbens relative to orbitofrontal cortex might underlie risk-taking behavior in adolescents. *J Neurosci, 26*(25), 6885.
67. AMA Amici Curiae at 32.
68. AMA Amici Curiae at 31 (citing Abigail A. Baird et al. (1999). Functional magnetic resonance imaging of facia affect recognition in children and adolescents. *J Am Acad Child Adolesc Psychiatry, 38*(1), 1.
69. AMA Amici Curiae at 35.
70. AMA Amici Curiae at 34.
71. L. Steinberg at 54; Dustin Wahlstrom et al. (2010). Neurobehavioral evidence for changes in dopamine system activity during adolescence. *Neurosci Biobehav Rev, 34*, 631 (hereinafter Wahlstrom).
72. Ibid.
73. APA Amici Curiae at 15.
74. Steinberg & Scott at 1016.

75. See Brief for the American Psychological Association, American Pychiatric Association, and National Association of Social Workers as Amici Curiae in Support of Petitioners *Miller v. Alabama*, 132 S. Ct. 2455 (2012) (hereinafter APA Amici Curiae).
76. AMA Amici Curiae at 26 (citing Laurence Steinberg. (2009). Adolescent development and juvenile justice. *Ann Rev Clin Psychol*, *16*(3), 47, 57.
77. Jason Chein et al. (2011). Peers increase adolescent risk taking by enhancing activity in the brain's reward circuitry. *Dev Sci*, *14*, F1, F8.
78. Ibid.
79. Franklin Zimring. (2000). Penal proportionality for the young offender. In Thomas Grisso, & Robert Schwartz (Eds.), *Youth on trial* (pp. 271, 280).
80. *Miller* at 2458 (citing *Roper* at 570) (internal quotations omitted).
81. Steinberg & Scott at 1015; Wahlstrom at 643.
82. AMA Amici Curiae at 35.
83. *Graham* at 73 (quoting *Workman v. Commonwealth*, 429 S.W.2d 374, 378 (Ky. 1968)).
84. Edward P. Mulvey. (March 2011). *Highlights from pathways to desistance: A longitudinal study of serious adolescent offenders*. Juvenile Justice Fact Sheet. Department of Justice.
85. Steinberg & Scott at 1016.
86. S.B. 9, 147th Gen. Assem., Reg. Sess. (Del. 2013); H.B. 23, 62nd Gen. Assem., Reg. Sess (Wyo. 2013); S.B. 9, 2011-2012 Reg. Sess. (Calif. 2012).
87. S.B. 5064, 63rd Gen. Assem. Reg. Sess. (Wash. 2014).
88. See, e.g., Marsha Levick. (2012). From a trilogy to a quadrilogy: *Miller v. Alabama* makes it four in a row for U.S. Supreme Court cases that support differential treatment of youth juveniles. *BNA Crim Law Rept*, *91*, 749.
89. *State distribution of youth offenders serving juvenile life without parole (JLWOP)*. Human Rights Watch, October 2, 2009, available at http://www.hrw.org/news/2009/10/02/state-distribution-juvenile-offenders-serving-juvenile-life-without-parole. (hereinafter HRW State Distribution).
90. H. B. 7035, 2014 Legislature. (FL 2014).
91. H. B. 7035, 2014 Legislature. (FL 2014).
92. Marsha L. Levick, & Robert G. Schwartz. (2013). Practical implications of Miller v. Jackson: Obtaining relief in court and before the parole board. *Minn J Law Ineq*, *31*, 369 (hereinafter Levick & Schwartz).
93. *Miller* at 2468.
94. Kent Faulk. (September 13, 2013). *Alabama supreme court sets out how juvenile killers are to be sentenced*. Alabama Media Group.
95. 79 Del. Laws c. 37 (2013) and 11 Del. C. § 4209A
96. 79 Del. Laws c. 37 (2013) and 11 Del. C. § 4209A
97. H. B. 4210, 81st Gen. Assem., Reg. Sess. (WVa 2014).
98. *Id.* at Article 11(c)(1)-(15).
99. *Id.* at Article 11(c)(6).
100. *Id.* at Article 11(c)(6); 11(d)(1).
101. *Id.* ("Unless they fall within an exception to the general rule, new constitutional rules of criminal procedure will not be applicable to those cases which have become final before the new rules are announced.")
102. Order of Judge Timothy J. Savage, *Songster v. Beard*, No. 04-5916 (September 6, 2012).
103. *Hill v. Snyder*, 10-14568, 2013 WL 364198 (E.D. Mich. January 30, 2013).
104. *In re Evans*, 449 F. App'x 284 (4th Cir. 2011).
105. *Craig v. Crain*, No. 12-30035, 2013 WL 69128 (5th Cir. 2013); *In re Morgan*, No. 13-11175-D, 2013 WL 1499498 (11th Cir. Apr. 12, 2013).
106. Pennsylvania and North Carolina now prohibit juvenile life without parole for murder in the second degree or lower. S.B. 850, 204th Gen. Assem. Reg. Sess. (Pa. 2012); S.B. 635, 148th Gen. Assem. Reg. Sess. (N.C. 2012).

107. H.B. 23, 62nd Gen. Assem., Reg. Sess (Wyo. 2013) ("An Act...eliminating life sentences without parole for juvenile offenders."); S.B. 9, 147th Gen. Assem., Reg. Sess. (Del. 2013).
108. H.B. 5221, February 2014 Reg. Sess. (Conn. 2014).
109. James Swift. (June 25, 2013). *Miller v. Alabama*: One year later. Juvenile Justice Information Exchange.
110. H.B. 541, 97th Leg., Gen. Sess. (Mo. 2013); S.B. 260, 2013-2014 Gen. Sess (Ca. 2013); H.B. 1271 2013-2014 Gen. Sess. (Co. 2013).
111. Terry A. Maloney. (2010). The false promise of adolescent brain science in juvenile justice. *Notre Dame Law Rev, 85*, 89; see, e.g., Claudia Wallis. (May 10, 2004). What makes teens tick? *Time*; Paul Thompson. (May 25, 2001). Brain research shows a child is not an adult. *Ft. Lauderdale Sun Sentinal*; Allstate Insurance Co. Advertisement (2007). Available at http://www.allstate.com/content/refresh-attachments/Brain-Ad.pdf; David Walsh. (2004). *Why do they act that way? A survival guide to the adolescent brain for you and your teen.*
112. See, e.g., Saki Knafo. (September 20, 2013). Here are all the countries where children are sentenced to die in prison. *Huffington Post*; (November 26, 2013). Juvenile life without parole. *Juvenile Law Center.*

SECTION FOUR

Psychiatry Subspecialties and Forensic Psychiatry

13

Forensic Issues in Hospital-Based Psychiatric Consultations

Rachel Shmuts, Robert M. Weinrieb, and Kajal R. Patel

Introduction

Psychosomatic medicine, also known as consultation-liaison psychiatry, is a subspecialty of psychiatry that deals with the interface of psychological, ethical, social, and legal issues arising in a general hospital setting. Because of the complex nature of this area of practice, authors, clinicians, and ethicists have proposed principles and models to guide the understanding, practice, and management of these complex issues.

In their work on bioethics, Beauchamp and Childress defined four cardinal ethical principles that exist clinical care: *non-maleficence, beneficence, autonomy*, and *justice*, which are commonly recognized by many fields of medical practice[1] (see Table 13.1). Lederberg added depth to these principles by proposing a situational diagnostic methodology to define and address the different components of multilayered, ethically complex cases.[2] His systematic approach to evaluating ethically important situations includes examinations of patient and family issues, such as mental illness both in the patient and key significant others, staff issues, family–staff relationships ("joint" issues), legal/institutional issues, and ethical issues. Hundert has proposed a model suggesting the basic values comprising ethical dilemmas: *liberty, justice*, and *fairness*, which must be weighed for the relative importance of each value in order to take some moral action.[3]

In practice, laws in local jurisdictions and individual aspects of each clinical case can further complicate the execution of proposed ethical guidelines and principles in the treatment and management of patients in the hospital setting. Therefore, psychosomatic

TABLE 13.1 Four cardinal ethical principles in clinical care[1]

Principle	Definition
Nonmaleficence	An obligation to avoid doing harm
Beneficence	An obligation to benefit patients and seek their good whenever possible
Autonomy	The patient's ability to make deliberated or reasoned decisions for oneself and to act on the basis of such decisions
Justice	Fairness and equal resources/access to care

Beauchamp TL, & Childress JF. (1979). *Principles of biomedical ethics*. New York: Oxford University Press.

medicine physicians and specialists need to be familiar with concepts related to these principles. Furthermore, practitioners must have knowledge of the laws associated with their local jurisdiction in order to make informed treatment decisions and recommendations for their patients and primary teams.

This chapter reviews the most common clinically relevant forensic and ethical questions encountered on the psychiatric consultation service: *decision-making capacity*, which covers discussion on topics of informed consent, patient autonomy, and right to refuse treatment; and *duty to warn/protect*, which will explore topics of patient confidentiality, safety, and criminality in the clinical setting. Information will be discussed within a case-presentation format to help further illustrate the complexity of ethical dilemmas faced by psychosomatic medicine physicians in their practice.

Decision-Making Capacity

Consent for any treatment revolves around three cognitive pillars: (1) provision of adequate information to patients by primary teams, (2) voluntariness, and (3) decision-making capacity. However, simply because a person has mental illness or cognitive impairment, it does not necessarily mean they lack the capacity to make decisions. This is also true for individuals who are involuntarily committed or institutionalized. Because medical decisions could potentially profoundly impact one's health and well-being, physicians must be alert to the presence of fear, coercion, misconception, somatic disease, medications, and mental illness in their patients, all of which could adversely affect judgment. It may sometimes be necessary for physicians to assess decision-making capacity repeatedly and carefully during an acute care stay. It is important to know that psychiatrists are not the only physicians who can assesses decision-making capacity; in fact, capacity may be assessed by any physician.

Medical care providers consider the term capacity as the threshold determination for informed consent. Capacity is clinically determined, whereas *competency*, its legal equivalent, is clearly distinguished from capacity, as it requires judicial determination. However, both terms are often used interchangeably in both practice and literature. Capacity is always presumed to be intact in a patient unless there is a specific concern indicating otherwise. There should be a compelling reason as to why a patient should indeed lack capacity to make a certain decision. If this is the case, a detailed assessment of decision-making capacity in the context of the specific task or decision in question should take place. There may be situations in which a team requests a "global" or capacity evaluation for all decisions in general. However, capacity evaluations only take place in reference to a specific decision or clinical situation, and if there are multiple decisions that need to be made, each decision requires its own capacity determination. Psychiatric evaluation for capacity is limited to medical and medically related decisions only (i.e. dispositional capacity when a patient is being discharged from the hospital), and it does not apply to decisions regarding finances, estates, and legal matters.

The legal standards for a patient's decision-making capacity may vary across jurisdictions. Most jurisdictions require the following four components: (1) the ability to communicate a choice; (2) the ability to understand the risks, benefits, and alternatives to the proposed treatment; (3) the ability to appreciate and apply this information to his or her medical condition; and (4) the ability to reasonably manipulate this information and his or her choice, taking into account his or her background and cognitive abilities.[4–6] When there is no urgency for the patient to make a medical decision and a patient lacks capacity to make that medical decision, a surrogate decision maker is sought in accordance with the state statutory hierarchy. In some states, particularly Pennsylvania, which has among the clearest statutes, assignment of a surrogate decision maker is predetermined according to priority and relationship, that is, spouse, adult children, siblings, other relatives, and even someone not related to the patient who knows the patient's values, morals, and preferences, in that order.[7] If a surrogate decision maker is not available, the court must be petitioned to decide whether treatment may be imposed over a patient's objection. This is of particular importance in situations in which there is no surrogate decision maker or if a proxy has questionable cognitive ability or is suspected of ulterior motives. Sometimes conflicts may arise regarding assignment of surrogate decision makers in which surrogates of equal priority (e.g., spouse versus adult child from a previous relationship) may disagree on a specific treatment or choice. If surrogate decision makers of equal priority are present, the decision must be made by majority rule. If these surrogates cannot agree to decide in a particular situation, then the interested parties must go to court to petition for a designated decision maker. The standard by which the surrogate makes a decision on behalf of the patient is called *substituted judgment*. Substituted judgment takes into account the patient's morals, values, and beliefs; or in essence, deciding how the patient would decide should he or she be deemed to possess the capacity to make the decision on his or her own. If nothing is known about the patient's views, then the decision should be made according to the best interest of the patient.

In order to assess whether a patient's capacity to decide on a specific medical intervention is intact, the treating physician or team must first and foremost provide him with enough information about the specific prescribed intervention. It is very important this information-providing discussion occurs before or at the time of psychiatric assessment, as patients who are not adequately informed about the medical recommendations may very well appear to lack capacity on the basis of not understanding the clinical situation. Indeed, such a patient may actually have full capacity to make a medical decision, but he or she has not been provided with enough information to manipulate it appropriately. For example, if a physician recommended lumbar puncture for a patient and the patient refused the procedure without first having heard an explanation of the risks, benefits, and alternatives of the procedure, then the patient lacks informed consent and will falsely appear to lack capacity. However, had a discussion taken place with the provider and the patient in which the risks, benefits, and alternatives of a lumbar puncture were described, the treating physician may have found that the patient in fact does have medical decision-making capacity to refuse the procedure. If the patient didn't have an adequate opportunity to have the medical situation explained to him or her by their provider, it may lead to an ethical infraction of a patient's autonomy to choose proper medical care by falsely assuming the patient does not have the mental wherewithal to make that choice. In the preceding example, if the physician forged ahead with the lumbar puncture against the patient's wishes, then that procedure would be considered *unauthorized and unjustified touching* in the eyes of the law, and the physician would be guilty of battery.

The exception to the above rule about obtaining informed consent applies in a life-or-death emergency, either in an adult who is unable to communicate, or in pediatric patients when a parent is not at the bedside. In these situations, physicians are not required to obtain informed consent prior to providing life-saving treatment, as informed consent (barring the presence of a living will or advance directive) and decisional capacity are assumed. When the patient is stable and/or cognizant, an informed consent discussion must take place, and capacity evaluation, if necessary or relevant, should be conducted.

It is also important for the patient to demonstrate consistency in the preferred choice long enough for that particular treatment choice to be administered or enacted. Capacity is a point-determination in time, and consistency may need to be evaluated with repeat capacity evaluations. Because capacity can change over time, if a patient is initially determined not to have capacity, and the underlying reason for this inability to decide improves, he or she may regain capacity, and complex involvement of family and potentially the legal system may not be warranted. It is implicit in the psychosomatic medicine consultant's goals, to attempt to come up with safe ways of restoring capacity to their patients whenever possible.

In practice, the stringency of the decision-making capacity evaluation varies directly with the seriousness of the likely consequences of the specific decision. This is referred to as the "sliding scale" approach.[8] This sliding scale is determined by the risk to benefit ratio of the treatment. A patient would thus require less capacity to make a decision about a low-risk, low-benefit procedure than if he or she were deciding about a high-risk, high-benefit procedure. For example, if a patient chooses to refuse a stool softener pill (low risk, low benefit), the need for his or her ability to demonstrate capacity would be less rigorous than if this same patient was refusing intubation for imminent respiratory arrest (high risk, high benefit).

In the following paragraphs, three specific clinical cases will be presented to illustrate some of the nuances of decision-making capacity.

Clinical Case #1

A psychosomatic medicine service was consulted to evaluate a 45-year-old woman who was admitted to the medical unit for abdominal pain. The work up revealed alcoholic pancreatitis as the etiology for her acute pain. After the treatment for her pancreatitis was complete, but before her ability to tolerate oral intake was assessed, the patient informed the primary team she wanted to leave the hospital. The team wanted to keep the patient in the hospital for observation and to perform a diet challenge. She began to refuse all further medical intervention from nursing and staff physicians, and she ate food despite her *nil-per-os* status. She was loud and oppositional. The psychiatry team was consulted to evaluate the patient's decision-making capacity to leave against medical advice (AMA).

On psychiatric exam the patient was standing at the nursing station, refusing to answer most questions. She said she wanted to go home and pay her bills. Her speech was pressured, her mood was "angry," and her affect irritable, but mood-congruent. Previous records revealed a historical diagnosis of Bipolar Affective Disorder but no significant treatment history. The patient adamantly denied any psychiatric history.

Questions for Consideration

1. Does this patient have any underlying or active primary psychiatric diagnosis that would preclude her decision-making capacity to leave AMA at this time?
2. Does this patient possess sufficient understanding about her medical condition to leave the hospital (defined as dispositional capacity), or should she be held against her wishes if it is determined she lacks capacity for this specific decision?

Case #1 Discussion

In the case of this patient with pancreatitis, there were no incontrovertible signs of mania or psychosis, and therefore she did not have clear underlying psychopathology that would result in her lacking capacity to leave AMA (question #1). In evaluating this patient's capacity to leave the hospital, one must consider the four major tenets of a capacity assessment—the patient's ability to: (1) communicate a consistent choice; (2) understand the clinical situation and risks versus benefits of the decision; (3) appreciate the situation; and (4) reason logically and be able to manipulate information to reach their decision. In this example, the patient clearly communicated a choice, was able to understand the risks and benefits as well as alternatives of the proposed intervention, and could apply this information to her condition. She was, however, not willing to manipulate this information and discuss her thought process regarding her choice. The patient wanted to leave before completion of her medical treatment, but the danger to her well-being by leaving AMA was considered minimal because the symptoms of her pancreatitis had largely resolved and she was tolerating oral intake without any complications. Upon weighing the potential medical risks of the patient's decision and her autonomy to leave the hospital, it was determined that the patient had dispositional capacity, and she was allowed to leave with appropriate medical follow up and a crisis plan in place.

Clinical Case #2

During a medical hospitalization, a high-functioning 65-year-old woman with no past psychiatric history was diagnosed with multiple myeloma. She wanted to leave the hospital AMA without initiating treatment for her cancer or allowing for arrangement of follow-up care, which included aggressive chemotherapy and radiation. The team documented in the chart in detail their discussions with the patient in which they outlined the nature of the cancer treatment, the risks and benefits of both accepting treatment and rejecting treatment, and alternative options. They clearly felt the patient's disease would worsen quickly, should she reject care.

The patient appeared cognitively intact and intelligent. She stated she had to leave the hospital because she needed to take care of her home, which she insisted was more important to her than receiving treatment at that time. She was able to verbalize the information that was provided to her by the team about the proposed treatment recommendations; however, she avoided further conversation about her diagnosis, treatment, or prognosis. Nonetheless, she remained adamant about wanting to leave. Although she believed she would survive without treatment, she was unable to explain how that could be possible.

Questions for Consideration

1. Is denial of illness affecting this patient's ability to make dispositional decisions?
2. If this patient lacks dispositional capacity, should treatment for her cancer and follow-up care by implemented against her wishes?

Case #2 Discussion

In this case, the patient was able to communicate her choice to leave AMA. She was also able to talk about the risks, benefits, and alternatives of the recommended treatment, but she did not appear to be able to or willing to rationally manipulate this information and apply it to her condition. It seemed a profound denial of illness played a role in this patient's inability to both appreciate her situation and demonstrate a logical thought process leading to her stated choice. Here, the risks of refusing treatment were severe enough (high benefit of treatment versus rapid advancement of cancer presumably leading to hastening of death) to warrant interpretation of the sliding scale of capacity. Based on this argument, and because of the potential for great adverse health impact through refusal of treatment, the patient was determined to lack capacity to leave the hospital AMA.

Having made a determination of this patient's incapacity to leave AMA, the first step in managing this case is to document the nature and *potential duration* of incapacity as well as to identify etiologies for incapacity. In this case, the patient does not appear delirious or demented. A careful assessment of other primary psychiatric disorders, like depression or anxiety, should be completed. Denial of illness and lack of insight in this patient appear to be motivating factors contributing to her choice, and these factors should be explored further. Once a reason for incapacity is identified, measures should be taken to try to restore the patient's capacity. This patient in particular may require multiple discussions to help translate the impact her illness will have on her life as well as her life expectancy. Having a family member or close companion present for these conversations may help increase her level of insight. Treatment of any underlying psychiatric illness with antidepressants or antianxiety medications may also assist in restoring capacity if these entities are influencing her thought process. Should all of these measures fail to restore capacity, an appropriate surrogate decision maker should be sought to make decisions on this patient's behalf, considering the patient's morals, beliefs, values, (i.e., substituted judgment).

Clinical Case #3

A 51-year-old woman who denied a past psychiatric history was admitted to the hospital for severe malnutrition and a flare of her long-standing ulcerative colitis (UC). On admission, her body mass index was measured to be 13 (normal is 18.5–24.9). Psychiatry was consulted because the patient began refusing total parenteral nutrition (TPN), which the primary team considered to be an urgently necessary life-saving treatment. The team was informed that in prior hospitalizations, the patient had also refused TPN for various reasons, including reporting a side effect of diarrhea, which the medicine team concluded was unlikely. On physical exam the patient was noted to be profoundly underweight with rotting teeth, temporal wasting, sallow skin, and inability to concentrate. Laboratory studies revealed a hemoglobin as low as 6.7 g/dL. Albumin and prealbumin were also very low, indicating severe malnutrition. She was found to be hyponatremic, hypocalcemic, and severely iron deficient. Her husband said she had extremely poor oral intake for years prior to admission, and medical work up did not reveal any obvious etiology for her limited nutritional intake. Assessments by multiple psychiatrists on the consultation team concluded the patient suffered from a severe eating disorder, for which she had no insight. She was intermittently agreeable to some forms of oral feeding and but refused to be fed via nasogastric tube. The primary team wanted the patient's psychiatric team to comment on her capacity to refuse life-saving medical care as well whether it would be safe to discharge her to home if her nutritional status and overall health sufficiently improved.

Case #3 Discussion

This provides another example of how lack of insight into one's own illness can have profound effects on a patient's medical condition. In this case, despite detailed collateral information that the patient's eating disorder had progressed over many years, she denied having any psychiatric complaints or history. She regularly attributed her physical condition to her underlying inflammatory bowel disease, which was inconsistent with its usual course, according to the treating team. Her decision to accept life-saving medical care was inconsistent, as she would sometimes consent to only certain plans of care, and other times refuse. She superficially acknowledged understanding of the severity of her illness and need for treatment, but provided illogical and disordered thinking to support her reasons for refusing certain interventions.

Ultimately, it was determined that the patient retained sufficient capacity to consent to medical care, but using the sliding scale of capacity, we determined she would need to demonstrate a much higher threshold of understanding to refuse life-saving interventions. She was therefore determined to lack capacity to refuse life-saving treatments and to decide her disposition.

Attempts were made to treat the patient's eating disorder through behavioral interventions, managed primarily by the nutrition service. Patient's meals were supervised and strictly monitored, and goals for maximal intake and completion of meals were set. The patient was in agreement with this plan, and by the end of her hospitalization complied with these recommendations. When it came time for the patient to be discharged, the psychiatry team felt the patient might benefit from inpatient eating disorder treatment. The patient would not sign in voluntarily, and her family did not feel comfortable committing her against her will. Explicit psychoeducation was provided to the patient's family about both her medical and psychiatric conditions, and they appeared to understand the severity of the situation. Because the patient was incapacitated to decide disposition, her husband was designated as the primary surrogate decision maker. In the end, working with the treatment team, the patient's family decided to take her home and adhere to strict behavioral supervision and agreed to take her to the emergency room or call 911 for psychiatric evaluation should the patient fail to cooperate with these plans.

Duty to Warn/Protect

In each of the cases described, the assessment of decision-making capacity involved careful consideration of the patient's safety, especially the cases in which the patient was medically compromised and wanted to leave AMA. However, there can also be instances in which hospital psychiatric consultants, as part of their general evaluation process, must consider not only the patient's safety but also the safety of persons in the patient's social sphere or immediate surroundings. In the remainder of this chapter, we will discuss approaches, strategies, and ethical considerations in the evaluation of patients who may be dangerous to others.

Confidentiality has been a central feature of the physician–patient relationship for thousands of years. As early as 430 B.C., confidentiality was codified in the Hippocratic Oath: "Whatever I see or hear, professionally or privately, which ought not to be divulged, I will keep secret and tell no one."[9] Over time this declaration of absolute confidentiality has given way to several exceptions and modifications that reflect the complex balance between the importance of privacy in the doctor–patient relationship and societal demands for public safety.

Mental health professionals have clinical, ethical, and legal responsibilities to assess the potential for future violence toward others when caring for patients in clinical practice.[10]

This assessment usually involves taking a thorough behavioral history of past violence and careful evaluation for any Axis I and II pathology, including personality disorders or traits. It is also crucial to evaluate a patient's enduring characteristics and his or her immediate environmental situation, which may mitigate or aggravate the likelihood of violence, and a general tendency toward impulsivity.

A caveat and common misconception among nonpsychiatric physicians and caregivers is that despite thorough and repeated assessments for the risk of violence, no one can wholly or accurately predict with a high degree of certainty how any individual will behave in a particular situation in the future. Oftentimes consultation psychiatrists are asked, "Will this patient commit suicide?" or "Will this patient hurt someone else?" It is in these situations that the psychiatrist should help reframe the primary team's question by explaining that there is no way to answer these questions definitively. Nonetheless, a risk assessment for violence may be performed to help determine the likelihood of violence rather than definitively predicting it. Because the strongest predictor of future violent behavior is past violent behavior, a comprehensive history and collateral information are the most effective methods to increase the sensitivity of a violence assessment.

After careful assessment for the potential for violence, the clinician should make an informed estimate of whether a threat exists. If it is determined that an imminent threat of future violence is unlikely, the clinician may simply maintain the patient's confidentiality and can continue to evaluate and treat the patient as clinically indicated. However, if it is determined that there is a reasonable potential for imminent future violence toward a specific individual, according to the landmark court decision *Tarasoff v. Board of Regents* by the Supreme Court in California in 1976,[11,12] the clinician is legally obligated under "duty to warn" to breach the patient's right to confidentiality and warn the third party (an individual outside the doctor–patient relationship) of the patient's intent to harm.

An extension of this law is the duty to protect the third party by informing the appropriate officials in addition to the target. Because *Tarasoff* translates into different laws in different jurisdictions, it is critical for practitioners to be aware of the legal requirements in their jurisdictions regarding their duty to protect. There are variations in when a duty exists, to whom the duty applies, what set of circumstances trigger the duty, and what actions discharge the physician's obligation. In states with statutes that govern the duty to warn/protect, the scope of the duty is generally limited to situations in which there is a specific threat to an identifiable third party, circumstances in which the patient has a known history of violence, and/or cases in which there is reasonable cause to anticipate violence. State laws may also outline specific measures that may need to be pursued to discharge a duty to warn. These measures include notifying law enforcement, hospitalizing a mentally ill patient, and warning the potential victim. It is important to note that some patients who present to emergency rooms or psychiatric evaluations repeatedly may make multiple threats against one or more targets at different points in time. Each and every time a risk of violence is assessed to be high; the duty to warn/protect applies and must be instituted with each individual threat.

Clinical Case #4

A 54-year-old woman with a diagnosis of borderline personality disorder was admitted to a surgical service after she was bitten in the neck by a dog. The patient claimed her neighbors deliberately released their dog into the patient's yard with the intent to hurt her. Upon asking the patient details of the incident, she explained that this event had occurred before, involving the same dog and the same neighbors. The patient expressed her anger toward the neighbors and stated she planned to "take matters into her own hands this time around." She described a plan to shoot the dog with a BB gun upon her discharge from the hospital. When asked whether she had thoughts of specifically hurting the neighbors, she denied any intent or plan, but she said she "could not predict what would happen in the heat of the moment." The patient further added that her neighbors were unpredictable and dangerous. On psychiatric exam, she appeared psychiatrically stable. She was compliant with her medications and regularly met with her outpatient psychiatrist.

Questions for Consideration

1. Is there duty to warn/protect animals?
2. Given the patient's homicidal ideation is toward the neighbor's dog, and she could not deny harm could potentially come to her neighbors, should this case invoke duty to warn/protect?

Case #4 Discussion

As highlighted by the case, clinical situations can be complex and can raise a host of ethical and legal dilemmas. Currently, there is no legal obligation to breech patient confidentiality in order to warn/protect animals, although this could very well change in the future. In this case, after a thorough clinical evaluation and an in-depth discussion with different members of the team, it was ultimately concluded that there was a duty to warn/protect the neighbors given the possibility that the patient could hurt the neighbors directly (or indirectly) in her attempt to kill their dog. Given the patient's description of her neighbor's behaviors toward her, it was felt the patient's neighbors were dangerous and retribution would be likely, which would therefore place the patient in physical danger after discharge. As a result, it was decided that rather than having hospital personnel warn the neighbors directly, which could ultimately identify the patient as a threat, the patient was informed that the police were told about the patient's plans to hurt her neighbor's dog, and action to warn/protect was therefore deferred to their judgment and protocol.

Criminality in the Clinical Setting: Disposition and Treatment

There is scarce literature available discussing and guiding the management of psychiatric patients when there is a clash of medical ethics and the law. Although medicine is practiced in a legal and regulatory context, the ethics of medicine can differ from the ethics of everyday life. The law, which incorporates parts of morality, can at times be at odds with medical ethics.

Clinical Case #5

A 34-year-old woman with a past psychiatric history of severe, recurrent major depressive disorder with psychotic features and multiple previous suicide attempts was brought into the emergency room after killing her children. She subsequently attempted suicide by overdose on medications. She was arrested, placed in police custody, and brought to the hospital for medical and psychiatric evaluation.

Questions for Consideration

1. Is this patient in need of urgent psychiatric care?
2. If so, what treatment is recommended? What is the best environment for her to receive psychiatric treatment?

Case #5 Discussion

The Emergency Medical Treatment and Labor Act (EMTALA) Section 1867 establishes requirements for medical screening examinations for medical conditions as well as necessary stabilizing treatment or appropriate transfer.[13] The source of the consultation is irrelevant, and the EMTALA rules must be followed whether emergency department physicians, the in-house medicine service, or the authorities request the evaluation. Despite the disturbing nature of this case and others like it, EMTALA dictates our immediate actions in emergency psychiatric assessment. In such a tragic case, the psychiatry resident involved was counseled by the attending physician supervisor to put aside his understandably strong feelings toward the patient and focus on performing a thorough psychiatric evaluation.

After the psychiatric resident on call examined the patient, he concluded the patient was in need of inpatient psychiatric care. Confusion ensued as to where and by whom that care should take place. In some past cases, the consultation-liaison service was advised by hospital attorneys to recommend and arrange the psychiatric treatment thought to be best for the patient, such as admitting the patient to a medical or surgical floor to manage her condition. Legal implications and responsibilities could be further explored while the patient is being stabilized. However, in this case, although it was felt inpatient psychiatric treatment in a locked unit was best, the hospital attorneys and the city's Office of Mental Health advised that police take the patient to jail, after which she could be transferred to a forensic psychiatric unit and evaluated by a psychiatrist employed by the judicial system. Based on these experiences, it is recommended to defer to the hospital's legal counsel and the city's Office of Mental Health (or comparable governing or regulatory body), and accept that patients in police custody should remain in police custody after being medically cleared. Just as in cases in which patients with comorbid substance abuse and psychiatric issues might best be served by treatment in a dual diagnosis unit, patients with mental illness and comorbid criminal behavior might also be served well in a forensic unit designed to address both predominant acute issues.

Conclusion

The cases discussed demonstrate the high level of complexity often encountered in the practice of consultation-liaison psychiatry. It is necessary to perform a thorough psychiatric evaluation despite the myriad pressures of the fast-paced environment of a busy hospital, and as much as possible, minimize errors of omission. The interface between psychiatric illness and the law is one of the most complex and interesting areas of medicine. This type of work can be emotionally and intellectually challenging, and psychosomatic medicine physicians are typically the clinicians possessing the most experience to appropriately meet the complex needs at the heart of these challenges.

References

1. Beauchamp TL, & Childress JF. (1979). *Principles of biomedical ethics.* New York: Oxford University Press.
2. Lederberg MS. (1997). Making a situational diagnosis. Psychiatrists at the interface of psychiatry and ethics in the consultation-liaison setting. *Psychosomatics, 38*(4), 327–338.
3. Hundert EM. (1987). A model for ethical problem solving in medicine, with practical applications. *Am J Psychiat, 144*(7), 839–846.
4. Appelbaum PS., Lidz CW, & Meisel A. (1987). *Informed consent: Legal theory and clinical practice.* New York: Oxford University Press.
5. Appelbaum PS. (2007). Clinical practice: Assessment of patients' competence to consent to treatment. *N Engl J Med, 357*(18), 1834–1840.
6. *Ibid.*
7. Pennsylvania Medical Society. http://www.pamedsoc.org/MainMenuCategories/Government/LawsAffectingPhysicians/AdvanceDirectives/Act169facts.aspx Accessed January 1, 2012.
8. Buchanan AE., & Brock DW. (1990). *Deciding for others: The ethics of surrogate decision-making.* Cambridge: Cambridge University Press.
9. Chadwick J, & Mann, WN. (1983). Hippocrates: The oath. In GER Lloyd (Ed.), *Hippocratic writings* (p. 67). London: Penguin Books.
10. Beck JC. (1998). Legal and ethical duties of the clinician treating a patient who is liable to be impulsively violent. *Behav Sci Law, 16*(3), 375–389.
11. Schuck PH, & Givelber DJ. (2003). *Tarasoff v. Regents* of the University of California: The therapist's dilemma. In RL Rabin, & SD Sugarman (Eds.), *Tort stories* (pp. 99–128). New York: Foundation Press.
12. *Tarasoff v. Board of Regents* of the University of California. 17 Cal. 3d425, 551 P.2d 334, 131 Cal. Rptr. 14 (Cal 1976).
13. CMS.gov Centers for Medicare and Medicaid Services Emergency Medical Treatment Act and Labor Act https://www.cms.gov/emtala/Download link for CMS-1063F. Retrieved January 1, 2012.

14

Forensic Issues in Geriatric Psychiatry

Joel E. Streim

Forensic psychiatry issues of relevance to older adults include those that pertain to the general adult population and those that are unique to adults in the late stages of life. As a subspecialty field, geriatric psychiatry has made substantial contributions that address important challenges in forensic psychiatry with specific relevance to older adults in the areas of testamentary capacity and undue influence, driving safety, the guardianship and proxy decision making at the end-of-life, and elder abuse and neglect. This chapter provides an overview of these topics, and a discussion of the forensic questions that commonly arise in geriatric health care settings when there are conflicts between health care goals related to elder autonomy and provider or caregiver responsibility.

Cognitive Impairment and Decision Making in Older Adults

The prevalence of cognitive impairment is higher among older adults than any other age cohort. Epidemiological studies have revealed a 22.2% overall prevalence of mild cognitive impairment or cognitive impairment not dementia[1] and 13.9% prevalence of dementia in community-dwelling elders over 70 years of age.[2] Among the various causes of dementia, neurodegenerative disease is the most common. One study found the prevalence of dementia owing to probable Alzheimer's disease is 3% in those 65 to 74 years of age; 18.7% in those aged 75–84; and 47.2% in those aged 85 years and older.[3] The prevalence of cognitive impairment and dementia is much higher in long-term care settings, such as assisted living facilities and nursing homes.

Cognitive limitations may occur in persons of any age, with etiologies ranging from congenital problems and developmental disabilities to traumatic brain injury, stroke, and neurodegenerative disorders. However, the older adult segment of the population is uniquely vulnerable to and accounts for most cases of neurodegenerative dementia, caused by such conditions as Alzheimer's disease, frontotemporal lobar degeneration, Lewy Body disease, and Parkinson disease. The cognitive impairment caused by most of these neurodegenerative diseases is insidious in onset and gradually progressive. This characteristically slow decline presents unique challenges in determining the point at which a person's cognitive capacity significantly impedes independent decision-making. In clinical practice, this poses a need to monitor declining cognitive function and its effects on activities of daily living, including the management of finances, in order to recognize the point in time when the person requires the assistance of a proxy, or the appointment of a guardian. In forensic practice, the gradual decline seen in many cases of dementia poses a challenge to develop thresholds for decision-making capacity, to identify those elders who are no longer able to effectively or safely function independently.

There is an extensive medicolegal literature on the clinical assessment of decision-making capacity that is beyond the scope of this chapter (and is addressed in other chapters in this book). However, it should be noted that geriatricians have found that most older adults with mild dementia can participate in medical decision making as defined by legal standards.[4] It has been suggested that the older adult's ability to describe salient reasons for a specific choice (i.e., ability to meet a reasoning standard), and ability to describe the implications of various choices (i.e., to demonstrate an appreciation of potential consequences), are both important in determining if dementia limits the person's understanding of diagnostic and treatment information. The field of geriatrics has also been compelled to address older adults' decisional capacity to complete advance directives and participate in end-of-life planning. Assessment tools have been developed for this purpose.[5]

In addition, the pressing need to conduct research on dementia, and in particular to enroll older adults in clinical trials for Alzheimer's disease treatments, has highlighted ethical and legal dilemmas in decisional capacity and surrogacy. This has prompted the field of geriatrics to define standards and establish methods for assessing the decisional capacity of cognitively impaired older adults specifically for the purpose of participating in dementia research.[6,7] In particular, the MacArthur Competence Assessment Tool for Clinical Research was designed to be customized to a variety of clinical trial designs,[8] and has been used to evaluate geriatric patients for Alzheimer's trials. The concept of assent has also been invoked in geriatric care and enrollment in clinical trials.[9] In cases in which an elderly person has been determined to lack decisional capacity and an appointed surrogate gives consent, the impaired individual may still communicate distress or displeasure with the treatment or study procedures.[10] In such cases, the verbal or nonverbal refusal, or evidence of affective distress or behavioral resistance, is interpreted as a lack of assent, or dissent, which—according to the views of most participants in ethics research on consent of the cognitively impaired—should trump the consent given by the surrogate.

Geriatric psychiatrists have also worked to refine the contemporaneous and retrospective determination of testamentary capacity in older adults.[11–13] Shulman and colleagues have pointed out that the classic case of Banks *vs* Goodfellow[14] established the task-specific nature of testamentary capacity versus the global mental status or cognitive functioning of the person. The criteria established in Banks include an understanding the nature of a Will; knowledge of the nature and extent of one's assets; knowledge of the persons who are natural heirs or have a reasonable claim to be beneficiaries; an understanding of the impact of the dispositive plan; being free of any delusions that influence the disposition of the assets; and the ability to communicate one's wishes clearly and consistently. Of most relevance to geriatric psychiatry is the need to recognize situations in which the testator fails to meet these criteria either because of impairment in cognitive function or because of the presence of psychosis that influences and distorts decisions involved in making a Will. It is common for persons with Alzheimer's disease and other neurodegenerative disorders to have characteristic delusions of theft or infidelity. It is also common for these older adults to have delusions or visual agnosia associated with the belief that a family member or friend is an imposter. The content of such delusions is uniquely different from the content of delusional beliefs typically held by persons with conditions such as chronic schizophrenia or mood disorders with psychosis, though older adults with mood disorders commonly experience persecutory delusions.

Vulnerability of Frail Elders: Undue Influence and Elder Abuse

It has been pointed out that determining the protection needs of an elder who is being abused or neglected often hinges on that person's decisional capacity and ability to fend for him or herself.[15] Conversely, living in a situation of abuse or neglect may significantly influence and alter the decisions that an older adult makes, including the decision to seek help or take legal action against the abuser. Older adults with physical and/or cognitive disability may express a choice to remain under the care or custody of an abusive caregiver because they fear possible retaliation for trying to sever the relationship, or because of anxiety in the absence of a secure fallback position that ensures the receipt of social support and physical assistance they require.

It is always important for health care professionals to safeguard the interests of infirm elderly patients. Many states now require physicians and other licensed health professionals to report suspect cases of elder abuse, which are then referred to protective service agencies for older persons. Those who are frail or have significant cognitive impairment may be particularly vulnerable to undue influence and other forms of elder abuse. Those who are disabled and dependent on others may feel obligated to submit to the expectations and demands of their caregivers, particularly in situations in which they feel vulnerable to abandonment, or don't have the financial resources to pay for the care they need. Frail older adults in such situations deserve careful clinical evaluation of both their cognitive function and the psychosocial context in which they live, to determine whether or not they need to be protected from undue influence or other abuse. In conducting such evaluations, health care professionals must take special care to distinguish situations that require special protection of an older person from those situations in which the older person is still capable of making independent decisions, based on her or his own wishes and preferences. Often, in clinical practice, the situation requires careful balancing of beneficent protection versus assurance of autonomy.

Responsibility for Assessing, Predicting, and Reporting Driving Safety

The task of recognizing when cognitive impairment poses safety risks extends beyond the assessment of decisional capacity to determinations of driving safety. Some states require health care professionals to report to departments of motor vehicles any health conditions that may impede safe driving; others assign the responsibility for reporting relevant health problems to the patient. Even when the patient is responsible for self-reporting, the health care provider still has the moral and medical-legal responsibility for recognizing the risk and informing patients that their condition may render them unsafe to drive. Failure to do so exposes the clinician to substantial liability if the patient is subsequently found to be at fault in a motor vehicle accident.

There have been numerous attempts to develop cognitive assessment tools to assist health professionals in their prediction of driving safety[16] but virtual and actual road tests remain the most reliable tools for determining whether driving is no longer safe.[17] Given the gradual progression of most dementing illnesses, a patient may be tested and found to be safe to drive early in the course of the illness; yet there is no established metric to determine appropriate time interval for reassessment. That is because the patient may reach the point of dangerousness on the road at any time in the period before a reassessment is conducted. It has not been possible to establish a reliable time interval between neurocognitive tests or on-road assessments for determining the moment at which the patient declines to the point of dangerousness on the road. Frequent serial assessments are impractical, leaving patients vulnerable to accidents, and leaving clinicians liable if they fail to report cases of dementia in the early stages when, in fact, some patients may still be able to drive safely for a period of months or even a few years.[18]

Nursing Homes and Conflicting Health Care Goals

Geriatric patients residing in nursing home settings have a very high prevalence of medical-psychiatric comorbidity, often associated with cognitive impairment and decline in functional status. Epidemiological studies in US nursing homes have found the prevalence of psychiatric diagnoses between 80% and 94%.[19–23] This has prompted the description of nursing homes as de facto institutions for older adults with mental disorders, though these facilities were never designed, staffed, or licensed for that purpose.[24] Nursing homes do not operate with psychiatrically trained staff nurses, nor do they have provisions typically found on acute hospital inpatient units, such as seclusion rooms or physical restraints. In fact, a nursing home reform movement that came of age in the 1980s has resulted in sweeping federal regulations and campaigns to transform the culture of nursing homes to make them less institutional and more homelike and person-centered. This translates into less restrictive environments that foster independence and promote the autonomy of older adults. Federal regulations explicitly enumerate the rights of nursing home residents, including those who have impaired cognitive function from conditions such as dementia.

In addition to those federal regulations designed to protect patient rights, there are regulations that hold nursing homes accountable for providing high-quality care, which includes ensuring the safety of nursing home residents. Although the initial intention of all these regulations was generally to improve the quality of care in nursing homes that receive Medicare or Medicaid funds (which includes most of the 16,000 nursing facilities in the United States.), the goals related to resident rights and assurances of patient safety often pose a conflict for nursing facilities and their staff. For example, nursing facility staff is expected on the one hand to promote resident autonomy and encourage independent ambulation, and on the other hand to protect nursing home patients by reducing the risk of falls and fall-related injuries. These goals are sometimes in direct conflict. For example, it is common to find a nursing home resident with both dementia and unsteady gait. In such cases, the risk of falls due to gait instability is compounded by the patient's cognitive deficits, which may include a lack of insight regarding the extent of his or her physical disability, lack of safety awareness, and disinhibited or impulsive behavior. Thus, allowing the resident to transfer from bed to chair or ambulate independently may place him or her at risk for an injurious fall; conversely, forcing the resident to wait to get out of bed or chair may be deemed too restrictive. Before Congressional passage of the Nursing Home Reform Amendments to the Omnibus Budget Reconciliation Act of 1987 (OBRA '87), nursing homes routinely used physical restraints, in many cases with the intention to prevent falls. However, OBRA '87 directed the Centers for Medicare and Medicaid Services (known by the acronym CMS and previously called the Health Care Financing Administration or HCFA) to issue regulations specifically stating that residents of nursing homes have the right to be free from physical restraints. Subsequent research in nursing home populations demonstrated that, in fact, restraints do not reduce fall-related injuries, and may actually increase the incidence of injuries. Even though it is now generally accepted that physical restraint use is inappropriate in nursing homes (except for acute emergency management), federal regulations covering patient rights and quality of care clearly state that resident rights must not be abridged by approaches to care, including alternatives to physical restraints as a method of fall risk reduction.

As a result of such conflicts, it may not be clear who is at fault when a patient falls in a nursing home. In cases involving a fall resulting in serious injury or death, the plaintiffs often claim negligence on the part of the staff and the facility. The defense may claim that, consistent with federal guidelines that define quality of care, the resident's goals and wishes were being respected by staff. These conflicts between the goal of preserving resident rights and promoting autonomy versus the goal of protecting residents from harm are seldom addressed directly in documented care plans. Thus, when these cases come to trial, there is often an important role for the geriatric or forensic psychiatrist to tease apart the standards of care in the context of sometimes conflicting federal mandates related to quality of care. From a practice perspective, the role of the geriatric psychiatrist as nursing home consultant can include discussions of goals for health and well-being, as well as clarification of risk tolerance with residents and family members or health care proxies; and assisting nursing home staff and administrators with incorporating the resident and family goals in the written plan of care that is required by federal regulations. Thoughtful, guided discussions and careful documentation may reduce the risk of nursing home litigation.

Forensic Implications of Evolving Criteria for the Diagnosis of Dementia

The American Psychiatric Association Diagnostic and Statistical Manual of Mental Disorders, Fifth Edition[25] (DSM V) has substituted "major neurocognitive disorder" for the DSM IV diagnosis of "dementia," and added "mild neurocognitive disorder" as a diagnosis for patients with mild but clinically significant cognitive deficits. The DSM V furnishes operational descriptions of deficits in various cognitive domains, with emphasis that goes well beyond the DSM IV focus on impairment in memory. Of particular importance to forensic psychiatry is the evaluation of executive function in older adults with major neurocognitive disorders. Executive function is highly salient to forensic psychiatry because it includes awareness of one's situation and the ability to recognize one's needs; the ability to deliberate and choose goals; and the ability to plan, initiate and execute tasks, with adequate agency and appropriate sequencing to achieve one's goals. Thus, the change in DSM definitions for diagnosing cognitive disorders is likely to increase attention to the range of cognitive deficits that are relevant to issues in forensic psychiatry, from testamentary capacity and undue influence to driving safety to elder abuse and guardianships. It will almost certainly shift the focus of expert reports and court testimony to more comprehensive evaluations of executive function and other cognitive domains.

Conclusion

The field of geriatric psychiatry addresses and informs many areas of relevance to the field of forensic psychiatry, and vice versa. This reciprocal relationship results in substantial overlap in the training of subspecialists in both fields, and consequent overlap in the functions performed by practicing geriatric and forensic psychiatrists. Geriatric psychiatrists-in-training learn about assessment of cognitive capacity and competency, undue influence, guardianship, abuse, neglect, protective services and guardianship, liability, and other legal concepts related to aging and mental health. They also must hone their skills in report preparation and expert testimony in court. Similarly, forensic psychiatrists-in-training learn from the geriatric clinician about cognitive decline and dementia, dependency, and proper care and treatment of the elderly. The most challenging cases may require the expertise of subspecialists from both fields. The practice of medicine has become increasingly complex, and the availability of new medical knowledge, new assessment tools, evolving diagnostic criteria, and new regulations and laws may require increased coordination of psychiatric subspecialists working together with other medical specialists.

References

1. Plassman BL, Langa KM, Fisher GG, et al. (2008). Prevalence of cognitive impairment without dementia in the United States. *Ann Intern Med, 148*, 427–434.
2. Plassman BL, Langa KM, Fisher GG, et al. (2007). Prevalence of dementia in the United States: Yhe Aging Demographics, and Memory Study. *Neuroepidemiology, 29*,125–132.
3. Evans DA, Funkenstein HH, Albert MS, et al. (1989). Prevalence of Alzheimer's disease in a community population of older persons: Higher than previously reported. *JAMA,262*, 2551–2556.
4. Moye J, Karel MJ, Azar AR, et al. (2004). Capacity to consent to treatment: empirical comparison of three instruments in older adults with and without dementia. *Gerontologist, 44*, 166–175.
5. Molloy DW, Silberfield M, Darzins P, et al. (1996). Measuring capacity to complete an advance directive. *J Am Geriatr Soc, 44*, 660–664.
6. Jeste DV, Palmer BW, Appelbaum PS, et al. (2007). A brief new instrument for assessing decisional capacity for clinical research. *Arch Gen Psychiatry, 64*, 966–974.
7. Jefferson AL, Lambe S, Moser DJ, et al. (2008). Decisional capacity for research participation in individuals with mild cognitive impairment. *J Am Geriatr Soc, 56*, 1236–1243.
8. Appelbaum PS, & Grisso T. (2001). MacArthur Competence Assessment Tool for Clinical Research (MacCAT-CR). Sarasota, FL: Professional Resource Press.
9. Overton E, Appelbaum PS, Fisher SR, et al. (2013). Alternative decision-makers' perspectives on assent and dissent for dementia research. *Am J Geriatr Psychiatry, 21*:346–354.
10. Black BS, Wechsler M, & Fogarty L. (2013). Decision making for participation in dementia research. *Am J Geriatr Psychiatry, 21*:355–363.
11. Shulman KI, Cohen CA, & Hull I. (2005). Psychiatric issues in retrospective challenges of testamentary capacity. *Int J Geriatr Psychiatry, 20*, 63–69.
12. Shulman KI, Cohen CA, Kirsh FC, et al. (2007). Assessment of testamentary capacity and vulnerability to undue influence. *Am J Psychiatry, 154*, 722–727.
13. Shulman KI, Peisah C, Jacogy R, et al. (2009). Contemporaneous assessment of testamentary capacity. *Int Psychogeriatrics, 21*, 433–439.
14. Banks *v.* Goodfellow. L.R.5 Q.B. 549, (1870).
15. O'Connor D, Hall MI, & Donnelly M. (2009). Assessing capacity within the context of abuse or neglect. *J Elder Abuse Negl, 21*, 156–169.
16. Dickerson AE. (2014). Driving with dementia: evaluation, referral, and resources. *Occup Ther Health Care, 289*, 62–76.
17. Hoggarth PA, Innes CR, Dlarymmple-Alford JC, et al. (2013). Predicting on-road assessment pass and fail outcomes in older drivers with cognitive impairment using a battery of computerized sensory-motor and cognitive tests. *J Am Geriatr Soc, 61*, 2192–2198.
18. Rapoport MJ, Naglie G, Herrmann N, et al. (2014). Developing physician consensus on the reporting of patients with mild cognitive impairment and mild dementia to transportation authorities in a region with mandatory reporting legislation. *Am J Geriatr Psychiatry, 22*, 1530–1543.
19. Chandler JD, & Chandler JE. (1988). The prevalence of neuropsychiatric disorders in a nursing home population. *J Geriatr Psychiatry Neurol, 1*, 71–76.
20. Parmelee PA, Katz IR, & Lawton MP. (1989). Depression among institutionalized aged: Assessment and prevalence estimation. *J Gerontol, 44*, M22–M29.
21. Rovner BW, Kafonek S, Filipp L, et al. (1986). Prevalence of mental illness in a community nursing home. *Am J Psychiatry, 143*, 1446–1449.
22. Rovner BW, German PS, Broadhead J, et al. (1990). The prevalence and management of dementia and other psychiatric disorders in nursing homes. *Int Psychogeriatr, 2*, 13–24.

23. Tariot PN, Podgorski CA, Blazina L, et al. (1993). Mental disorders in the nursing home: another perspective. *Am J Psychiatry, 150*, 1063–1069.
24. Streim JE. (2012). Clinical psychiatry in the nursing home. In DG Blazer, & DC Steffans (Eds.), *Essentials of geriatric psychiatry* (2nd ed., pp. 351–379). Washington, DC: American Psychiatric Publishing.
25. American Psychiatric Association. (2013). *Diagnostic and Statistical Manual of Mental Disorders* (5th ed.). Arlington, VA: American Psychiatric Publishing.

15

Inpatient Forensic Psychiatry

Clarence Watson

The clinical treatment of persons with mental illness in the context of the criminal justice system is an especially complex undertaking. The swirl of competing legal, medical, and administrative interests surrounding any given forensic patient transforms the typical doctor–patient relationship into one that is fraught with potential legal consequences. In the inpatient forensic setting, the treatment provided is scrutinized from multiple perspectives: the patient, clinicians, defense counsel, prosecuting attorneys, judges, and the relevant governmental correctional authorities to which custody of the patient has been charged. Accordingly, the usual tensions associated with psychiatric hospitalization take on new dimensions, as the ramifications of treatment affect not only clinical concerns, but also the administration of justice.

Historically, persons with mental illness deemed too violent or criminally disturbed were placed in institutions once referred to as criminal lunatic asylums[1] One of the earliest institutions treating the "criminally insane" was the Royal Hospital of Bethlem (Bethlem Hospital) in London. Originally founded in 1247 as a priory, Bethlem Hospital was noted to have confined "six lunatics" by 1400 and that "the inventory of the instruments kept on the premises for their treatment is curious—'six chains of iron, with six locks; four pairs of manacles of iron, and five pairs of stocks'."[2] The Criminal Lunatics Act of 1860 established the first British institution specifically designated for the treatment of mentally ill criminals, Broadmoor Criminal Lunatic Asylum in Berkshire.[1]

Following the model of Bethlem Hospital, the Pennsylvania Hospital opened in 1752 as the first mental hospital in colonial America.[3] Throughout the nineteenth century, there was significant growth in the number of mental hospitals in the United States, with the majority being state funded.[4] Over the centuries, much progress has been made from the early days of asylums toward modern day patient-centered care initiatives for the treatment of persons with mental illness. Today, psychiatric treatment of patients in forensic hospitals is delivered with an eye toward the balance of the preservation of patients' rights with the demands of the criminal justice system.

The Inpatient Forensic Psychiatric Hospital

Typically, inpatient forensic psychiatric treatment is provided in a freestanding maximum-security forensic hospital or a specialized forensic unit at a state hospital. Unlike the usual routine of a clinician determining the appropriateness of hospital admission and the timing of discharge, admissions and discharges of forensic patients are most often directed by the court system. The duration of hospitalization in forensic settings is usually significantly longer than that of hospitalization in civil settings. Unlike civil hospitalizations, forensic hospitalizations involve not only the goal of resolving psychiatric symptoms, but also involve addressing the referring courts' concerns in correlated legal matters.

Because of the patient's legal involvement and the court's interest in resolving pending legal matters, there is regular oversight of the patient's course of treatment by the referring judge and the attorneys involved. In addition, the relevant jurisdiction's correctional agency usually retains legal custody of the forensic patient during hospitalization, and accordingly, that agency also has an interest in the course of the patient's treatment. Depending on the nature of the legal issues at hand, the degree of confidentiality that forensic inpatients can expect is limited by their legal circumstances and the attendant judicial and correctional interests. As a consequence, the provision of psychiatric and psychological reports to referring courts and clinical updates to correctional agencies, regardless of patients' consent, is customary.

Treatment services that forensic hospitals typically provide include the following: competency to stand trial restoration and evaluation programs; presentence evaluations; psychiatric stabilization of post-trial convicted individuals who have been found guilty but mentally ill (GBMI); psychiatric stabilization of convicted individuals who have decompensated while incarcerated; and, treatment of post-trial acquittees who have been found not guilty by reason of insanity (NGRI).

The Inpatient Forensic Population

Generally, the inpatient forensic patient population is a heterogeneous group that shares the commonality of the criminal justice system's involvement. Some forensic patients are pretrial detainees, whereas others are post-trial convicts and serving criminal sentences. The range of pending and substantiated criminal charges that hospitalized forensic patients carry is broad. It is not uncommon for detainees charged with nonviolent offenses and detainees accused of serious violent offenses, including sex offenses, to receive treatment together within the same inpatient setting. In addition, NGRI acquittees may also receive treatment in forensic hospital settings until they are no longer considered to pose a risk of danger to the community.

Although the courts usually initiate entry into the forensic treatment unit, correctional agencies may also arrange for the hospitalization of incarcerated individuals suffering acute psychiatric symptoms when a higher level of treatment than can be provided in the correctional setting is necessary. Psychiatric care is routinely available in correctional facilities. As some have pointed out, jails and prisons have collectively become the largest providers of inpatient mental health services in the United States[5]; however, the severity of an inmate's illness dictates the necessity of hospitalization. The authority of a correctional institution to transfer prisoners for psychiatric hospitalization is not without limitation. The U.S. Supreme Court, concerned with the potential stigma of psychiatric hospitalization, ruled in *Vitek v. Jones* (1980) that procedural protection of prisoner rights must be followed before such transfers can occur.[6]

DiCataldo developed a typology of inmates and pretrial detainees transferred from correctional institutions to a secure forensic psychiatric hospital between 1990 and 1996.[7] The eight-group typology outlines the various types of challenges that inmates can represent within the correctional setting. The types are as follows (Ref. 7, p. 270):

1. Psychotic-Disruptive Offender: Inmates with acute psychotic symptoms that interfere with functioning in a correctional setting
2. Malingering-Instrumental Offender: Inmates who report psychiatric symptoms or threaten self-harm in order to be transferred from the correctional setting to a clinical setting, which they view as more comfortable or more advantageous to their pending criminal matter
3. Depressed-Suicidal Offender: Inmates who experience acute depressive symptoms owing to a psychological stressor, such as the loss of an important personal relationship or receipt of a lengthy prison sentence
4. Anxious-Distressed Offender: Inmates who are new to the correctional setting and often express fear about being victimized by other inmates
5. Violent-Exploitative Offender: Inmates with histories of institutional violence who are placed in administrative segregation, and report psychiatric symptoms to be moved from segregation, or suffer psychological decompensation as a result of prolonged segregation
6. Self-Abusive-Disruptive Offender: Inmates who typically suffer from severe personality disorders and engage in unremitting patterns of self-injurious behaviors to cope with the stress of incarceration
7. Hostile-Protesting Offender: Inmates with identifiable grievances against the correctional institution or the court system, who engage in self-injurious behavior (i.e., hunger strikes) to draw attention to their complaints
8. Fixated-Delusional Offender: Inmates with long prison sentences who have become quietly psychotic but have been able to function within the correctional setting. They are typically close to the completion of their prison sentences, but their psychotic symptoms raise concerns about their safety in the community.

As with the inpatient civil patient population, clinical concerns in forensic hospitals regarding suicidality, patient aggression, and treatment adherence abound. In fact, an amplified sense of despair related to looming legal consequences is not an uncommon experience for forensic inpatients, which heightens the risk of self-injurious behaviors and physical aggression.[8] Accordingly, clinicians delivering care in forensic hospital settings must regularly consider patients' particular legal circumstances, including the seriousness of charges, trial status, and recent sentencing, in order to adjust treatment interventions in the face of shifting psychological stressors. Patient-centered therapeutic interventions involving a combination of medication management, individual and group psychotherapy, and recreational therapy may be helpful in reducing psychiatric symptoms related to such stressors.

Restoration of Competency to Stand Trial

An important function of inpatient forensic hospital programs is to provide psychiatric and psychological treatment to individuals who have been found to lack the mental capacity to proceed in their criminal matters. Whether it is for the trial itself, acceptance of a plea agreement, or sentencing matters, individuals whose mental functioning is so impaired by psychological disturbances that it interferes with their ability to competently participate in their legal matters will be deemed incompetent to proceed. *Dusky v. U.S.* (1960) delineates the constitutional requirement that defendants must possess the ability to consult with their attorneys and possess rational and factual understanding of their pending criminal proceedings.[9] Accordingly, defendants who are unable to demonstrate those mental capacities are likely to be found incompetent to proceed and will likely require treatment in a competency restoration program.

Estimates indicate that up to 60,000 defendants are referred for evaluation of competency to stand trial annually in the United States and that 30% of those individuals are found incompetent.[10] Interestingly, defense attorneys doubt the mental capacity of their clients in 8% to 15% of felony cases, but mental health assessments are sought in less than half of those cases.[11] Studies indicate that of the defendants referred for competency evaluations, 45% to 65% with psychotic disorders, 23% to 41% with mood or organic disorders, and 12.5% to 36% of persons with intellectual disability are found incompetent.[12] It is also estimated that, at any given time, individuals hospitalized for competency restoration account for approximately 4,000 inpatient psychiatric beds in the United States.[13]

Nationally, competency restoration inpatient treatment programs vary in their approach, but medication management, educational counseling, and multidisciplinary treatment teams are central components. Medication management focused on the alleviation of psychiatric symptoms impairing competency-related functioning is universally offered in these programs. According to a survey of 151 state psychiatric hospitals offering competency restoration treatment, most ranked medication as the most prevalent intervention, 88% used didactic or psychoeducational group interventions, and 41% provided competency restoration manuals to patients.[14]

The educational component of competency restoration programs can vary greatly. Some programs offer extensive curriculums with didactic lectures focused on relevant aspects of criminal legal matters. Some programs offer experiential approaches, such as mock trials in which patients participate. Media, such as movies and television shows with courtroom scenarios, have also been utilized to enhance educational interventions. Noffsinger proposed that a model competency restoration program would include the following: (1) an objective competency assessment upon admission; (2) individualized treatment programming; (3) multimodal, experiential competency restoration educational experiences; (4) an educational component; (5) an anxiety reduction component; (6) additional education interventions for defendants with low intelligence; (7) periodic reassessment of competency; (8) medication treatment; and, (9) treatment decision capacity assessments and involuntary treatment when appropriate.[15]

As noted in Noffsinger's model program, persons with low intellectual functioning often require additional educational services to accomplish the requisite degree of mental capacity to stand trial. Cognitive and adaptive functioning deficits associated with intellectual disability (previously mental retardation in DSM IV) can become major hurdles in demonstrating competency-related tasks. As mentioned previously, between 12.5% and 36% of defendants with intellectual disability have been found incompetent to stand trial.[16,17] Restoration programming must be equipped to assist this population in gaining competency-related skills that may never have been previously possessed. In that sense, a restoration program would assist the defendant with intellectual disability in acquiring competency skills instead of restoring those skills. Special care must be taken with this population that the parroting of legal concepts does not pass for authentic competency-related skills. Accordingly, thorough competency reassessments following educational interventions are recommended.

Another area of concern for individuals with intellectual disability undergoing competency restorative efforts is the probability of restorability. This concern is also present for incompetent defendants suffering from neurocognitive disorders, such as Alzheimer's disease, or treatment-resistant psychotic disorders. Although 75% to 90% of incompetent defendants are usually restored within 6 months of inpatient treatment,[18], Mossman identified two groups of incompetent defendants that have below average probability for restorability: (1) chronically psychotic individuals with histories of prolonged inpatient hospitalizations; and, (2) individuals with irremediable cognitive disorders.[13] For these groups and other defendants for whom competency restoration efforts have been unsuccessful, indefinite inpatient hospitalization for competency restoration is not possible.

In *Jackson v. Indiana* (1972), the U.S. Supreme Court ruled that indefinite hospitalization for the purpose of competency restoration is unconstitutional and prohibited.[19] Specifically, the Court ruled that incompetent defendants "cannot be held more than the reasonable period of time necessary to determine whether there is a substantial probability that he will attain competency in the foreseeable future. If it is determined that this is not the case, then the State must either institute the customary civil commitment proceeding that would be required to commit indefinitely any other citizen, or release the defendant." (Ref. 19, p. 738). Although most states have responded to *Jackson*'s mandate through statute or practice, an alarming variation among state jurisdictions' definition of "the reasonable period of time necessary to determine" restorability has been noted.[20]

One potential obstacle to successful competence restoration is the refusal of treatment by the incompetent defendant. The psychiatric symptoms that interfere with an incompetent defendant's recognition of his mental illness can also interfere with his accurate perception of his competency status and need for restoration services. Consequently, the incompetent defendant who views himself as competent may refuse medications prescribed for restoration purposes. When such situations arise, clinicians must consider whether the involuntary administration of medication is indicated. When there is a substantial risk of imminent danger present in such cases, the usual grounds for and procedures associated with involuntary treatment may be followed.

There are situations, however, in which the incompetent defendant refuses medications for competency restoration but does not pose a risk of danger. In general, defendants have a constitutionally protected right to refuse medications. However, the U.S. Supreme Court in *Sell v. U.S.* (2003) ruled that forced medications for the purpose of competency restoration in the absence of a dangerousness risk is constitutionally permitted "only if the treatment is medically appropriate, is substantially unlikely to have side effects that may undermine the fairness of the trial, and, taking account of less intrusive alternatives, is necessary significantly to further important governmental trial-related interests."[21] As with other situations involving refusal of psychiatric treatment, the initiation of procedures for medication over a patient's objection should be a matter of last resort. The effort to engage a resistant patient in treatment may be especially difficult in the context of looming legal concerns, but it is a necessary step that may also assist with fostering a therapeutic alliance.

Hospitalization of Post-Trial Defendants

Depending on the jurisdiction, defendants who are adjudicated GBMI or NGRI of their criminal charges may be remanded to a forensic inpatient hospital for further observation and treatment. In the case of a GBMI conviction, the defendant may be admitted to the forensic hospital for a period of time to ensure psychiatric stability before serving the remainder of the mandatory sentence in prison. In the case of an NGRI finding, the acquittee may be remanded to a forensic inpatient hospital for ongoing treatment until hospital clinicians and the presiding court agree that the acquittee no longer poses a dangerousness risk.

Treatment during those forensic hospitalizations focuses on psychiatric concerns that would be expected with typical inpatient psychiatric hospitalizations. Symptoms of mood, anxiety, and psychotic disorders are treated in a similar manner as in civil hospitals with a combination of medication management, individual psychotherapy, and group therapy. Suicidal behaviors and physical aggression are also major clinical concerns, given the elevated occurrence of these behaviors in correctional populations.[22,23]

Further, clinical treatment in inpatient forensic settings must address more than the psychiatric symptoms associated with a patient's particular diagnosis. Complex feelings of remorse, anger, hopelessness, and stress related to the reality of incarceration, isolation from family and friends, perceived interpersonal impact of the precipitating criminal act, and residual frustration with the legal process may complicate the patient's clinical presentation.[8,24,25] Psychotherapeutic interventions that allow preservation of patients' dignity while coping with the significant stressors related to their criminal justice involvement is critically important in these settings.

Ethical Considerations

Primum non nocere or first, do no harm, forms the basis of physicians' ethical obligation to their patients. In the inpatient forensic setting, there are situations that conflict with patients' interests, and accordingly, it is essential that treating psychiatrists inform their patients of these potential conflicts during the course of treatment. One area of conflict arises with questions of confidentiality. Since patients are typically court-ordered to forensic hospitals for legally related treatment objectives, such as competency restoration, there is often an expectation grounded in statutory law that reports regarding the treatment will be generated for the court. Although the customary doctor–patient confidentiality is limited in those situations, that does not absolve the psychiatrist from the duty to inform the patient of the confidentiality limitations or from the duty to avoid unauthorized disclosures.

In addition, it has been recommended that treating psychiatrists avoid conducting forensic evaluations of their patients. The host of problems related to attempts to commingle treatment provider and objective forensic evaluator roles has been well published.[26] Depending on the jurisdiction, it may be difficult to adhere to this recommendation in forensic hospitals when the referring court or the applicable statute requires treating clinicians to provide forensic evaluations to the court for their patients. If possible, arrangements should be made to have a hospital clinician who is not directly involved in the inpatient's treatment conduct the forensic evaluation. When such an arrangement is not possible, it is important to inform the patient of the treating psychiatrist's dual role in the same manner that issues of confidentiality are discussed.

Conclusion

Inpatient forensic psychiatry represents, perhaps, the purest representation of the intersection of psychiatry and the criminal justice system. The unique and formidable landscape of inpatient forensic psychiatry fully encompasses the numerous facets of the demands of psychiatry and the criminal justice system. Whether pretrial or post-trial, felony or misdemeanor, genuine or malingered symptomatology, treating clinicians and inpatient forensic evaluators must utilize a full array of clinical skills while remaining cognizant of the impending legal implications. The multidisciplinary approach often encountered in the inpatient forensic setting, involving medication management, psychological and neuropsychological testing, psychotherapy, and educational interventions, provides the specialized attention required by constitutionally derived rights owed to mentally ill persons entangled in the criminal justice system.

The role of the inpatient forensic psychiatrist requires the constant monitoring and balancing of varied clinical and legal objectives, which are always at play, but are sometimes inharmonious. A special challenge for the inpatient forensic psychiatrist is to establish and maintain therapeutic alliances with his or her patients, who may view hospitalization as an extension of an unfair and overreaching legal system. With the absence of legal authorities in the hospital setting, such as judges, attorneys, and police officers, it is the forensic psychiatrist who is usually perceived by patients as the only available authority figure with whom to address legal grievances. Accordingly, it behooves the inpatient forensic psychiatrist to have a firm understanding of the jurisdiction's legal process and to maintain a keen awareness of therapeutic boundaries that patients may find inconvenient.

References

1. Theobald HS. (1924). Places for care of lunatics. *The Law Relating to Lunacy, 1*, 184–189.
2. Renton AW. (1897). Chapters in the English law of lunacy: Reform in asylum administration. *Green Bag*, 9, 387–392.
3. Prosono M. (2003). History of forensic psychiatry. In R Rosner (Ed.), *Principles and practice of forensic psychiatry* (2nd ed., pp. 14–30). London: Arnold.
4. Gold LH. (2010). Rediscovering forensic psychiatry. In: RI Simon, LH Gold (Eds.), *Textbook of forensic psychiatry* (pp. 3–42). Washington, DC: American Psychiatric Publishing.
5. Lamb HR, & Weinberger LE. (2005). The shift of psychiatric inpatient care from hospitals to jails and prisons. *J Am Acad Psychiatry Law*, i(4), 529–534.s
6. Vitek v Jones, 445 U.S. 480 (1980).
7. DiCataldo F. (1999). A typology of patients admitted to a forensic psychiatric hospital from correctional settings. *J Am Acad Psychiatry Law, 27*(2), 259–271.
8. Hillbrand M, & Young JL. (2008). Instilling hope into forensic treatment: The antidote to despair and desperation. *J Am Acad Psychiatry Law, 36*(1), 90–94.
9. Dusky v United States, 362 U.S. 402 (1960).
10. Melton GB, Petrilla J, Poythress NG, & Slobogin C. (2007). *Psychological evaluations for the courts: A handbook for mental health professionals and lawyers* (3rd ed.). New York, Guilford Press.
11. Bonnie RJ, Poythress NG, Hoge SK, & Monahan J. (1996). Decision making in criminal defense: An empirical study of insanity pleas and the impact of doubted client competence. *J Crim Law Crim, 87*(1), 48–62.
12. Mossman D, Noffsinger SG, Ash P, et al. (2007). AAPL practice guideline for the forensic psychiatric evaluation of competence to stand trial. *J Am Acad Psychiatry Law, 35*(Suppl), S3–72.
13. Mossman D. (2007). Predicting restorability of incompetent criminal defendants. *J Am Acad Psychiatry Law, 35*(1), 34–43.
14. Pinals DA. (2005). Where two roads meet: Restoration of competence to stand trial from a clinical perspective. *N Engl J Crim Civil Confine, 31*, 81–108.
15. Noffsinger SG. (2001). Restoration to competency practice guidelines. *Int J Offender Ther, 45*(3), 356–362.
16. Reich J, & Wells J. (1985). Psychiatric diagnosis and competency to stand trial. *Comprehensive Psychiatry, 26*(5), 421–432.
17. Warren JI, Fitch WL, Dietz PE, & Rosenfeld BD. (19910). Criminal offense, psychiatric diagnosis, and psycholegal opinion: An analysis of 894 pretrial referrals. *Bull Am Acad Psychiatry Law, 19*(1), 63–69.
18. Morris DR, & DeYoung NJ. (2014). Long term competence restoration. *J Am Acad Psychiatry Law, 42*(1): 81–90.
19. Jackson v Indiana, 406 U.S. 715 (1972).
20. Rosinia N. (2012). How "Reasonable" has become unreasonable: A proposal for rewriting the lasting legacy of *Jackson v. Indiana*. *Wash U L Rev, 89*, 673–703.
21 *Sell v. U.S.*, 539 U.S. 166 (2003).
22. Hayes LM. (2005). Suicide prevention in correctional facilities. In: CL Scott, & JB Gerbasi (Eds.), *Handbook of correctional mental health* (pp. 69–88). Washington, DC: American Psychiatric Publishing.
23. Weinstein HC, Kim D, Mack AH, Malavade KE, & Saraiya AU. (2005). Prevalence and assessment of mental disorders in correctional settings. In CL Scott, JB Gerbasi (Eds.), *Handbook of correctional mental health* (pp. 43–68). Washington, DC: American Psychiatric Publishing.

24. Kapoor R. (2008). "Filled with desperation": Psychotherapy with an insanity acquittee. *J Am Acad Psychiatry Law, 36*(4), 563–566.
25. Papapietro DJ. (2008). Commentary: Psychotherapy in a forensic hospital. *J Am Acad Psychiatry Law, 36*(4), 567–571.
26. Strasburger LH, Gutheil TG, & Brodsky A. (1997). On wearing two hats: Role conflict in serving as both psychotherapist and expert witness. *Am J Psychiatry, 154*(4), 448–456.

16

Correctional Psychiatry

Its Influence on the Forensic Psychiatrist

Jeffrey L. Metzner, Kenneth L. Appelbaum, and Robert L. Trestman

Correctional psychiatry played an essential role in forensic psychiatry becoming formally recognized as a subspecialty of psychiatry by the American Board of Medical Specialties (ABMS) in 1992. As discussed in chapter Rappeport's Preface, the American Academy of Psychiatry and the Law (AAPL), which had its first annual meeting in November 1969, agreed to co-sponsor the American Board of Forensic Psychiatry (ABFP), along with the American Academy of Forensic Sciences and the Forensic Sciences Foundation, Inc., in 1976. The ABFP subsequently developed a board certification process that became the de facto subspecialty certification for forensic psychiatry. However, to achieve mainstream medical/psychiatry recognition as a subspecialty, AAPL and the American Psychiatric Association (APA) jointly initiated efforts to have forensic psychiatry formally recognized as a subspecialty of psychiatry by the ABMS. A requirement for subspecialty recognition by the ABMS included the existence of fellowship programs that had a unique and identified target population. The ABMS accepted the correctional population and the state hospital forensic population as meeting this requirement. The first American Board of Psychiatry and Neurology (ABPN) forensic psychiatry board examination was administered in 1994. The last step in this long process occurred in 1997 when the Accreditation Council on Graduate Medical Education (ACGME) first certified forensic psychiatry training programs in 1997.[1]

Historically, most forensic psychiatrists had little involvement as treatment providers in jails or prisons before the development of ACGME-approved fellowship programs, although they were frequently involved in forensic evaluation of pretrial detainees (e.g., competency to proceed and/or sanity assessments, presentence evaluations, and sex offender assessments). Forensic psychiatric evaluations of prison inmates included parole assessments of dangerousness risk and need for treatment if paroled. It was ironic that many forensic psychiatrists did not have experience providing clinical treatment in a jail or prison because they commonly provided opinions relevant to incarceration. For example, presentence psychiatric evaluations often addressed treatment recommendations with little awareness by the forensic evaluator whether the prison system had the recommended services.

Psychiatrists did not work in jails or prisons as treatment providers for many reasons. Such reasons included the rural location of many facilities, the nontherapeutic nature and institutional culture of such settings, facility inadequacies (e.g., lack of basic office and programming space), low pay, and inadequate mental health staffing. There was also the allure of academic or private practice settings. Many of these deficient conditions began to change in the mid-to-late 1980s because of successful class action litigation that included court orders and consent decrees specifically designed to remedy these issues.[2] Further, the growing dominance of managed care made private practice less attractive for many psychiatrists. When these factors were combined with the continued downsizing of state hospital systems and an increasing population of inmates with serious mental illnesses, correctional facilities became more common places of employment for psychiatrists. This chapter describes the evolving role of the correctional psychiatrist in forensic psychiatry.

Impacting the Correctional Health Care System

The evolution of correctional psychiatry has not occurred in a vacuum. Many other initiatives have evolved simultaneously. The American Medical Association (AMA) was instrumental in the early years of this endeavor. The AMA exerted significant organization efforts during the 1970s to provide technical assistance to jails regarding correctional health care systems through its Project on Jail Health Care.[3] The National Commission on Correctional Health Care (NCCHC) was established in 1983 by the AMA and other organizations (including the AAPL and the APA) concerned with ensuring adequate health care to inmates. The NCCHC eventually developed standards for health care services in jails and prisons. It also developed an accreditation process that parallels, although less vigorously, the work of the Joint Commission with hospitals and community health care systems. During the first two decades of its existence, the NCCHC created medical and psychiatric standards currently published as separate documents for jails and prisons.[4,5] Beginning in 2008, the NCCHC additionally published separate standards for mental health services in correctional facilitiess[6]; the broader health care standards continue to address mental health care services as well. Forensic psychiatrists have significantly influenced the NCCHC, which has included three psychiatrists (Henry Weinstein, M.D., Charles Meyer, Jr., M.D. and Joseph Penn, M.D.) each serving a term as chair of the Board of Directors of the NCCHC and actively participating in development of policies and health care standards.

Building on the structure of the NCCHC standards for health care services, a Task Force of the APA published a report entitled "Psychiatric Services in Jails and Prisons," which provided guidelines for such services in these facilities.[7] The APA's Council on Psychiatry and Law has also produced a resource document on the use of restraints and seclusion in correctional facilities.[8] Both of these documents have aided correctional psychiatrists in effectively advocating for adequate psychiatric services by referencing nationally recognized guidelines pertinent to staffing resources and policies and procedures.

Class-action litigation and intervention by the Civil Rights Division of the US Department of Justice through the Civil Rights of Institutionalized Persons Act of 1980[9] have also provided important opportunities for the forensic psychiatrist to shape the correctional mental health system.[10] Forensic psychiatric evaluations of the adequacy of a correctional mental health system, which should be based on existing national guidelines/standards, have served central roles in these litigations. At times, forensic psychiatrists address evolving areas of practice that lack clearly defined standards (e.g., placement and/or treatment of prisoners with serious mental illnesses in locked-down settings such as administrative segregation). At other times, they provide valuable consultation when community standards such as confidentiality during interviews and sharing of protected health information are challenged or compromised in practice. In such circumstances, the forensic psychiatrist can help define an appropriate standard of care based on extrapolation from acceptable community practices. For example, community standards do not promote locking a person with a serious mental illness in a room for 23 hours per day for weeks to years. The task of the correctional psychiatrist under such circumstances is to work with custody staff to implement an adequate psychosocial rehabilitation model in a safe manner for both prisoners and staff.[11]

Forensic psychiatrists have also played an active role in monitoring court orders and/or consent decrees on mental health services in jails and prisons. This monitoring generally helps correctional mental health care systems to develop resources (e.g., obtaining necessary staffing allocations and physical plant resources), and provides useful technical assistance.

Influencing the Correctional System

In the early 1980s, mental health and health care staffs often described themselves as "guests in the House of Corrections." This perception had a substantial limiting effect on attempts to improve correctional health care. However, by the early 1990s it was clear that health care was an essential component of the correctional system and not just an afterthought. Administrative reorganization at the institutional and central office level reflected this recognition (e.g., creation of an Associate Warden for Health Care position at individual prisons and a systemwide central office director of health care and mental health care). Health care staff, including psychiatrists, were now included in many institutional and central office administrative meetings that provided them with opportunities to use their expertise to positively affect the correctional system.

Similar to a psychiatric liaison model (in contrast to a psychiatric consultation model), forensic psychiatrists were now able to interact with custody staff to develop policies and procedures on inmate management that went beyond health care per se. This has been particularly fruitful for inmates with serious mental illnesses in locked-down settings (e.g., administrative segregation and disciplinary segregation housing units). Such inmates are often overrepresented in these settings for reasons that include inadequate mental health services. They suffer harm when lockdown and isolation causes their psychiatric conditions either to deteriorate or not improve. An evolving standard of care in response to this problem includes mental health input into the disciplinary process concerning mitigating circumstances when inmates with serious mental illnesses commit disciplinary infractions.[12,13] Leadership by forensic psychiatrists in advocating for exclusion of inmates with serious mental illnesses from such environments, or drastically changing the conditions of confinement, has resulted in significant benefits. Benefits of psychiatric leadership include improved access to adequate treatment for inmates, a safer working environment for staff, and fewer management issues for administration because of the enhanced availability of treatment. Position statements developed by forensic psychiatrists within the APA during 2012 and the Society for Correctional Physicians during 2013 have facilitated such successful advocacy.[14,15]

The psychiatrist also should have active involvement in formal and informal training of nonmental health and custody staff on identification and referral of prisoners with mental illness and suicide prevention. These activities provide the psychiatrist with another opportunity to make the correctional environment less punitive and more therapeutic.

Educational Opportunities

Many forensic psychiatry fellowship programs have obtained funding through partnerships with local jails and/or state departments of corrections. The educational opportunities for the forensic fellow include learning more about psychiatric treatment, working with a multidisciplinary team (e.g., correctional officers, other mental health and health care professionals, probation and parole officers), learning a system's approach to mental health treatment, doing forensic examinations, and training staff about mental health issues.

Treatment opportunities include the ability to follow a patient long-term, to work with patients who have challenging personality disorders or paraphilias, and to help custody staff implement cognitive-behavioral-based management plans for inmates with significant disruptive behaviors. In addition, many inmates have long-standing substance use disorders that need to be addressed. Much can be learned from them, especially after establishing a therapeutic alliance. Working with persons under supervision in the criminal justice system provides the forensic fellow ample opportunity to become clinically knowledgeable about dangerousness and suicide risk assessment instruments.

Working effectively with a multidisciplinary team often requires the forensic fellow to learn new skills to overcome "turf" barriers and to function in correctional cultures that otherwise may encourage punitive responses and disrespectful environments. Forensic fellows need to understand services from a correctional mental health system perspective. Challenges they will face may include being told just what to do (e.g., which patients to see—and frequently in settings that do not allow for adequate sound privacy), often by a scheduling clerk, regardless of the circumstances (e.g., not enough time allotted for such services). Lack of a systems perspective can result in clinical problems such as compromised assessments, lack of continuity of care, and untimely follow-up. Close supervision is needed by the forensic fellowship program director to ensure that the forensic fellow is not put into situations that reinforce bad clinical practices. This entire area of clinical ethics, boundary violations, and human rights is one encountered head-on in correctional settings. It is an evolving area and one that may lead to extraordinary growth in clinical and administrative skills. Appropriately designed and implemented training programs incorporate supportive supervision and guidance for the fellow in this process.

Dual agency issues are an example of potential ethical problems for the correctional psychiatrist who provides direct patient care and is requested to perform various forensic (e.g., parole board evaluations) or quasi-forensic assessments (e.g., psychiatric assessments specific to alleged disciplinary infractions). Such problems can be minimized by the correctional psychiatrist not doing a forensic examination on inmates under his/her clinical care. Similar to psychiatrists practicing in a small town, this may not always be possible if there is only one psychiatrist working at the correctional facility. In such circumstances, the informed consent process provided to the inmate before initiating treatment should include this potential limit of confidentiality as well as others unique to a correctional system, such as learning about a plan for an impending facility riot.

Physical plant limitations often result in the correctional psychiatrist being asked or told to evaluate and/or treat inmates in a setting that does not allow for adequate sound privacy for confidentiality purposes. The proper chain of command should be followed to remedy such circumstances, which invariably will be successful if the psychiatrist is clear and persistent in educating appropriate custody staff concerning this need.

Participation in quality improvement (QI) processes helps the forensic fellow learn a system's approach to correctional mental health care. Many psychiatric residents lack adequate exposure to QI processes and do not directly participate in QI studies. Active participation in QI studies helps forensic fellows improve their clinical practices and often serves as a precipitant for clinical research projects.

Forensic fellows have many opportunities to do forensic examinations in jails and prisons. Depending on the jurisdiction, jail-based psychiatrists may perform forensic examinations on pretrial detainees. These evaluations may include competency to proceed, legal sanity, presentencing assessments for diagnosis and treatment recommendations, and civil commitment. Forensic evaluations for prison inmates may be requested for parole board purposes, mitigation assessments for disciplinary hearings about alleged rule infractions, and hearings on transfer to a psychiatric inpatient unit and sex offender commitments.

The Next Generation of Correctional Psychiatrists

There are many current benefits for forensic psychiatrists who work in correctional settings. Those who practice as experts at deposition or trial can meet requirements for set amounts of time spent in the practice of clinical psychiatry by delivering direct care in a jail or prison. Correctional psychiatry also provides a substantial contribution toward ABPN-required Maintenance of Certification. Further, the practice environment within many correctional systems is like a staff-model health maintenance organization, requires no coding or billing, no preauthorizations from insurers, and offers a stable and reasonable compensation package.

Looking to the future of health care in the United States, population medicine, integrated and coordinated care, and responsible use of limited resources are becoming ever more important. Practicing in many correctional settings already provides a learning environment to hone the practices and skills needed to achieve excellence in that evolving community system. Given current political and judicial limitations and culture, the incarceration rate for persons with serious mental illness will likely remain high. Future correctional psychiatrists will require the skills to provide care to disadvantaged and ill patients, who are generally very appreciative of that care. They also must develop the skills for collaborative, interdisciplinary practice. Such skills will benefit their patients, most of whom will return to their communities, and enhance the ability of forensic psychiatrists to have a full scope of practice with a substantial evidence basis.

Conclusion

Correctional psychiatry is an evolving area ideally suited to forensic psychiatrists. A forensic psychiatry fellowship is not a requirement for practice within jails or prisons, but it will enhance the skills, knowledge, and perspective needed for this work. From educational experiences, to the clinical satisfaction of working with diverse and compromised patients, to the population health perspectives, to the administrative and leadership opportunities, correctional psychiatry is an excellent arena within which forensic psychiatrists may work and grow,

References

1. American Academy of Psychiatry and the Law. Fellowship Programs in Forensic Psychiatry. Available at http://www.aapl.org/fellow.php Accessed January 4, 2014.
2. Metzner JL. (2002a). Class action litigation in correctional psychiatry. *J Am Acad Psychiatry Law, 30*, 19–29.
3. King, LN. (2006) Doctors, patients, in the history of correctional medicine. In: M. Puisis (Ed.), *Clinical Practice in Correctional Medicine* (2nd ed., pp. 3–11). Philadelphia: Mosby Elsevier.
4. National Commissioner on Correctional Healthcare. (2008a). *Standards for health services in jails*. Chicago: National Commission on Correctional Health Care.
5. National Commissioner on Correctional Healthcare. (2008b). *Standards for health services in prisons*. Chicago: National Commission on Correctional Health Care.
6. National Commissioner on Correctional Healthcare. (2008c). *Standards for mental health services in correctional facilities*. Chicago: National Commission on Correctional Health Care.
7. American Psychiatric Association. (2000). *Psychiatric services in jails and prisons: A task force report of the American Psychiatric Association*. Washington DC: American Psychiatric Association.
8. Metzner JL, Tardiff K, Lion J, et al. (2007). Resource document on the use of restraint and seclusion in correctional health care. *J Am Acad Psychiatry Law, 35*, 417–425.
9. Department of Justice. Rights of persons confined to jails and prisons. Available at http://www.justice.gov/crt/about/spl/corrections.php Accessed 2 January 2014.

10. Metzner JL (2009). Monitoring a correctional mental health care system: The role of the mental health expert. *Behav Sci Law, 27,* 727–741.
11. Metzner JL, & Dvoskin JA. (2006). An overview of correctional psychiatry. *Psychiatr Clinics N Am, 29,* 761–772.
12. Krelstein MS. (2002). The role of mental health in the inmate disciplinary process a national survey. *J Am Acad Psychiatry Law, 30,* 488–496.
13. Metzner JL. (2002b). Commentary: The role of mental health in the disciplinary process. *J Amer Acad Psychiatry Law, 30,* 497–499.
14. American Psychological Association. Fellowship Programs in Forensic Psychiatry. Available at http://www.psychiatry.org/advocacy--newsroom/position-statements Accessed 4 January 2014.
15. Society for Correctional Physicians. Fellowship Programs in Forensic Psychiatry. Available at http://societyofcorrectionalphysicians.org/resources/position-statements Accessed 4 January 2014.

17

Managing Malpractice Risks During Psychopharmacologic Treatment

Joseph N. DiGiacomo and Robert L. Sadoff

The number of psychiatric malpractice cases has increased dramatically over the past several decades. Patients have become increasingly litigious and lawyers more creative in finding reasons to blame psychiatrists for unsuccessful treatment.

Managed care has also significantly affected the rise in psychiatric malpractice litigation. Third-party payers have the power to limit the quality of psychiatric care. Such limitations often challenge the treating psychiatrist's recommended course of treatment; consequently, when substandard care is authorized, the risk of a malpractice claim rises.

Consider the increasing variety of psychotropic agents and standards of care that must be followed when medication is prescribed. A prudent practitioner must be aware of the side effects of each medication, the effects of various combinations of such medications, and the contraindications for the use of the various medications in specific situations. Failure to follow proven standards and guidelines can harm a patient and ultimately lead to a malpractice action.

One of the fastest growing types of malpractice litigation concerns the utilization of various medications for different psychiatric conditions. This chapter presents and examines case studies from the authors' forensic experience, highlighting standards of care in the use of psychiatric medications and conflicts at the interface of psychiatry with other specialties over the utilization of psychiatric medications in combination with other types of medication.

Standards of Care

When considering standards of care with regard to malpractice risks, the practitioner should be aware of the four necessary elements for a successful malpractice lawsuit. These four conditions are often referred to as *the four D's*: duty, dereliction, deviation, and damage. The practitioner has a duty to the patient. If the psychiatrist is derelict in his or her duty to the patient and that deviation from the standard of care is a direct cause of damage to the patient, the necessary elements for a malpractice suit are in place. A malpractice finding cannot rely merely upon a deviation from the standard of care; the deviation must be the proximate cause of damage to the patient for a successful malpractice claim to be established.[1] Thus, even if the psychiatrist made an error in prescribing medication to the patient, but that error was harmless to the patient, no malpractice has occurred. The practitioner is not expected to have acted in an ideal fashion with respect to the use of medication, but any action must be deemed reasonable. Similarly, variations in the use of psychotropic and other medications will be viewed as acceptable as long as their use was reasonable and did not harm the patient. Consequently, the psychiatrist should always use the concept of risk/benefit ratio analysis when selecting psychotropic medications for a patient. The psychiatrist should also discuss the effects and side effects of such medications and combinations of medications with the patient.

The use of psychopharmacological agents to treat mental and emotional illnesses has grown dramatically over the past several decades. Training in psychiatry currently devotes a significant amount of time to teaching psychopharmacology, brain physiology, and organic mental conditions. Psychotropic medications have been developed for a number of different psychiatric conditions, including: schizophrenia, depression, bipolar disorder, anxiety disorders. and obsessive/compulsive disorders. Various classifications of antidepressants and neuroleptics have given the treating psychiatrist a number of options from which to choose both individual medications and various combinations of medications. Combinations of various medications may prove dangerous to the patients in that they may be incompatible or cause very serious and harmful side effects (e.g., Demerol and MAOIs cannot be administered concurrently). There are a rising number of specialists in the field of psychopharmacology research, especially those conducting basic research on the effects and side effects of new medications. The field has grown so rapidly and with such complexity that psychiatrists often need to consult a guidebook on psychopharmacologic agents or consult with a specialist in psychopharmacology.

Side effects of various medications may be classified as frequent, infrequent, or rare. In the early days of using psychopharmacologic agents, an unwritten rule was to advise patients of serious side effects if the side effect had an incidence of 1% or greater, or to advise the patient that the side effect is minimally harmful if the incidence of that side effect were 5% or greater. Some psychiatrists chose not to divulge various side effects that might deter the patient from taking the medication. These practitioners claim that this was a "therapeutic privilege"; if they were to tell the patient of the serious side effect, the patient might be frightened to such a degree that recommended medication would not be taken.

As patients acquired more rights under our legal system, including the right to adequate treatment and the right to refuse treatment (especially treatment involving psychotropic medication that may lead to harmful side effects), psychiatrists have become willing to discuss all potential negative effects of the medication of patients and to allow patients to make their own decisions about whether to take the medication. This openness has come to be standard in the prescribing of medication for the seriously mentally ill, and allows the patient some feeling of control over the treatment. The previously paternalistic approach of the psychiatrist who tells the patient, "I am your doctor and you are the patient—I know best, and you'll do what I say," is no longer acceptable, let alone practical. Most patients want to know about their illness and medications in order to take greater responsibility for their treatment. As a result, compliance rates are much higher for those patients who are given adequate explanation of their illness and the medications that are prescribed.

One of the problems that arises with such explanations concerns the way in which psychiatric patients are treated in outpatient practice. Most patients under managed care will see a nonpsychiatrist for psychotherapy on a regular basis, and see the psychiatrist for "medication management" only briefly and infrequently. In many cases, the psychiatrist does not have sufficient time to develop the type of psychotherapeutic relationship that allows in-depth explanation of the effects and side effects of psychotropic medication. Whatever the psychiatrist's role within the managed care treatment program, the psychiatrist must take adequate time, at least initially, to explain the effects and side effects of a given medication and be available to the patient for a telephone consultation in the event negative responses result from the medication.

Psychiatrists may have difficulty in treating patients, not only in outpatient settings under managed care conditions, but also when a patient is hospitalized. For inpatients, psychiatrists must be aware of frequent, infrequent, and rare side effects of various medications. They must be extremely vigilant in their suspicion of unusual conditions in patients receiving medication. An early problem for psychiatrists using psychotropic medications was the unfamiliarity with unusual effects and the acceptance that bizarre symptoms were often related more to the psychiatric illness than to the medication used to treat that illness.

The following areas must be considered in which a psychiatrist may encounter difficulty when utilizing psychotropic medications:

- Medication side effects: infrequent and rare side effect
- Interface conflicts for psychiatrist with other specialties over the utilization of psychiatric medications in combination with medication for physical conditions
  - Problems with combinations of psychotropic medications
- Explaining therapeutic effects and side effects of various medications to the patient and to family members when appropriate
- Obtaining informed consent for use of various medications

Case Example of an Infrequent Side Effect

A psychiatrist is sued for malpractice and damages by a 34-year-old for untreated trazodone (Desyrel) induced priapism of 26 hours duration.

Admitted to a rehabilitation center with a diagnosis of dysthymia, recurrent major depression, and long-standing opioid dependence, he had been taking seven bags of heroin daily and abusing alcohol for 3 years. He failed several previous rehabilitation efforts. His psychiatrist prescribed fluoxetine (Prozac), 20 mg per day, and trazodone (Desyrel), 100 mg at night for sleep. Several days later, trazodone was increased to 200 mg. The patient complained his penis was swollen and painful to the ward nurse, 2 days later. The night dose of trazodone was withheld and diphenhydramine (Benadryl), 50 mg was given. The next day the psychiatrist discontinued trazodone because he thought the priapism was related to trazodone. He recommended ice packs, pain relievers, and Vistaril for insomnia.

Four hours later, the patient was still complaining of pain in the penis, and doclofenac (Voltaren) and ibuprofen (Motrin) were prescribed. His chart indicated *"Erection due to the side effect of Desyrel."* Eight hours later, the patient still complained of scrotal and penile pain. The family practitioner was called bu no further orders were received. Twelve to 16 hours later, his chart documented continuing complaints of genital pain and swelling, unrelieved by naproxen (Naprosyn). Twenty-four hours after the first complaint, he still had pain in the genital area and difficulty in initiating urination. He was agitated, with difficulty in walking and unable to lie down. He refused to take any more medications.

He was seen 26 hours after the original complaint of penile pain in a community hospital emergency room. Priapism secondary to trazodone was diagnosed. He was given medication to reduce the erection. He was unresponsive to further irrigations, ultimately requiring both a Winters and corpora spongiosum to cavernosum shunt.

Months later he was unable to achieve a satisfactory erection even with injectable medication. A detailed evaluation by a urologist noted a high inflow of blood to the penis with venous leaks on duplex doppler ultrasound, and indicated the impotence had a "strong organic" component. The impotence did not respond to surgical corrective procedures.

The patient sued the rehabilitation center and doctors for malpractice for failure to initiate definitive therapy within a reasonable time period for trazodone-induced priapism. The staff was aware of the association of priapism with trazodone, but 26 hours elapsed before any definitive intervention was attempted.

Priapism is now recognized as a an infrequent, but not rare, side effect of trazodone.[2–4] The treating psychiatrist should advise the patient that priapism could be a possible side effect, and should be anticipated and treated as soon as it is noted. Rapid and efficient treatment of this condition is necessary to avoid long-term damage to the patient. Excessive delay, over 4 hours, in providing effective treatment for this condition may be grounds for a successful malpractice suit for negligent practice. The issue of informed consent and knowledge by the treating psychiatrist of the risks in using various medications in particular patients must be assessed; and if the side effect is noted, it must be treated forthwith.

Case Example of a Rare Drug Side Effect

A psychiatrist is sued for malpractice and damages by a patient who developed a serum sickness syndrome secondary to fluoxetine.

A 48-year-old woman sought treatment because of a 30-year history of dysphoria. The psychiatrist elicited symptoms sufficient to meet the diagnostic and statistical manual of mental disorders criteria for major depression. The patient was not suicidal. The psychiatrist prescribed fluoxetine, 20 mg every other day to be followed by a 20 mg daily dose after two weeks. He discussed the side effects of fluoxetine, ordered baseline labs, and saw the patient for three sessions on a bimonthly schedule.

The patient canceled her fourth appointment, but refilled her prescription for Prozac and was seen 2 weeks later. She described a lifting of the depression and an absence of side effects. A new prescription for fluoxetine was written at this visit and the patient was to report again in 2 weeks. She canceled her subsequent appointment because she was going to be out of town. After talking to the patient on the telephone, the psychiatrist determined that she was not depressed and presented with no adverse side effects to fluoxetine. The patient refilled the prescription for fluoxetine three more times. She did not contact her psychiatrist again. Six weeks later, the patient's husband notified the psychiatrist that his wife was in the hospital.

The patient had developed a rash with nausea, joint pain, and fever approximately 2 months after starting the fluoxetine. A diagnosis of serum sickness-like syndrome was made. She was treated with prednisone, diphenhydramine, and an antiemetic and discharged 2 days later. She was seen in another emergency room 4 days after discharge with blotches without edema or urticaria. She was given prednisone, 120 mg per day which was tapered and discontinued in a week. Approximately 2 weeks after the original hospitalization, the patient became confused with increasing agitation and "hysterical behavior" and admitted to a psychiatric facility. A prednisone-induced mania was diagnosed. After a brief hospitalization, both the serum sickness and mania cleared. The psychiatrist was sued for the serum sickness-like syndrome resulting from fluoxetine use. Counsel for the psychiatrist argued that the diagnosis of fluoxetine-induced serum sickness was presumptive, as the patient had been on other medications more frequently associated with serum sickness (i.e., antibiotics and nonsteroidal anti-inflammatory agents [NSAIDs]). The case was settled for "nuisance value."

Rare drug side effects, demonstrated in this patient, are of the type that cannot be anticipated by the treating psychiatrist. Because the incidence of serum sickness is rare with the use of fluoxetine, it is unlikely that psychiatrists would mention it as a potential side effect. It is also unlikely that most psychiatrists would be aware that serum sickness could develop from the use of fluoxetine (unless the psychiatrist was well acquainted with the literature or had previous experience with serum sickness as a side effect of fluoxetine). However rare, serum sickness-like syndrome is a side effect that has been reported and should be considered in the event such symptoms arise in the patient receiving fluoxetine.[5–8]

Malpractice Issues Involving Conflicts at the Interface of Psychiatry with Other Specialties

A Malpractice Action for Failing to Monitor Renal Function in a Patient on Lithium Therapy

A patient was treated by a psychiatrist with lithium carbonate for manic depressive illness for 25 years. Clinically stable and she maintained a lithium level in the therapeutic range of 0.8–1.0 mEq/L. Her father died in a state hospital with a manic depressive illness. Her general practitioner (GP) was treating her for migraine type headaches and assumed responsibility for the management of her lithium therapy. He detected a thyroid enlargement on physical examination, which was managed by an endocrinologist. The last renal studies were done about 1 year before and the blood urea nitrogen (BUN) was reported as normal. (The reading was 22 mg/dL with a lab normal range of 6–20.)

The patient was hospitalized 4 months later and routine preoperative lab studies indicated a BUN of 33 mg/dL and a creatinine of 2.8 mg/dL. The GP's records did not document the finding. Six months later, the doctor noted she was depressed, "not thinking logically, confused, refused to see a psychiatrist." She finally agreed to see a psychiatrist, who did an evaluation and sent a letter to her GP. The psychiatrist increased the dose of lithium to get the blood level in the therapeutic range. He sent an order slip for lithium levels and renal function tests to the GP whose lab did the testing. The lithium level was 1.7 mEq/L and the lithium dose was reduced. The renal function tests were not reported. Approximately 4 months later the GP did his own routine labs in the yearly evaluation and informed the psychiatrist that the BUN was in the range of 45–60 mg/dL with a creatinine of 5–5.4 mg/dL. A nephrologist concluded the patient developed renal failure secondary to "chronic tubulointerstitial nephropathy." She refused to stop lithium but eventually agreed to start on carbamazepine.

The psychiatrist and family practitioner were sued for failure to monitor renal studies, which resulted in renal failure. The psychiatrist was convinced the GP was responsible for monitoring renal and thyroid function. The GP averred the psychiatrist did not ask him to monitor the renal function. In their depositions, the doctors agreed they were communicating with each other but the issue of monitoring the creatinine and BUN was never discussed.

The litigation was further complicated because the etiology of the renal failure was unclear. The patient had been abusing analgesics. She also had Sjögren's syndrome, which can produce renal failure.[9,10] A traumatic etiology was suspected because the abrupt rise in the BUN and creatinine occurred after a severe automobile accident. The discussion focused on whether the psychiatrist should be dropped from the case because the family practitioner was responsible for the physical workup and evaluating renal function.

This case involves the precept of the duty to monitor and reflects the complexities of assigning liability to a psychiatrist when other physicians and/or hospital are involved. The issue of communication between and among doctors and hospital personnel is extremely important. The psychiatrist must avoid lapses in ordering the necessary labs for renal and thyroid results when prescribing lithium therapy. An article, "I wish I had seen this test result earlier!" discussed "test result management." In this study, the faculty was compared with house staff on test result tracking. The faculty and house staff did well keeping records of the test ordered and reviewing all incoming test results, but poorly with a system to detect if patients had missed their test. Psychiatrists cannot use the excuse that they never received the results from the labs they ordered. A test result management or tracking system can be an invaluable tool when monitoring lithium therapy.[11,12]

In addition, communication failure between the psychiatrist and the GP is a plaintiff lawyer's dream. The attorney will focus on the interaction between the professionals involved and attempt to divide loyalties. The plaintiff's attorney doesn't care which physician the jury finds at fault, as long as one of them is held responsible. Thus, the combination of a result tracking system and a clear assignment of tasks can prevent this type of error.[13,14]

A Malpractice Action Involving a Psychiatrist and an Addictionologist

A 45-year-old woman was evaluated by a psychiatrist because of numbness in her left arm, episodic spells of sweating, difficult breathing, and numbness on the top of her head. The symptoms "vanished" on 3 mg per day of alprazolam (Xanax). She attributed her symptoms to an automobile accident. Post-traumatic stress disorder was diagnosed, with phobia to crossing streets or riding in a motor vehicle. However, there was a history of major depression 7 years before. There was no history of drug or alcohol abuse, but her father, who worked in construction and had never missed a day of work, drank a great deal. Alprazolam relieved her symptoms, but she was unhappy being addicted to and dependent on pills.

The psychiatrist, attempting periodically to reduce the alprazolam, prescribed an antidepressant, psychotherapy, and behavioral therapy for the phobia. Stressful events, including ongoing litigation over the automobile accident, necessitated remaining on medication. It was noted she had an excellent response to the alprazolam on many occasions. Following the resolution of the auto accident litigation, she underwent talk therapy with a psychologist who also diagnosed panic disorder with agoraphobia. She had not taken the antidepressant but remained on alprazolam.

She read a newspaper article indicating alprazolam was addictive. She contacted the reporter, who reported her story. She claimed that her psychiatrist had addicted her to alprazolam. She went to a family practitioner, a self professed addictionologist, who specialized in detoxification. After a brief history and no consult with the treating psychologist, the addictionologist noted, "substance abuse, admitted for detoxification." Alprazolam was discontinued abruptly and the patient developed a full-blown panic/anxiety syndrome and was unable to walk. During the 10-day detoxification, a psychiatric consultant to the detoxification center interviewed the patient and diagnosed general anxiety disorder and conversion reaction with a dependent personality. He recommended the use of anxiolytics. He saw her after discharge but she did heed any of his recommendations.

The patient sued the psychiatrist for "addicting me to Xanax." Her expert was the addictionologist, who contended that alprazolam is addictive. He opined she should not have been put on alprazolam because her father was an alcoholic and alcoholism was in her genes. The patient's records indicate episodes of panic attacks 13 years ago, which subsided on a combination of amitriptyline and perphenazine (Triavil). The addictionologist testified that he was unfamiliar with the pharmacokinetics and pharmacology of alprazolam, other than that it was reported to be addictive. After several years of litigation, the judge sided with the defense just prior to the trial.

With respect to cases involving habituation, addiction, or dependency on drugs or medications (prescribed or illegal), the psychiatrist must consider all factors involving the patient when prescribing psychotropic medication. This case is important because it underscores the difference in attitude and approach toward medication use, which often exists between psychiatrists and nonpsychiatric physicians, especially those specializing in addiction medicine. The psychiatrist is expected to be aware of the total condition of the patient, including the issues of dependency, addiction, or habituation for prescription medications and illegal drugs. The physician specializing in addiction medicine may be limited in his or her approach when he or she does not consider the total needs of a patient. The use of anxiolytics, especially benzodiazepines, in those who have a history of drug dependence or a family history of addiction, may be appropriate if used cautiously and monitored regularly. Simply because a person has a history of drug dependence or family history of addiction or alcoholism, does not necessarily preclude the use of benzodiazepines for the treatment of anxiety.

Case Example of a Psychiatrist Failing to Diagnose a Medication Complication

A psychiatrist was sued for malpractice for failing to diagnose and attend to a medical complication stemming from the use of psychiatric medications.

An 83 year-old woman was admitted to a psychiatric hospital because of threatening, acting-out, belligerent behavior, sleep disturbance and visual hallucinations. She was restless, agitated and unable to remain seated. She refused to continue the psychiatric interview. Her affect was labile with outbursts of yelling and screaming. She was "oriented times two" and "memory was fair."

She was addicted to diazepam (Valium) and a barbiturate for many years. She incurred a fracture of L4 about 20 years before the current admission. The fracture was felt to be related to an unstable gait secondary to her medications. She had a history of congestive heart failure and pulmonary edema associated with agitation and belligerent behavior. She also had thyroid problems, glaucoma, coronary artery disease, and diabetes.

The patient was detoxified, and started on an antidepressant and a behavior modification program. She refused psychological testing, a CAT scan, and an echocardiogram. During her hospitalization, she complained about pain in her back and legs. The yelling and complaining continued for 3 days. The psychiatrist evaluated her daily and thought the behavior could be functional but wanted to rule out any organic cause. The on-call medical physician thought of "the unlikely possibility of a hip fracture" and recommended an x-ray of the hip. An internist came by the following day and did not feel an x-ray was indicated because the history of back complaints was of longstanding and the patient was unwilling to subject herself to tests. The following day an x-ray revealed a hip fracture. As the primary treating doctor in a psychiatric hospital, responsible for carrying out the diagnostic and treatment recommendations, the psychiatrist was sued but later dropped from the litigation before trial.

The psychiatrist attending in a psychiatric hospital and nonpsychiatric physicians were sued because of medical complications that were not attended to by either physician. The psychiatrist has the responsibility of caring for the medical needs of the patient. His role is to coordinate the total treatment for the patient by proper referrals and consultations to other specialities. It is important for the doctor to establish a team approach to treatment whereby the decision-making process is shared. It is also an example of a psychiatrist giving in to the demands or refusals of a patient. There are times when the psychiatrist must insist on various tests or treatment modalities that are essential to the proper management and treatment of the patient. A number of lawsuits have occurred in which the claim was made by the plaintiff that the doctor abrogated his or her responsibility by allowing the patient to make an inappropriate and incompetent decision or by allowing a layperson, such as a parent or spouse, to make the decision. The outcome depends upon the facts of the case. In some cases, the psychiatrist will be seen to have negligently relinquished his or her decision-making role in favor of the patient's demands. In other cases, such relinquishment will be seen as appropriate because a decision was not critical to the health of the patient. In yet other cases, the psychiatrist will appear to have done all that was reasonable to provide treatment for the patient who then refused care recommended.

The courts have allowed that psychiatrists need not take control over their patients in order to effectively treat them. At the same time, the courts have maintained that the psychiatrist must do what is reasonable to provide treatment to the patient; however, in the absence of an emergency or imminent threat of harm, the patient may refuse the treatment offered by the psychiatrist if the patient is deemed competent to refuse. In this case, because the 83-year-old woman had a prior history of a spinal fracture, the consideration that she experienced the fractured hip 20 years later was not unreasonable.

As the primary physician in the psychiatric hospital, the psychiatrist had a clear duty to follow through with the medical recommendations to obtain an x-ray. Though the patient refused, the psychiatrist should have considered the risks and benefits of the testing. The psychiatrist should not have passively allowed the patient to make the decision, especially because the decision was not in the patient's best interest. The psychiatrist might have invoked the help of a family member or petitioned the court to declare the patient incompetent and then proceeded with the testing or treatment.

Case Example of Medical Responsibility in a Managed Care Facility

A 40 year-old woman was in outpatient therapy with a psychologist for marital problems. She became increasingly anxious and depressed, which was attributed to the therapy exploring the dynamics of her marriage. The psychologist, participating in a managed care arrangement, felt his patient met criteria for dysthymia and possibly major depression. He spoke to the managed care firm's consulting psychiatrist on the phone. The psychologist summarized his findings and diagnosis and recommended the psychiatrist prescribe fluoxetine.

On the day of the psychiatric evaluation, the patient showed up 30 minutes late to a 45-minute evaluation. The psychiatrist did a 15-minute intake and prescribed half of a 20 mg fluoxetine pill daily. He did not arrange for follow-up evaluation, assuming fluoxetine was a drug with a good safety profile and the psychologist would monitor the medication.

The patient told the psychologist that she was pleased with the effects of fluoxetine, but her anxiety had become "different" and more unpleasant. The psychologist increased the fluoxetine to a whole pill (20 mg daily). Several days later, the patient uncharacteristically left home, went to a motel, and ingested a large number of diphenhydramine tablets. She was found the next morning and taken to a local emergency room. In the process of the psychiatric evaluation, she was told she had an akathesia secondary to fluoxetine. She attributed her "uncharacteristic" suicide attempt to the fluoxetine-related akathesia and sued the psychiatrist for malpractice and damages. She did not sue the psychologist. The psychologist maintained, at deposition, that he had not recommended a specific antidepressant to the patient, nor had assumed responsibility for monitoring the medication. The psychiatrist agreed to a small settlement.

Psychiatrists working in a managed care situation may be open to this type of lawsuit if they do not take time, initially, to explain the risks, side effects, and benefits of the medication to the patient.[15,16] This cannot be done effectively in 15 minutes. The psychiatrist needs time to develop a relationship with a patient and to explore other medication issues that may be relevant. Follow-up is essential and cannot be left to a psychologist or nonmedical clinician. Also, psychologists should not recommend increasing the dose of a medication without first consulting the psychiatrist. In no case should a psychiatrist prescribe medication without first examining the patient. Inadequate treatment may lead to negligent treatment and subsequent lawsuits.

Malpractice Litigation Involving Drug Interaction

An attorney sues his psychiatrist for malpractice and damages for not informing him of a potential interaction. Without going into great detail about what occurred, the patient was prescribed a combination of fluoxetine for depression and a neurologist later prescribed carbamazepine (Tegretol) for what he felt was a seizure disorder.[17,18] Very little at that time was known of the interaction incompatibility between these two medications. Because of the lack of knowledge and little research that was conducted on the interaction, the lawsuit filed by the patient against the psychiatrist did not go forward. The psychiatrist is not legally responsible for knowing about drug interactions that are, at the time of the treatment, controversial or even unknown. That would be unreasonable; the law requires the psychiatrist to practice only in a reasonable manner.[19,20]

Conclusion

The complexities of psychotropic interactions pose a significant challenge to the practicing psychiatrist to avoid harm to the patient and subsequent malpractice litigation. With increasing numbers and types of psychotropic medication for various psychiatric illnesses, psychiatrists have been faced with a challenge of providing adequate care (not ideal care) in a safe and effective manner. The practicing psychiatrist utilizing newer medications must stay abreast of the literature and the research studies involving the medications utilized in psychiatric practice. Failure to consider side effects, both usual and unusual, and toxic effects of combinations of medication may prove to be harmful to the patient and could result in a malpractice lawsuit.

The psychiatrist must assess the risk management probabilities with the use of each medication and combinations of medications. The risk increases especially for the difficult patient who has been resistant to standard and commonly used medications and requires a newer medication or combination of various medications. An effective method of managing difficult cases is to seek consultation from an experienced colleague. Is the benefit worth the risk? The answer lies in the experience of the therapist and the primary concern of doing no harm to the patient. Putting the patient's welfare first in difficult cases will mitigate the malpractice risk.

This chapter is presented as an example of the ability of psychopharmacologists to work with forensic psychiatrists when malpractice lawsuits become a possibility. The forensic psychiatrist can advise the psychopharmacologist about the reasonableness of the practice of psychiatry, and the risk/benefit ratio in the use of various medications and combinations of medications, and can advise the treating physician to keep up with the literature and the research on the medications that he or she is prescribing.

As the practice of psychiatry becomes more technological, chemical, and scientific, the risk of untoward or unexpected or unforeseen reactions will increase. The psychiatrist is not legally responsible for unforeseen occurrences or those that have not been reported in the literature or by his own experience. However, the psychiatrist is legally responsible for those cases in which damage occurs to the patient because the treating psychiatrist was derelict in his duty to research the recent literature pertaining to the use of such medication. If the medication use was a direct cause of the damage to the patient, the psychiatrist may be sued in malpractice for "dereliction of duty." Thus, the utilization of forensic issues and forensic psychiatric consultation in psychopharmacology has become a reasonable procedure.

Acknowledgment

This chapter is adapted from a paper published by the authors in *Essential Psychopharmacology*, 3:1, 1999, p. 65–91. Reprinted with permission by Hatherleigh Medical Education. www.hatherleigh.com

References

1. Asch DA, & Parker RM. (1998). Sounding board: The Libby Zion case. *N Engl J Med, 318*, 771–775.
2. Scher M, Krieger IN, & Juergens S. (1983). Trazodone and priapism. *Am J Psychiat, 140*, 1362–1363.
3. Warner MD, Peabody CA, Whiteford HA, & Hollister LE. (1987). Trazodone and priapism. *J Clin Psychiat, 48*, 244–245.
4. MeadJohnson Pharmaceutical Division: Letter. October 1985.
5. Medical Economics. (1995). Desyrel. Physicians' Desk Reference (p. 520). Medical Economics, New York City, NY.
6. Teicher MH, Glad C, & Cole J. (1990). Emergency of intense suicidal preoccupation during fluoxetine treatment. *Am J Psychiat, 147*, 207–210.
7. Spier SA, & Fontera MA. (1991). Unexpected deaths in depressed medical inpatients treated with fluoxetine. *J Clin Psychiat, 52*, 377–382.
8. Ereshefsky L, Alfaro CL, & Lam YWF. (1997). Treating depression: potential drug interactions. *Psychiat Ann, 27*, 244–258.
9. Harvey AT, & Preskorn SH. (1996). Cytochrome P450 enzymes: interpretation of their interactions with selective serotonin reuptake inhibitors. Part I. *J Clin Psychopharm, 16*, 273–282.
10. Harvey AT, & Preskorn SH. (1996). Cytochrome P450 enzymes: interpretation of their interactions with selective serotonin reuptake inhibitors. Part II. *J Clin Psychopharm, 16*, 345–354.
11. Jefferson, JJ. (2010). A clinician's guide to monitoring kidney function in lithium-treated patients. *J Clin Psychiat*, 2010;71(9):1153–1157.
12. Poon EG, et al. (2004). "I wish I had seen this test result earlier!": Dissatisfaction with test result management systems in primary care, *Arch Intern Med, 164*, 2223–2228.
13. Schou, M. (1988). Effects of long-term lithium treatment on kidney function. *J Psychiat Res, 22*(4), 287–298.
14. Markowitz GS, et al. (2000). Lithium nephrotoxicity. *J Am Soc Nephrol, 11*, 1439–1448.
15. Greenblatt D, Preskorn SH, & Cotreau MM. (1992). Fluoxetine impairs clearance of alprazolam but not of clonazepam. *Clin Pharmacal Ther, 52*, 479–486.
16. Lemberger L, Rowe H, & Bosomworth JC. (1988). The effect off fluoxetine on the pharmacokinetics and psychomotor responses of diazepam. *Clin Pharmacal Ther, 43*, 412–419.
17. Moor NC, Lerer B, Meyerdorf£ E, et al. (1985). Three cases of carbamazepine toxicity. *Am J Psychiat, 142*, 974–975.
18. Hershey LA. (1986). Hepatic reaction to carbamazepine. Letter to Editor. *J Clin Psychopharmacal*, 6, 251.
19. Ketter TA, Post RM, et, al. (1991). Principle of clinically important drug interactions with carbamazepine. Part I. *J Clin Psychopharm, 11*, 198–203.
20. Ketter TA, Post RM, & Worthington K. (1991). Principle of clinically important drug interactions with carbamazepine. Part 11. *J Clin Psychopharm, 11*, 306–312.

18

Forensic Psychiatry and Addiction Psychiatry

Richard F. Limoges

Thinking in addiction psychiatry and in forensic psychiatry differs in fundamental ways that are important to appreciate. Addiction psychiatrists employ what might be called "therapeutic medical thinking," whereas forensic psychiatrists utilize "forensic or legal medical thinking." The essential difference is most clearly seen in the matter of the purpose for which a diagnosis will be used. The addiction psychiatrist diagnoses the patient in order to formulate a treatment plan and a prognosis so that all may be in agreement with the nature of the disorder and its treatment, and the treatment will be consistent, relevant, and accepted.

The forensic psychiatrist makes a diagnosis in order to identify and accurately describe the nature of the condition at issue and, more importantly, to describe and discuss the relevant behavioral and cognitive sequelae of this condition and how it relates to the legal questions being posed. Here, the goal is not necessarily agreement. Although two forensic psychiatrists may examine the same patient, and even agree on the diagnosis, they may come to strikingly different conclusions and opinions about the significance and relevance of their findings and how these findings apply to the legal question.

It is also important to appreciate how the language and terminology differs in the two specialties and to be aware of a new vocabulary; one that is spoken in legal matters, not medical. For example, a physician may think of a narcotic as an opiate-derivative drug, but legally it is any scheduled chemical that is prohibited or used in violation of government regulations. Thus marijuana and cocaine are legally narcotics. Medically, use or abuse of a chemical is not the same thing as dependence or addiction to that same chemical, One may become dependent on a regular and unchanging amount of a scheduled medication such as the benzodiazepines, never increase the dose, and yet undergo a withdrawal period if stopped abruptly. This is not addiction, which is yet another phenomenon. Addiction is characterized by craving; increasing use; sneaking, lying, and subterfuge; and increasing amounts of time and money devoted to obtaining the substance. Addiction is a term that is poorly defined both legally and medically, and yet the term is bandied about all the time, leading to imprecise thinking. Addiction and alcoholism are not terms that will be found in the Diagnostic and Statistical Manual, Fifth Edition.[1] Rather, the current diagnostic category is "Alcohol Use Disorder."

Insanity is another problematic word. This term has utterly no medical meaning and yet is used all the time. Legally however, insanity has a very precise and exact meaning, but one that varies from jurisdiction to jurisdiction. Another term that can be misunderstood is the concept of *voluntariness*, which differs in medicine and law. In law, drinking is considered to be voluntary, with the single exception of when a person unknowingly ingests an intoxicating substance. In addiction psychiatry, the concept of voluntariness is widely rejected, and drinking or drug using is seen as the result of craving, compulsion, or even perhaps neurobiological activity in the brain.

The psychiatrist who specializes in the diagnosis and treatment of addiction disorders is expected to know the effects of various intoxicants, the phenomenology of addiction, neurotransmitters, receptor sites, neuroanatomy of the brain, treatment modalities, medical co-morbidity, prevention, and approaches to populations with special characteristics. In addition, the well-prepared addiction psychiatrist needs to know the basic principles of forensic psychiatry, or how medical knowledge of the field of addiction psychiatry and that of forensic psychiatry are interwoven in many ways. The importance of the legal and forensic aspects of addictions are not emphasized and seldom taught. These matters are usually relegated to one small chapter at the back of most textbooks of addiction medicine or addiction psychiatry.

History

Over many years, concerns in psychiatry have changed. Broadly speaking, the discipline has moved from the concept of the eighteenth century "Mad Doctor" who attempted to treat florid psychoses, to Superintendents who ran mental hospitals, to "Alienists" whose concern was a careful examination, description, classification, and nosology of mental illness, and then to the new field of psychoanalysis, or inquiry into individual psychic pain and suffering caused by unconscious drives and neurotic conflicts, with an emphasis on psychoanalytic techniques and in-depth therapy over long periods of time.[2]

However, present day psychiatry increasingly places more emphasis on behavior, and has moved away from theories of neurotic conflict or lengthy analytic treatment. Emphasis has shifted to modification of behavior in the present, rather than primarily formulating an understanding of how such behavior may have developed in the past. As examples of this, what used to be the Department of Psychiatry at several respected medical schools is now variously called the Department of Human Behavior, the Department of Behavioral Science, or the Department of Behavioral Health.

More than most areas of psychiatry, that of addictions is often concerned with behavior having legal dimensions. The element that ties these two disciplines together is an emphasis on human behavior, including knowledge of both the influence of chemicals on behavior as well as the consequences that may arise in not conforming one's behavior to the requirements of the law. Knowledge of the basic tenets of forensic psychiatry is helpful to the addiction psychiatrist, as the behavioral manifestations of addictions often lead to legal consequences, which have not been viewed traditionally as of medical concern. The predominant corpus of addiction psychiatry's concerns has been physiological effects of chemicals on the body and mind, habituation and its treatment, issues of withdrawal and detoxification, the appropriate use of medication to treat overdoses and serious withdrawal states such as delirium tremens, ways to help with cravings and promote abstinence, prevention, and monitoring.[3]

Addiction psychiatry emphasizes the importance of long-term involvement in one or another therapeutic modality over time to achieve, maintain and preserve sobriety. The forensic psychiatrist does not have this concern. The task is to impartially evaluate a person and the legal case and formulate an opinion in order to aid the court or trier of fact to reach a determination concerning a particular act at a moment in time. The forensic psychiatrist makes it clear at the beginning that the examination confers no doctor–patient relationship and this is not a therapeutic evaluation for any kind of treatment. Although the ultimate goal is different, the addiction psychiatrist can gain much by considering the method and approach of the forensic psychiatrist, which is to carefully verify and corroborate as much as possible the history the person gives from the very beginning by interviewing other people, reviewing hospital and other records, and by employing standardized testing if helpful.

Whereas the forensic psychiatrist does this in order to have opinions be credible in court, the addiction psychiatrist must address the patient's initial distorted clinical data and confirm the offered narrative as well. Addiction psychiatrists often treat patients who face more legal consequences than do most other psychiatrists. Such consequences, or the imminent possibility of serious consequences, may often motivate a person to enter therapy but also to withhold essential information about continuing problematic, and possibly illegal, behavior that might be clinically important, such as distribution or stealing.

These denials and omissions can mislead the clinician who is not mindful of the potential legal issues that are almost always present. The need for objective correlation of the patient's narrative is one of the ways in which a forensic approach assists the addiction psychiatrist. An understanding of this forensic approach, which may seem to run counter to the classic therapeutic stance, will assist the addiction psychiatrist to work through the initial denial, distorted thinking, self-deception, projection, and minimization the new patient inevitably displays. The physician must assess whether or not the patient wants to be sober or drug free, or whether he just wants to minimize or avoid the consequences of drug or alcohol use, much as the person the forensic psychiatrist evaluates seeks to avoid the possible legal consequences of criminal actions. The psychiatrist in either situation must assume that the patient/client is not initially forthcoming.

The forensic psychiatrist depends upon corroborative and correlative information obtained from other people, records, and documents. The wise addiction psychiatrist will also interview concerned others at the beginning of therapy and seek previous treatment records as well as police records. Permission should be sought to obtain independent data at the very beginning of treatment. The general psychiatrist is taught to accept the patient's narrative as reality and to work with that as the basis for therapy. This approach does not work in either addictions or forensics.

The forensic psychiatrist has no duty to accept and believe what is related initially, and in fact is obligated to be skeptical of all narrative and to verify what the examinee is relating. The addiction psychiatrist must tread a narrow middle ground; tentatively accepting the patient's story knowing it is incomplete and perhaps deceptive, but requiring permission to interview involved third parties who may have a different point of view, as well as useful information. This should be done at the outset in order to make the point that the addiction psychiatrist is thorough but supportively skeptical, and not necessarily willing to accept everything at face value. In the long run this tentative position is helpful, as the psychiatrist will not collude with the patient in his defenses, but rather have the means and basis to challenge distortions in a helpful and therapeutic way.

As with the forensic psychiatrist, it is important for the addiction psychiatrist to obtain previous treatment records, especially those from hospitals and rehabs, if any, and to ask the patient to clarify discrepancies. Asking for permission to speak to previous therapists is often essential. If a patient refuses such permission, then the clinician is made aware early on that there are unknowns and secrets. This must be dealt with carefully at the beginning of therapy, as the position of the doubting therapist is a difficult one, but information is much more easily gathered while initially developing the patient's comprehensive past history. Early on, the psychiatrist can clear up missing facts and misstatements and then begin to develop the doctor–patient relationship. The patient knows then that his doctor will not be easily duped, and that his narrative may be questioned.

Example of Addiction in a Man with ADD and OCD

Recently, a pleasant athletic man in his early 30s was referred for help for his stated attention deficit disorder and obsessive-compulsive personality disorder. He said that his behavior of either forgetting to do things or else being caught up in rituals was compromising his relationship with his fiancée. He was quite distressed. He said that currently, his parents were supporting him, but this support was coming to an end. He told me he was diligently looking for a job but that various sports injuries in the past prevented much physical activity at present. Despite his earnest demeanor, I wondered why he had been sent to an addiction psychiatrist, and so I sought a telephone consultation with his parents, while he was in the room with me. I soon learned from them that he had indeed sustained various sports injuries for which he was taking opiates; he had been prescribed stimulants for his ADD, and took benzodiazepines for sleep. Most importantly he had recently been an inpatient in a rehab facility because of his problematic and worrisome drinking.

He agreed with all these facts, but said he considered his drinking to be in the past, he had been prescribed the stimulants, and he indeed did take opiates for pain, but only occasionally. Therefore, none of this seemed important to him, and he thought it was not worth bringing up. He did not seem to be dissembling, merely skipping information he thought trivial. I told him and his parents that his difficulty must be dealt with in its entirety and that I must know every relevant fact and concern. Only then would I have enough information to address his issues. The forensic psychiatrist must maintain the position of corroborating statements that don't sound quite right, and the addiction psychiatrist must do the same.

Working with an Attorney

Civil Matters Involving Addicted Individuals

Since addictions bring up many legal issues, attorneys will often consult with the addiction psychiatrist in cases that involve addiction or alcohol in some way. Civil cases involving chemical dependence, addiction, or intoxication often include dram shop cases, domestic disputes, will challenges, validity of a signed contract, custody cases, or divorces. These all may benefit from the knowledge of the addiction psychiatrist. There are many ways to assist the attorney in what is essentially a foreign environment for the physician. Benefit accrues in both directions. In addition to bringing expertise to help attorneys in areas in which they may not be knowledgeable, the addiction psychiatrist in turn will learn the legal parameters of the attorney's case. This can help the addiction psychiatrist's contribution to be more salient and meaningful.

When the addiction psychiatrist is called upon to assist the attorney, it must be clear what this role is to be. Is it to be an expert witness, a fact witness, or no witness at all but rather retained as a consultant to the attorney and not expected to write a report or to testify? In the last capacity it is because the consultant possesses a great deal of knowledge about chemical dependence. The expectation is to be as an advisor about certain aspects of the case. All the clinical material will be reviewed with the attorney to see what facts are important and relevant, then advise the attorney what more materials are necessary, such as employment or school records. Hospital records will be reviewed in order to guide the attorney through important medical issues that may emerge. Suggestions may be offered for the attorney to consider in light of the totality of the case, and perhaps to opine about whether it looks like there is a case to take forward at all, in light of all that has been considered. The psychiatrist might point out important aspects the attorney has not considered because he did not recognize their significance.

Malpractice Cases

In a different setting, the addiction psychiatrist might be called upon as a consultant to assist in the defense of a malpractice case in which a physician has been accused of "causing a patient to become addicted," a not uncommon allegation. Here, the addiction specialist has to blend medical knowledge and expertise with the legal elements and procedures the lawyer must work within. First the plaintiff's allegations are reviewed, along with medical history and records. Then the attorney and the physician assess the medical vulnerability of the defendant physician. Assistance here can take the form of helping the attorney formulate questions for depositions and for cross-examining the witnesses at trial, to warn of medical pitfalls and to advise about the significance of facts and data.

In order to assess the nature and extent of the claimed harm, in this instance causing an addiction, the expert must perform a thorough psychiatric evaluation, review and consider all pertinent documents and other information, ask for missing documents or call attention to those that are not available, obtain collateral information from others to corroborate facts and details, request results of all studies and tests, and perhaps suggest other measures such as psychological testing or neuroimaging if the claim warrants. It is extremely important to obtain all the medical records.

The expert must be familiar with the needs of the attorney and the court. The addiction psychiatrist here is well advised to be familiar with the skills the forensic psychiatrist utilizes in writing a report, because this document is different from a clinical report to a consultant. It is not meant to summarize treatment or to inform a colleague, or to prepare for an academic presentation such as grand rounds. Ideally it is carefully crafted and includes a list and description of all materials considered.

Testamentary Issues, Capacity and Competency

Another matter in which the addiction psychiatrist may be invited to assist, but in a very different way, is in the matter of a will challenge. Here, the validity of a will is being challenged by a claim that the testator did not have the mental capacity to write the will at the time it was written. The issue here is the state of mind of the testator at the time the will was written, and whether or not the person understood the process and what the desired outcome would be. Issues of alcoholism, addiction, intoxication, clouded thinking, or undue influence may be alleged. The addiction psychiatrist is asked to apply knowledge of ways in which chemicals might have affected the decedent's thinking. Multiple collateral interviews are helpful, along with hospital records, bank records, tax records, correspondence, and, if available, newspaper articles, obituaries, e-mail, and social media, in order to assess whether or not the testator was of sound mind at or around the time the will was written. In addition, what evidence is there, if any, to support the claim of alcoholism or drug dependence, and to what extent did they influence or distort the testator's thinking? The addiction psychiatrist is not being asked to make a diagnosis, because a diagnosis is secondary to the issue of competency, but on the other hand can help explain the situation if incompetency or lack of capacity is determined.

Contracts; Competency in Addicted Individuals

In another context, the addiction psychiatrist might be asked to offer an opinion about the validity of a contract, if signed while the person was in the throes of active alcoholism or addiction. The question to be examined is the state of mind of the signer of the document at the time he signed it. Collateral and corroborative material at or around the time of the signing again is most helpful.

Example of Competency to Contract for Divorce

In a divorce case the husband could not accept that his marriage was over. He persisted in the fantasy that his wife still loved him. During this time he was in the throes of a serious opiate addiction, but to casual observation he seemed to be functioning normally. One day, while he was in a beclouded condition, his wife abruptly presented him with a property settlement and demanded that he sign it. He stated that he could not accept even then that she was serious, and he further said that he believed she would never cause him any harm. Although he signed the document, later he stated he never read its contents because he trusted his ex-wife, and so did not know what it said or what he agreed to. Only later, once he was in recovery, did he realize that he had signed away his entire estate, past and future, and that he had agreed to give her absolutely everything he possessed.

The addiction psychiatrist was asked to ascertain, as much as possible, the husband's state of mind at the time of signing, and how his thinking was influenced by his considerable opioid addiction, in order to assist the attorney to show the court that this was not a valid, knowing, and informed settlement contract. Again, collateral and corroborative material at or around the time of the signing was most helpful. It is wise to remember that the task of the addiction psychiatrist in this matter is a descriptive one, shedding as much light as possible on state of mind at a past event.

Dram Shop Case

Another matter in which the addiction psychiatrist may be asked to participate is in a dram shop case. Here the task of the addiction psychiatrist is to opine as accurately as possible whether or not the subject patron of the bar in question was "visibly intoxicated" at the time he was served additional alcohol, and whether or not the bartender should have refused service, thus preventing the events that precipitated the suit. The person whose condition is in question may be dead, so the psychiatrist's opinion must be based on as much other information as it is possible to glean. It can be expected that there will be conflicting narratives one must evaluate. In addition, the addiction psychiatrist can be asked to opine and describe what effect a given amount of alcohol might have on a person's thinking, reasoning, personality, motor functioning, coordination, speech, flushed skin, impulsivity, judgment, or aggressivity.

Custody Cases

A custody dispute is another matter in which the addiction psychiatrist might be asked to participate, which can be one of the most difficult issues possible. Often each estranged and embittered parent claims that the other is an alcoholic or drug addict and therefore should be denied custody or visitation rights. In such a situation, if one decides to participate, the psychiatrist must insist on being retained by the court and not by either side. This arrangement permits the psychiatrist to examine both parents.

Criminal Matters

In criminal cases the addiction psychiatrist can be called upon to be of assistance but in a different way. Addictions, intoxication, or being under the influence of a drug or chemical, or claiming amnesia or a blackout are not complete defenses to a crime, but discussion of these phenomena may help place a criminal act in context and be useful at sentencing. The addiction psychiatrist who becomes involved in a criminal case needs to know general criminal court procedure.

Here the addiction psychiatrist can be of help in informing and educating the court about the effects a given chemical may have on a person's behavior at the time of the crime, and how the ingestion of such a chemical might have influenced the defendant's judgment, perception, impulse control, or thinking.

If retained by the prosecution, the addiction psychiatrist can be of assistance in helping to respond to a claim of "blackout" or alcoholic amnesia, a claim that is made by a significant number of defendants. The defendant claims no knowledge or memory for the acts the prosecution has charged, and may therefore maintain no knowledge or conscious control over what happened at the time. The absence of memory does not signify or imply a lack of cognitive functioning or an inability to act rationally at the time of the crime, nor does it suggest that the criminal act itself did not take place (see chapter 30).

A basic tenet of the legal view of alcoholism that is at variance with the literature of alcoholism and addiction is that intoxication is always viewed as voluntary. Alcoholism and addiction are conceptualized quite differently from the legal view, bearing in mind the previous discussion that these terms have no diagnostic meaning but continue in the lexicon as useful concepts or "shorthand." Drinking may be driven by cravings and strong urges. After the first drink the alcoholic no longer has the ability to predictably and consistently control intake or to stop drinking. Usually the drinking episode is stopped one way or another by an external event. Nevertheless, the law holds that the first drink is always voluntary and the defendant knows when drinking begins both of past inability to control the amount consumed as well as its ensuing consequences. Therefore, knowing what is likely to happen, the choice is made to drink anyway. In addition to the discussion of the phenomenology of pathologic ingestion of alcohol or chemicals of abuse, testimony concerning unanticipated reactions to drugs or medicines can be of great assistance to the court.

Example of Criminal Behavior in an Addicted Individual

A young man presented in serious difficulty. He was a senior in high school and bound for college. He was an Eagle Scout and an exemplary model student held out to others as what one can accomplish as the only child of a single mother on extremely modest means. He did not drink, nor did he use drugs. He was devoutly religious and very conservative in clothing, activities, music, and recreation. Nevertheless, shortly before graduation, he was charged with calling his high school late at night to make terroristic bomb threats, and his voice was confirmed on tape. This was a devastating event, one that would imprison him and ruin his life, and one not easily explained.

In brief, a history showed that during the time in question he had been suffering from a severe cold or flu for many days. He described that, in order to not miss school, he began to take a proprietary cold remedy. On inquiry it was ascertained that this remedy contained dextromethorphan and pseudoephedrine. He was impatient and so began to take a lot of it. On the night in question he had a fever and had not eaten. He did not know it, but he had taken enough pseudoephedrine to produce insomnia and so he was up all night. In addition, the amount of dextromethorphan he ingested produced hallucinations, delusional thinking, dissociation, and euphoria. In the morning he had no recollection of what he had done and thought he had a bad dream. When this information was presented to the prosecution, it changed the whole nature of the case. It was not possible to overlook a bomb threat, but the consequences were far less catastrophic.

An addiction psychiatrist may be called upon in a driving under the influence case, to challenge the results of breath or blood tests, or to offer alternative causes. Because a person has been found to be driving with a blood level above 0.08 mg/dL in most states, this does not necessarily mean that person has an Alcohol Use Disorder, using current terminology, even though driving had been affected and influenced. Often enough time has passed that testimony can be offered to show the court what the defendant has done to address the problematic drinking. This should be supported with documentation of participation in an appropriate regimen. This could involve an inpatient or outpatient rehab program, participation in a 12-step program, random urine monitoring, and documented meaningful and appropriate therapy, Although this testimony might be offered at the trial phase, it is more often given as mitigation at sentencing, to offer to the judge that the defendant has assumed responsibility for driving under the influence and is taking measures to remedy the situation.

Administrative Matters

Addiction psychiatrists are often involved in the treatment of licensed professionals such as attorneys, physicians, nurses, and others in the health care professions. Here it is essential to know the regulatory and administrative context in which each of them must function. The licensing authorities will have certain requirements for the patient, and these requirements often involve the treating psychiatrist as well. Various state boards will request information that requires careful consideration of the privacy laws, HIPAA, CFR 42, Part 2, and so forth on the part of the treating physician. Often the physician must be both the treating physician and the monitor as well, which compromises treatment severely. If reports are required, the addiction psychiatrist must know what laws apply that safeguard sensitive information. Many states have intermediary monitoring and advocacy programs separate and apart from licensing boards, and it is wise to know how they work. Sometimes in the workplace these monitoring functions are performed by medical review officers, whose sole function is to monitor drug-testing programs and to investigate the relevance and significance of positive findings.

Disability Issues

The addiction psychiatrist may be asked to assist the patient or the patient's lawyer in filing a disability claim. One must keep in mind that clinical disability is not legal disability. A disability policy is a legal document that specifies what disability means in a specific context. It will contain exclusions, exemptions, definitions, conditions, limits, and other specifiers. If one is asked to participate, it is essential to obtain a copy of the disability policy and see how it defines disability, and what conditions apply. The patient may need to seek legal counsel in complicated or contested cases. Should disability be awarded and the person remains under care, the psychiatrist can expect that the insurance company will ask for reports on a periodic basis. It is well to keep in mind that such information will be used in part to determine whether or not the state of disability continues. Careful consideration must be given to these reports, as much can depend on the wording.

Conclusion

Many psychiatrists fear and dread involvement with legal matters and avoid it at all costs, usually because of a lack of familiarity with the field. It should be evident that there are many valuable and meaningful ways to contribute and share expertise with their forensic colleagues. If indeed, as was noted at the beginning, psychiatry is more and more the study of behavior, then psychiatrists are obligated to have at least rudimentary knowledge of the kinds of behavior that have legal consequences, and be willing to participate in that process. Knowledge of the legal system, forensic approaches, and procedure and customs can make what might seem to be terrifying much more understandable and perhaps even a new and intriguing area of medicine.

References

1. American Psychiatric Association. (2013) *Diagnostic and statistical manual of mental disorders* (5th ed., pp. 483–589). Arlington, VA: American Psychiatric Association.
2. Shorter E. (1997). *A history of psychiatry: From an era of the asylum to the age of Prozac*. New York: John Wiley & Sons.
3 Sinha R. (2013). The clinical neurobiology of drug craving. *Curr Opin Neurobiol, 23*, 649–654.

SECTION FIVE

Forensic Psychiatry and Other Professions

19

Forensic Psychiatry and Psychology

Fraternal Twins of Courtroom Science

Eric Y. Drogin and
Frank M. Dattilio

Biological science informs us that identical (monozygotic) twins form when a single fertilized egg (ovum) splits in two. Fraternal (dizygotic) twins develop from two separately fertilized eggs, and are no more alike than individual siblings born at different times. This scientific fact neatly mirrors the relationship between forensic psychiatrists and forensic psychologists—alike in many ways, but they also share in distinct differences. It is clear that psychiatry first appeared approximately 100 years before the birth of professional psychology,[1] but the subspecialties of *forensic* psychiatry and psychology have both been in existence for approximately four decades, such that both are considered relative neophytes in their respective realms of medicine and psychology.

Little has been published on the relationship between forensic psychiatrists and psychologists or their co-existing status as experts in the field of courtroom science. Existing studies tend to cast this relationship in terms of a dichotomy, highlighting the specific similarities—and, far more prominently, the differences—that exist between the two disciplines. Most recently, an article published by Dattilio[2] entitled "Toward a Good Fit between Forensic Psychologists and Psychiatrists" surveyed the professional literature and credited Perlin[3] with addressing the chasm that has existed between perceptions of forensic psychiatrists and psychologists since their mutual professional debuts. Perlin noted that at that time considerable conflict was evident, pertaining mostly to matters of perceived turf. Sadoff[4] later offered a more diplomatic view of differing perspectives, emphasizing the notion that "part of the armamentarium of the forensic psychiatrist is the availability of a good forensic psychologist who is able to apply the skill of clinical psychology to legal issues," and adding that "a psychologist has an equally important role to play with a lawyer both in evaluation, examination and consultation, as well as functioning as an expert witness in court" (p. 107).

To be sure, there are certain inevitable ramifications of the fact that these fraternal twins were raised in different professional households. For better or for worse, psychiatrists—by virtue of their recruitment processes and professional training environment—are typically not as imbued with what attorney and forensic psychologist Richard Redding[5] has identified as the "psychology of political correctness" in a book of the same name. Additionally, by dint of education and training, the primary "truth finding mechanisms" between adherents of each profession can differ substantially, for although "medicine proceeds from a diagnostically focused 'medical model,' it is the psychologist—with an educational grounding in statistical analysis—who will be most inclined to conduct formula-driven hypothesis testing" (p. 107).[6]

The notion that forensic psychiatrists and psychologists can serve together as an effective *team* in consulting with attorneys in criminal as well as civil cases has long flourished outside of the professional literature—in courtrooms, law offices, and correctional institutions across the country—and has recently been underscored by the publication of a *Handbook of Forensic Assessment: Psychological and Psychiatric Perspectives* that acknowledged in its Foreword that "these specializations draw considerably on their respective disciplines, yet share much of the relevant law, science, ethics, and practice that guide the best practice of forensic mental health assessment" (p. vii).[7]

Complementary Differences

Forensic psychiatry and psychology complement each other in various ways, in a fashion very similar to the coexistence of ophthalmology and optometry, where the work in question is closely related, yet distinct. These distinct differences actually foster a harmonious multidisciplinary relationship that allows the two, when working together, to function as one.

Forensic psychiatry is a branch of medicine that focuses on the interface of law and mental health, and which stakes out one area in particular in which psychologists are not competent to practice: the domain of psychotropic medications. Forensic psychiatrists are uniquely qualified to gauge and explain the effects such compounds have on the human body chemistry and physiology, and any resulting impact on behaviors that underlie both criminal and civil matters. Although forensic psychiatrists—as do forensic psychologists—often obtain additional training and experience related to various other interfaces of mental health and the law, their most distinct form of expertise lies within the domain of biologically based evaluations and treatments. Forensic psychiatrists possess a general medical knowledge about the mechanics of the human body and how medical illnesses or diseases may impact on human behavior, and in some cases their specifically medical expertise may also allow them to opine on matters of toxicology (e.g., blood and body chemistry levels), as well as the results of certain forms of scans (e.g., EEG, fMRI, PET).

By contrast, forensic psychologists maintain unparalleled expertise in areas not usually covered at any significant level of detail by psychiatric training programs. These areas include psychodiagnostic testing, research design, and neuropsychological assessment. Forensic psychologists are trained in the intricate process of administration and scoring of standardized cognitive and personality tests. They are also uniquely skilled in understanding the utility of such tests, and are required to be competent to answer questions with regard to the statistical properties of such measures when an understanding of such characteristics becomes an issue in criminal and civil matters. Examples include the classification of intellectual functioning and the significance of the inevitable variability of available scores in capital homicide cases. Most forensic psychiatrists are neither educated about nor familiar with the nuances of the standardization of such measures or their true relevance to resulting interpretations. There has, however, been considerable encouragement as of late for forensic psychiatry training programs to offer additional course work on the interpretation of psychological test-driven appraisals.[8]

Hence, forensic psychologists are trained to withstand questions on instrumental reliability and validity with respect to the full range of psychodiagnostic instruments employed. Vigorous cross-examination on such topics as standard error of measurement, competence intervals, and normative populations will eventually ensue—if not in one's next courtroom appearance, then in one soon to follow. Experts who utilize psychodiagnostic tests and appraisals but are unfamiliar with core psychometric principles expose their reports to negative scrutiny. Such scrutiny may imperil work product generated for retaining counsel, haphazardly affect the fate of litigants, and even run the risk of incurring allegations of unethical behavior. In much the same vein, forensic psychologists would face similar scrutiny if they were to attempt to assert that they are experts on psychopharmacology or certain brain scans, falling into the trap of being unable to answer intricate questions pertaining to the pharmacokinetics of medication or the synergistic effects that compounds may have on one another.

Case Example

A classic example of the harmonious work between the forensic psychiatrist and psychologist is best portrayed by the following.

Mr. B was a 73-year-old married father of three and grandfather of six who had a long history of being a successful businessman in the community. He had no history of criminal behavior, nor any involvement with illicit drug or alcohol abuse/dependence. It was during his retirement years that he started to invest his savings in some risky stock and over a period of approximately 2 years lost much of his money. He became very disparaged and depressed and started to experience thoughts of anger and rage about large corporations that would take advantage of tax situations and compound their earnings to ridiculous proportions. After reading stories in the newspaper about large corporations and their high profit margins, he targeted an heir of a large national corporation who reportedly inherited $500 million from the family's enterprise. Mr. B suddenly got the notion that he should go and kidnap this heir and hold him for ransom. Despite the fact that this was something completely out of character for him, he began to make plans in which he rented a van, bought a disguise (fake mustache and hairpiece) and took a taser gun and drove to the heir's house to abduct him. In the process, the abduction failed and a short time later Mr. B was apprehended by the police when security cameras around the heir's compound captured an image of him and the license plate of the van he had rented. As a result, he was taken into custody by authorities. Mr. B's criminal defense attorney and family believed that he was laboring under some type of mental illness since his behavior was completely out of character for him after 72 years of being a good husband and father and a law-abiding citizen.

The initial psychiatric examination failed to reveal anything out of the ordinary, and as a result, the psychiatrist recruited a forensic psychologist to examine the defendant to determine whether or not there may be any organic factors underlying his personality dynamics and his actions in the instant offense. A complete neuropsychological battery was conducted that yielded unremarkable results. However, extensive personality testing shed light on the fact that this man was laboring under a delusional disorder that appeared to be spiked by a reaction to having lost his life's savings in a very short period of time. The result of the psychological evaluation was substantial in helping the defense team petition the court for consideration of a guilty but mentally ill plea, which aided the defendant in avoiding a lengthy prison term.

There are countless examples of this type of collaborative efforts in which forensic psychiatrists and psychologists work together as a team to render opinions in such complex cases.

Examples from the Literature

As noted, there has been a recent increase in articles in the professional literature on the differences between forensic psychiatry and psychology.[2,9] What is more important to emphasize is how they can work *together* and *complement* each other's efforts. The aforementioned *Handbook of Forensic Assessment: Psychological and Psychiatric Perspectives*,[19] was edited by both forensic psychologists and psychiatrists, and each chapter was authored by a team that included at least one forensic psychiatrist and at least one forensic psychologist, with the explicit goal of addressing the differences as well as similarities of each discipline's approach to the subject matter at hand. The collaboration between forensic psychologists and psychiatrists in this book depicts the respective disciplines and how they draw from their knowledge to work in a harmonious fashion addressing the various issues in the field of forensic science.

This *Handbook*'s topical coverage includes—among others—the following examples, focusing upon evaluations conducted in both criminal and civil matters.

Competence to Stand Trial

A progression of federal cases addressing the utility and appropriateness of involuntary medication of defendants during trial has resulted in a standard[10] that provides an excellent pretext for psychiatric consultation, given the need to determine, among other things, "that the proposed medication would be substantially likely to render the defendant competent without causing side effects that would interfere with his ability to work with his attorney" (p. 9).[11] Assessment protocols that may be undertaken by psychologists include the Competency Screening Test, the Interdisciplinary Fitness Interview, the Georgia Court Competency Test, and the MacArthur Competency Assessment Tool—Criminal Adjudication (pp. 14–17).[11]

Sentencing

The psychiatrist's review of medical records may constitute a primary component of a comprehensive sentencing assessment, as "birth records may document difficulties during delivery that may have caused an anoxic brain injury and a resulting developmental disorder, such as fetal alcohol syndrome," whereas "medical records establishing the neurological consequences of such an injury, including the permanence of the injury, personality changes, and impulsivity, will be relevant" (p. 53).[12] Assessment protocols that may be undertaken by psychologists include the Wechsler Adult Intelligence Scale, the Minnesota Multiphasic Personality Inventory, the Hare Psychopathy Checklist, and the Violence Risk Appraisal Guide.[12]

Sexual Offender Recidivism

The psychiatrist's ability to engage in medically oriented procedures may play a significant role in such evaluations, given that "the method with perhaps the longest history of use with sex offenders is perhaps phallometry, made possible by the measurement of penile tumescence in a laboratory setting as an objective measure of sexual preference," involving "physiological changes in blood flow in the penis in response to various stimulus modalities" (p. 107).[13] Assessment protocols that may be undertaken by psychologists include the Millon Clinical Multiaxial Inventory, the Screening Scale for Pedophilic Interests, the Minnesota Sex Offender Screening Tool, and the Hare Psychopathy Checklist (pp. 106–112).[13]

Competency to Consent to Treatment

Key to gauging an examinee's competency to consent to treatment is a proper understanding of the medical ramifications of such treatment. Psychiatrists may be uniquely poised to determine "the acuity of the medical condition" and the ramification of "high-risk procedures," and to grasp fully "the risks, benefits, and alternatives to treatment…as this will be an essential element of the evaluation" (p. 506).[14] Assessment protocols that may be undertaken by psychologists include the Competency Interview Schedule, the Assessment of Consent Capacity for Treatment, the Hopemont Capacity Assessment Interview, and the MacArthur Competence Assessment Tool—Treatment (pp. 509–510).[14]

Guardianship

Ensuring a prominent role for the psychiatrist in guardianship evaluations is an unavoidable recognition that "the examinee's alleged disability may be the result of any number of medically related causes. Is there a chronic physical or psychological condition—or some interrelated presentation in which, for example, depression is potentiated by chronic pain? What is the examinee's current medication status… What is the examinee's history of utilization of medical services, and how is this likely to affect his or her rehabilitation prospects..." (p. 523).[15] Assessment protocols that may be undertaken by psychologists include the Community Competence Scale, the Competency Interview Scale, and the Decision-Making Instrument for Guardianship (p. 529).[15]

Psychological Autopsy

"Psychological" though this form of forensic inquiry may be, it carries with it in most cases a pronounced medical and pharmacological component, with a need to investigate "prescription medications" and the "interaction effects of legal and/or illegal compounds" as well as, more generally, the nature and case-specific efficacy of "medical illnesses and treatments," respectively (pp. 599–602).[16] Psychiatrists possess a unique and potential vital skill set in this regard. Interpretation of previously obtained psychological test results will provide an essential role for forensic psychologists, as will the mastery of template protocols for reviewing "psychological history" that were initially developed by and for psychologists.[16–18]

For far too long, the fraternal relationship of these two indispensable specialties has been undermined in the professional literature by "a discipline-specific focus on either psychology or psychiatry—at the expense of identifying the other's unique and complementary contributions."[19]

References

1. Shorter E. (1997). *A history of psychiatry: From the era of the asylum to the age of Prozac.* New York: Wiley.
2. Dattilio FM. (2011). Toward a good fit between forensic psychiatrists and psychologists. *J Psychiatry Law, 39*, 689–696.
3. Perlin ML. (1977). The legal status of the psychologist in the courtroom. *J Psychiatry Law, 5*, 41–54.
4. Sadoff RL. (1980). Working with a forensic psychologist. In G. Cooke (Ed.), *The role of the forensic psychologist* (pp. 106–110). Springfield, IL: Charles C Thomas.
5. Redding RE. (2009). *The psychology of political correctness.* Washington, DC: AEI Press.
6. Drogin EY, & Barrett CL. (2010). *Evaluation for guardianship.* New York: Oxford University Press.
7. Heilbrun K, & Wettstein RM. (2011). Foreword. In EY Drogin, FM Dattilio, RL Sadoff, & TG Gutheil (Eds.), *Handbook of forensic assessment: Psychological and psychiatric perspectives* (pp. vii–ix). Hoboken, NJ: Wiley.
8. Scott, C. (2012, September). Response to letter to the editor. *Am Acad Psychiatry Law Newslett*, 24–25.
9. Grisso, T. (1993). The difference between forensic psychiatry and forensic psychology. *Bull Am Acad Psychiatry Law, 21*, 133–145.
10. *Sell v. U.S.*, 539 U.S. 166 (2003).
11. Stafford KP, & Sadoff RL. (2011). Competence to stand trial. In EY Drogin, FM Dattilio, RL Sadoff, & TG Gutheil (Eds.), *Handbook of forensic assessment: Psychological and psychiatric perspectives* (pp. 3–23). Hoboken, NJ: Wiley.
12. Atkins EL, & Watson C. (2011). Sentencing. In EY Drogin, FM Dattilio, RL Sadoff, & TG Gutheil (Eds.), *Handbook of forensic assessment: Psychological and psychiatric perspectives* (pp. 49–78). Hoboken, NJ: Wiley.
13. Witt PH, Dattilio FM, & Bradford JMW. (2011). Sex offender evaluations. In EY Drogin, FM Dattilio, RL Sadoff, & TG Gutheil (Eds.), *Handbook of forensic assessment: Psychological and psychiatric perspectives* (pp. 97–120). Hoboken, NJ: Wiley.

14. Foubister N, & Connell M. (2011). Competency to consent to treatment. In EY Drogin, FM Dattilio, RL Sadoff, & TG Gutheil (Eds.), *Handbook of forensic assessment: Psychological and psychiatric perspectives* (pp. 503–519). Hoboken, NJ: Wiley.
15. Drogin EY, & Gutheil TG. (2011). Guardianship. In EY Drogin, FM Dattilio, RL Sadoff, & TG Gutheil (Eds.), *Handbook of forensic assessment: Psychological and psychiatric perspectives* (pp. 521–542). Hoboken, NJ: Wiley.
16. Dattilio FM, & Sadoff RL. (2011). Psychological autopsy. In EY Drogin, FM Dattilio, RL Sadoff, & TG Gutheil (Eds.), *Handbook of forensic assessment: Psychological and psychiatric perspectives* (pp. 593–611). Hoboken, NJ: Wiley.
17. Sadoff RL, & Dattilio FM. (2012). Formal training in forensic mental health: Psychiatry and psychology. *Int J Law Psychiatry, 35*, 343–347.
18. Dattilio FM, Sadoff RL, Drogin EY, & Gutheil TG. (2011). Should forensic psychiatrists conduct psychological testing? *J Psychiatry Law, 39*, 477–491.
19. Drogin EY, Dattilio FM, Sadoff RL, & Gutheil TG. (2011). Preface. In EY Drogin, FM Dattilio, RL Sadoff, & TG Gutheil (Eds.), *Handbook of forensic assessment: Psychological and psychiatric perspectives* (pp. xi–xii). Hoboken, NJ: Wiley.

20

Forensic Psychiatric Ethics

A Return to the Ivory Tower

Claire Pouncey

Stone's 1984 Challenge to Forensic Psychiatry

In 1984 Alan Stone challenged forensic psychiatry with his position that the nature of forensic psychiatric expert work is inherently unethical. Speaking "from the vantage point of the ivory tower," and appealing to "the basic premise of the purists" that there is no real factual or moral knowledge in psychiatry, he concludes that defining the ethical boundaries of forensic psychiatry is conceptually impossible.[1] He claims to support this conclusion with four different lines of reasoning[I]: He references philosophical questions about fact and value, free will and determinism, mind and brain, and the unity of the self to argue that without certain answers to these metaphysical questions there cannot be an ethic of forensic psychiatry. My discussion here will appeal to both the philosophy Stone cites, to existing work in bioethics generally, and to forensic psychiatric ethics in particular, to argue that the ethics of forensic psychiatry is not only possible, but can be enhanced by one of the "purists" that motivated Stone's nihilism.

Stone's view from the ivory tower must have obscured the fact that we function as social and moral agents despite the four metaphysical indeterminacies to which he refers. Although philosophy challenges us to question the metaphysical bases of our human experiences, those experiences in no way depend on answering the questions. We treat each other as if we are agents with free will, which is the very basis of moral and legal accountability, and the setting for forensic psychiatric work. We also liberally and tacitly "presuppose a conception of the person as an enduring, defining, and integrated metaphysical identity"[2] regardless of

I. Stone articulates five lines of reasoning, but I take his distinctions between fact and value, and science and morality, as versions of the same question.

whether we try to or succeed at arguing a holistic conception of personal identity. Other inhabitants of Stone's ivory tower, including sociology of science and philosophy of science, had conclusively accepted by 1984 that facts and values are constitutively intertwined.[3–5] Still other inhabitants, such as cognitive science and philosophy of mind, had already recognized that we utilize a presupposed relationship between mind and brain, even if the ontology captured by our limited linguistic tools does not describe that relationship clearly.[6] Accordingly, I will show that Stone failed to consider the medical ethics literature available at the time, and he failed to explicate at least one of his academic resources in a scholarly way.

The Academic Setting for Stone's Argument

Stone fails to acknowledge the available scholarship in bioethics in 1984, with the notable exception of the Hippocratic oath and its injunction to avoid harm to the patient above all else. Stone argues that any assessment on behalf of a forensic evaluee will necessarily bias the psychiatrist in a way that counteracts the legal purpose he is meant to serve, and if he primarily serves the legal system he risks legal harm to the patient.[1]

One might have expected Stone to reference the 1979 Belmont report, published by the National Commission for the Protection of Research Subjects of Biomedical and Behavioral Research. Drawing on Beauchamp and Childress's seminal *Principles of Biomedical Ethics*, also published in the late 1970s, the Belmont report articulated three core ethical considerations for both patient care and human subjects research: respect for persons (as agents capable of self-determination), beneficence/nonmaleficence toward patients and research subjects, and justice.[7] The Belmont report recognized that "even avoiding harm requires learning what is harmful; and, in the process of obtaining this information, persons may be exposed to risk of harm." The moral problem is one of justifying and minimizing the risks research presents, not a fixed rule never to inflict physical harm. It does not speak to a physician's responsibility to avoid sociopolitical harm. What is more, the Belmont report extends the political concept of justice to medicine. Although the report interprets justice primarily as "fairness" in the distribution of research risks and protection of vulnerable subjects, the conceptual link between justice and medicine was well established by the time Stone voiced his concerns.[II] Despite this precedent, Stone remained pessimistic that forensic psychiatrists could "square the ethical imperative of the healing profession [to do no harm] with the adversarial goals of criminal prosecution."[1]

Neither did Stone consider the 1980 revision of the American Medical Association's (AMA) Principles of Medical Ethics, which included the following preamble in order to reconcile "the dynamic tension between professional standards and legal requirements":

> The medical profession has long subscribed to a body of ethical statements developed primarily for the benefit of the patient. As a member of this profession, a physician

II. Reference 8. Clements CD, Ciccone JR. (1984). Ethics and expert witnesses: The troubled role of psychiatrists in court. *Bull Am Acad Psychiatric Law, 12*(2), 127–136. Clements and Ciccone aptly note the same year Stone published his paper that "The central question concerning the role of psychiatrists in court revolves around the understanding of the terms 'expert' and 'justice' and has not been addressed."

must recognize responsibility to the patient first and foremost, as well as to society, to other health professionals, and to self.[9]

Stone seems to assume that forensic expert work entails a doctor–patient relationship, a premise widely disputed in the literature (and discussed more fully in the following), yet does not engage with the question of how a forensic psychiatrist, or any doctor for that matter, can reconcile competing social and professional obligations. He indicates that forensic psychiatrists inappropriately take up either the legal cause of the patient or that of the legal system at the patient's expense, when the AMA Principles suggest that such dilemmas may be both unavoidable and common.

The American Psychiatric Association (APA) adopted the AMA principles and provided annotations that make them more specific to the work of psychiatrists. In response to the 1980 AMA revision, the APA revised its Principles of Medical Ethics with Special Annotations for Psychiatry in 1981.[10] To illustrate, one annotation of the Section 1 prescription to respect human dignity and rights specifies not only that "A psychiatrist should not be a participant in a legally authorized execution," but that "Public education as carried out by an ethical psychiatrist would not utilize appeals based solely on emotion, but would be presented in a professional way and without any potential exploitation of patients." Section 2, which requires honesty and professionalism, says "The psychiatrist should diligently guard against exploiting information furnished by the patient and should not use the unique power afforded him/her by the psychotherapeutic situation to influence the patient in any way not directly relevant to the treatment goals." Section 4 enjoins us to protect confidentiality and privacy within the constraints of the law. Section 7 encourages psychiatrists "to serve society by consulting with executive, legislative, and judiciary branches of government," with the caveat that "Psychiatrists should always be mindful of their separate roles as dedicated citizens and as experts in psychological medicine." In sum, the APA's *Annotations* explicitly anticipate and consider the biases Stone feared forensic experts would never be able to avoid.

Many articulate voices from forensic psychiatry have responded to Stone since 1984. Various authors have argued that Stone's concerns about an expert harming an evaluee in a professionally relevant manner are unwarranted, since expert evaluations do not establish a doctor–patient relationship.[11,12] Furthermore, the psychiatrist is not the one who makes the legal decision at issue.[13–15] Others have resisted Stone's accusation that expert work constitutes "prostitution" of the psychiatric profession,[13] and that forensic psychiatrists are just "hired guns" whose assessment inevitably supports the side that pays them.[16] Appelbaum emphasized that forensic psychiatrists can uphold respect for evaluees as persons (in keeping with the bioethics tradition), and argued that experts can and must be truthful in reports and testimony.[11] Many more articles, and at least three comprehensive books[17–19] have been written specifically to articulate standards and guide ethical behavior in forensic expert work.

Forensic psychiatry as a profession has responded as well. The American Academy of Psychiatry and the Law (AAPL), largely in response to Stone, formally proposed "Ethics guidelines for the practice of forensic psychiatry" in 1987, and revised them twice since then.[20] The AAPL explicitly recognizes that forensic psychiatrists have "competing duties to the patient and to society" and attempts to supplement the APA Annotations to accommodate the unique ethical challenges of forensic psychiatric work. In doing so, AAPL uses the principle of transitivity to suggest that forensic psychiatry is a medical practice: If the AAPL guidelines are continuous with the APA Annotations, and the APA Annotations are continuous with the AMA Principles, then the ethics of forensic psychiatry is part of medical ethics in general, and forensic psychiatry is not qualitatively different from patient-centered psychiatry. The directives endorsed by the AAPL are (1) protecting evaluees' confidentiality to the greatest extent possible, (2) obtaining consent to do evaluations when the outcome may cause *social* harm to evaluees, (3) being honest with all parties and striving for objectivity in one's reasoning process,[III] and (4) having the appropriate professional qualifications to do forensic psychiatric work. In other words, the AAPL contradicts Stone's conclusion that it is conceptually impossible to delineate the ethics of forensic psychiatry, and that there is no way to uphold the mandates of medical ethics in the context of forensic work.

Responding to Stone from the Ivory Tower

As mentioned, Stone adopted "the basic premise of the purists," the claim that forensic psychiatrists are incapable of providing conclusive scientific conclusions about mental illness or disability, and also incapable of speaking authoritatively about human values. Stone invokes the philosopher Immanuel Kant as one of the "purists" he cites, an unusual move in medical ethics generally, since Kant's work tends to be theoretical, abstract, and difficult to apply to daily life.[18] Stone dismisses Kant's widely studied moral framework, the Categorical Imperative (CI), as "more convincing as an abstract statement than as a useful moral guide," yet he uses Kant's lesser work, *Anthropology from a Pragmatic Point of View*, to support his own position that psychiatry is incapable of providing real insight into psychological function. Stone is correct that Kant's CI cannot answer specific questions about ethical psychiatric practice, but the same can be said about moral theory in general, which is not intended to prescribe specific actions for particular situations.

In contrast to Stone, and in keeping with his own adoption of Kant's work as authoritative, I argue that Kant's description of the CI in the *Groundwork for the Metaphysics of Morals* provides three useful conceptual tools for understanding forensic psychiatric ethics.[21] These tools are his conception of the moral community, his notion of intrinsic moral worth, and his particular conception of autonomy and its antithesis, heteronomy.

Kant provides the CI as an account of what it is to behave ethically, or to "act in accordance with duty" in his words. He provides three formulations for the CI, one of which specifies that every person be recognized to have moral worth and human dignity, and thus be considered an end in herself rather than a means to some other aim. We have seen that this "moral worth" formulation is recognized by forensic psychiatric ethics,[11] and in medical ethics more generally.[7,22] The moral worth of persons is specified in all of the formal ethical guidelines discussed previously, and constitutes part of the conception of autonomy widely used in medical and research ethics.

III. The original guidelines called for objectivity, but were softened in 2005 to "striving for objectivity."

Another formulation of the CI reminds us that ethical behavior in any setting occurs within a community of moral agents, all of whom have moral worth. This is relevant to discussions about whether forensic psychiatry, especially expert witness work, constitutes the practice of medicine, and if so, whether forensic psychiatrists are bound by the same rules and guidelines as other psychiatrists and practitioners of other medical specialties. Philosophers who have weighed in on this question have argued that forensic psychiatrists are both members of the broader society[23] and the community of medical practitioners,[24] and as such are bound by the moral rules that apply to these broader communities. In other words, all moral agents are members of Kant's "realm of ends," or the moral community construed in the broadest possible terms. Within that "realm," the subcommunity of physicians is bound to further rules and guidelines specific to the practice of medicine. Subdividing further, psychiatrists hold themselves to the principles of ethics prescribed by the AMA and, in their Annotations, have anticipated ways the AMA guidelines may be applied in psychiatric care. And with respect to psychiatrists who participate in forensic work, the AAPL specifies ethical concerns that forensic psychiatrists must strive to avoid.

Kant's third formulation of the CI ties the first two together and provides some direction for what constitutes ethical action. The agents that comprise the moral community (in its broadest construal) must be "law-givers unto themselves," in the sense that they must hold themselves to act in accordance with duty. To identify what actions are mandated or prohibited by the CI, an agent must identify the principle by which he acts, and consider whether he would want everyone else to act in accordance with it. Kant's well-known example of the application of the "universal law" formulation of the CI considers whether it is ethical to lie: If everyone lied, we would have no basis for communication or belief. We would never be able to trust whether any utterance were ever true. Therefore, we have a moral duty to tell the truth. To summarize, moral agents comprise a moral community whose members "Act only according to that maxim whereby [they] can at the same time will that it should become a universal law."[21]

Putting the three formulations together, Kant concludes that "A rational being belongs to the kingdom of ends as a member when he legislates in it universal laws while also being himself subject to these laws."[21]Note the specification that moral agents are "rational," a word that perks the ears of moral philosophers and psychiatrists alike. Kant thinks that humans are only *imperfectly* rational, since we err in belief and in deed; he acknowledges that we mere mortals make errors of judgment, and that we act wrongly whether we intend to or not. Kant introduces *autonomy* as a technical term to describe the capacity that permits one to be a full member of the moral community and to be a moral lawgiver to oneself, that is, to act according to the universal law, rather than acting in one's own interests.

Kant can be criticized as overly stringent in thus claiming that ethical action precludes the satisfaction of any self-interest, but as argued by Secker,[25] we don't have to be Kantians to use Kantian concepts, as long as they make sense for the social world in which medicine is practiced. The bioethics literature has done something like this in appropriating autonomy as one of the core principles of medical ethics. Beauchamp and Childress describe autonomy as "self-rule that is free from both controlling interference by others and from limitations, such as inadequate understanding, that prevent meaningful choice.

The autonomous individual acts freely in accordance with a self-chosen plan, analogous to the way an independent government manages its territories and sets its policies."[22] We see the influence of Kant here in the references to "self-rule" and "understanding," as well as in the analogy to law, although the meaning of autonomy in bioethics differs from Kant's conception of autonomy. The notion of autonomy promulgated in the bioethics literature focuses on respecting the patient's innate ability and right to make his own (health care) decisions. In contrast, Kant's project is to characterize what constitutes morally right action.

The Kantian concept I want to appropriate for forensic psychiatry is his notion of *heteronomy*, the antithesis of Kantian autonomy. Heteronomy is the state of affairs that occurs when one lacks autonomy, and thus does not identify and act in accordance with moral law. This occurs when an agent factors self-interest into her decision making, and it occurs when she simply chooses not to act morally. Heteronomy also occurs when a person lacks the rational capacity to participate in the moral community, when one is mentally incapable of abiding by the CI.

Stone's references to Kant in 1984 missed the heart of the matter. The job of the psychiatrist is to help persons who have intrinsic moral worth but who lack autonomy in the strict Kantian sense. Psychiatry aims to aid heteronomous persons, whose limitations of rationality or will prevent them from fully participating in the moral community, in order to restore their moral autonomy. One job of the forensic psychiatrist is to determine whether and when heteronomous action is caused by rational limitations (e.g., mental illness) or deliberate nonparticipation in the moral community (e.g., criminal activity). Without psychiatric training, forensic experts would not be in a position to assist in legal proceedings in this way. The Kantian question is whether the psychiatric forensic expert, as a full moral agent participating in the larger moral community, could will as universal law that mental health experts use their medical training to assist the larger community in identifying and characterizing heteronomy.

Stone, I suspect, would say not, given his position that there is no psychiatric truth to be shared with the larger moral community, and because he believes forensic psychiatrists cannot avoid putting other interests before the moral law. However, I think a strong case can be made that the forensic psychiatrist's maxim (to characterize heteronomy for civic purposes) is, indeed, universalizable in the Kantian sense.

Although I do not have the space to make such an argument here, the moral codes to which forensic psychiatrists are already bound reflect an assumption that we *can* will as universal law that forensic psychiatrists assist the courts to characterize heteronomy. As discussed, justice is one of the three pillar principles that have shaped bioethics since the 1970s. Both the AMA and APA specify that physicians must respect the Kantian ideals of honoring the moral worth of persons, acting with honesty and integrity, and protecting private health information, while also acting as civic participants and improving the community. In their latest revisions, both the AMA *Principles* and the APA *Annotations* proscribe physician participation in torture and executions. The AAPL *Guidelines* acknowledge competing medical and social obligations, and reiterate the importance of (1) honoring the moral worth of forensic evaluees by protecting confidentiality and obtaining consent, (2) being honest and striving for objectivity, and (3) being duly qualified as a detector of heteronomy. Unlike Stone, these sources all accept that physician obligations to the patient and to the larger community may conflict, and that there are ways to do forensic work in an ethical manner.

Conclusion

In this chapter I, like many others, have used the provocative "ivory tower" perspective of Alan Stone as a point of departure. Whereas Stone cited the philosophy of Immanuel Kant to conclude that the forensic psychiatric work performed "in the trenches" is inherently unethical, I have used Kant's moral philosophy to argue that even according to Kant's strict standards for moral behavior, forensic psychiatry is not inherently unethical. I would need a much longer discussion to argue the stronger claim that forensic psychiatric work is ethical, given the heterogeneity of settings for it and of the persons who practice it. But I have shown that in the 30 years since Stone voiced his pessimism, medical and psychiatric codes of ethics have aligned in ways that contradict his stance, not only in practice, but in the spirit of one of the philosophical academic "purists" on which Stone bases his position. My purpose here has been to demonstrate that even within the ivory tower, "forensic psychiatric ethics" is not self-contradictory or vacuous. Although metaphysical questions about mind and brain, free will, and the role of values in science will always be debatable, even Kant agrees that life goes on despite our metaphysical conundra.

Certainly, there is more to be done in the academic study of the ethics of forensic psychiatry. Within the Kantian framework I present, if we take autonomy and heteronomy seriously, forensic psychiatry will have to grapple with questions raised by the recovery movement, which always favors patient self-determination, except in very limited situations.[26] If we take seriously the notion of a comprehensive moral community, forensic psychiatry will have to reconcile regional differences in legal and moral attitudes and practices. Beyond my discussion here, the ethics of forensic psychiatry has mostly focused on expert work, whereas forensic psychiatrists work in many other venues.[20] At this point in time, academic work in the ethics of forensic psychiatry lags behind research methods and findings that have advanced bioethics generally, despite the important scholarship Stone's flawed argument spurred. Although there is still work to be done, Stone provoked sustained, directed efforts in the ethics of forensic psychiatry, which will surely continue. In consequentialist (rather than Kantian) terms, then, perhaps the ends justify Stone's means.

References

1. Stone AA. (1984). The ethical boundaries of forensic psychiatry: A view from the ivory tower. *Bull Am Acad Psychiatry Law, 12*, 209–219.
2. Radden J, Sadler JZ. (2010). *The virtuous psychiatrist: Character ethics in psychiatric practice.* New York: Oxford University Press.
3. Barnes B, Bloor D. (1977). *Interests and the growth of knowledge.* Boston: Routledge & Kegan Paul.
4. Feyerabend PK. (1975). *Against method.* London: NLB.
5. Kuhn T. (1962). *Structure of scientific revolutions.* Chicago: University of Chicago Press.
6. Davidson D. (1970). *Essays on actions and events.* Oxford, UK: Clarendon Press.

7. National Commission for the Protection of Research Subjects of Biomedical and Behavioral Research. (1979). *The Belmont report: Ethical principles and guidelines for the protection of human subjects of research*, 10.
8. Clements CD, Ciccone JR. (1984). Ethics and expert witnesses: The troubled role of psychiatrists in court. *Bull Am Acad Psychiatric Law, 12*(2), 127–136.
9. American Medical Association. (2000). Principles of medical ethics. In Council on Ethical and Judicial Affairs (Ed.), *Code of medical ethics—Current opinions, 2000–2001* (14th ed.). Chicago: American Medical Association.
10. American Psychiatric Association. (2013). *Principles of medical ethics with annotations especially applicable to psychiatry*. Arlington, VA: American Psychiatric Association.
11. Appelbaum PS. (1997). A theory of ethics for forensic psychiatry. *J Am Acad Psychiatry Law, 25*, 233–247.
12. Modlin HC. (1984). The ivory tower v. the marketplace. *Bull Am Acad Psychiatric Law, 12*, 233–236.
13. Weiner BA. (1984). Ethical issues in forensic psychiatry: From an attorney's perspective. *Bull Am Acad Psychiatric Law, 12*, 253–261.
14. Zonana HV. (1984). Forensic psychiatry: Critique of a critique. *Bull Am Acad Psychiatric Law, 12*, 237–241.
15. Dike CC. (2008). Commentary: Is ethical forensic practice an oxymoron? *J Am Acad Psychiatry Law, 36*, 181–184.
16. Diamond BL. (1990). The psychiatrist expert witness: Honest advocate or 'hired gun'? In R Rosner, & R Weinstock (Eds.), *Ethical practice in psychiatry and the law* (pp. 75–84). New York: Plenum.
17. Rosner R, & Weinstock R (Eds.) (1990). *Ethical practice in psychiatry and the law*. New York: Plenum.
18. Candilis PJ, Weinstock R, & Martinez R. (2007). *Forensic ethics and the expert witness*. New York: Springer Science.
19. Sadoff RL. (2011). *Ethical issues in forensic psychiatry: Minimizing harm*. New York: Wiley-Blackwell.
20. American Academy of Psychiatry and the Law. (2005). *Ethics guidelines for the practice of forensic psychiatry*. Bloomfield, CT: American Association for Psychiatry and the Law.
21. Kant I. (1993/1785). *Grounding for the metaphysics of morals* (3rd ed.) Indianapolis: Hackett.
22. Beauchamp T, & Childress JF. (1983). *Principles of biomedical ethics* (2nd ed.). New York: Oxford University Press.
23. Radden J. (2001). Boundary violation ethics: Some conceptual clarifications. *J Am Assoc Psychiatry Law, 29*, 319–326.
24. Foot P. (1990). Ethics and the death penalty: Participation by psychiatrists in capital trials. In R Rosner, & R Weinstock R (Eds.), *Ethical practice in psychiatry and the law* (7th ed., pp. 207–217). New York: Springer Science.
25. Secker B. (1994). The appearance of Kant's deontology in contemporary Kantianism: Concepts of patient autonomy in bioethics. *J Med Philos, 24*(1), 43–66.
26. Pouncey CL, & Lukens JM. (2010). Madness versus badness: The ethical tension between the recovery movement and forensic psychiatry. *Theoret Med Bioethics, 31*, 93–105.

21

Forensic Sleep Medicine

Sleepwalking, Automatisms, Scientific Evidence, and the Law

Mark R. Pressman

> ...the courtroom is not the place for scientific guesswork, even of the inspired sort. Law lags science, it does not lead it.[1]

Sleep walking and its related disorders have been reported to be associated with violence and otherwise criminal acts going back hundreds if not thousands of years.[2] The description of the motor and cognitive behavior of ancient sleepwalkers is often similar to modern diagnostic descriptions but contaminated by religious, superstitious, and medical beliefs of the time. Additionally, *sleepwalking* was often a catchall term for what would now be several diagnostically and physiologically distinct disorders. Not all things that go bump in the night are sleepwalking, then or now. The modern differential diagnosis of "nocturnal wandering" includes sleepwalking as well as other diagnoses, such as epilepsy, alcohol intoxication, and REM Behavior Disorder must also be ruled out.[3] Thus, ancient diagnoses of sleepwalking may lump together numerous disorders that have been separated by modern sleep medicine.

Since ancient times, research and knowledge of sleep science and sleepwalking and related disorders has proceeded by fits and starts. However, with the availability of digital technology there has been a dramatic increase in published research—and our understanding of sleepwalking—in the last 10 years. However, legal approaches to automatisms and sleepwalking have continued to lag dramatically behind modern sleep science with nineteenth century legal principles often applied.

Despite the differing explanations over the cause of sleepwalking, it has generally been held that the sleepwalker who commits a criminal act is not criminally liable. The 1313 Council of Vienne[10] stated:

> If a child, madman or sleeper killed someone he was not culpable.

Diego de Covarrubias (1512–1577) as translated from the Latin by Walker:

> It follows of course... that a person who was asleep at the time of the homicide is not at fault, for the obvious reason that he was asleep when he killed his victim; such one lacks understanding and reason, and is like a madman.... For this reason the misdeed of a sleeper is not punished, unless it happens that in his waking state he knew very well that in his sleep he would seize weapons and attack people. For then if he did not take care to prevent himself from doing harm in his sleep to someone, certainly he should be punished, although not in the usual way.

A Scottish jurist, McKenzie (1678),[4] noted that "such as commit any crime whilst the sleep, are compared to infants."

Issac Ray, in his landmark volume, *Treatise of Mental Jurisprudence of Insanity*, discusses forensic aspects of somnambulism.[5]

> §508. As the somnambulist does not enjoy the free and rational exercise of his understanding, and is more or less unconscious of his outward relations, none of his acts, during the paroxysms, can rightfully be imputed to him as crimes. (p. 509)

The sometimes violent nature of sleepwalking since Victorian times has often been attributed to Freudian/psychodynamic ideas of trauma and the purpose of dreaming. Indeed, these concepts persist to this day in some areas of psychiatry.

Major Landmarks in Sleep Science

The diagnosis and understanding of the pathophysiology of sleepwalking has changed dramatically in the last 50 to 60 years.

Discovery of Rapid Eye Movement Sleep

Until the 1950s, somnambulism and related disorders were thought to be secondary to dreaming. However, there was no physiological description of dreaming. In 1953 Aserinsky and colleague for the first time noted, based on a laboratory recording, that dreaming was associated with very specific changes in physiology.[6] Rapid eye movement (REM) sleep was distinctly different than other types of sleep. Brain wave activity resembled wakefulness, although the sleeping subject was not awake and bursts of rapid eye movements were notable. Several years later it was noted that when these physiological signs were present they were joined by a third biological marker of dreaming, namely, the absence of voluntary muscle tone (electromyography) except for the extraocular muscles responsible for rapid eye movements.[7,8] However, this finding was not immediately applied to the theory of sleepwalking as enacted dreaming. Only later was it determined that if voluntary muscle tone was absent during REM sleep, then dreamers could not walk or other complex behaviors were not possible. Thus, the actions of a sleepwalking individual could not be attributed to REM dreaming. More recently this has become more complicated. It is still held that sleepwalkers are not acting out REM–sleep related dreams, but they may indeed recall dream-like imagery.[9] Sleep terrors have always been associated with a frightening image. However, this image tended to be static and lacked features of REM–sleep related dreaming. It is possible that some sleepwalkers also have frightening images at the start of their episodes that are not related to REM dreaming.

In 1985 REM Behavior Disorder (RBD) was first described.[10] In this disorder the neural mechanisms that inhibit muscle tone at the level of the motor neurons do not function properly. The result is that dreams actually are enacted, as was hypothesized incorrectly for sleepwalking 50+ years ago. The differential diagnosis between sleepwalking and RBD is actually fairly easy, and rarely has RBD been implicated in legal cases.

First Polysomnograms (Sleep Studies)

The dramatic implications of REM sleep atonia were not appreciated until the first modern sleep research laboratories were established and studied known sleepwalkers. The first published research studies in 1964 shattered all prior notions of sleepwalking as enacted dreaming.[11,12] Sleepwalking as well as the related disorder sleep terrors did not occur during the easily identified state of REM sleep. Rather, the occurred during periods of deep sleep characterized by high amplitude delta waves. Thus, sleepwalking was noted to be a disorder of NREM (non–rapid eye movement) sleep, not REM sleep.

Forensic Applications

With the description of the evaluation of sleepwalkers in the sleep laboratory, "objective" sleep study evidence started to be presented in court as part of the sleepwalking defense.[13,14] Defense experts continue to present this type of evidence, although the effects of evidence-based medicine and reliable sleep science have largely countered this evidence. First, sleep studies are often performed for forensic purposes months or even years after the date of the violent episode.[15,16] Current sleep science suggests that complex episodes of sleepwalking are the result of a perfect storm of genetics, priming factors, and triggers.[16] It is impossible to recreate these factors in the sleep laboratory. In fact, it is well known clinically that even frequent sleepwalkers will not sleepwalk in the sleep laboratory. Second, sleep studies may document potential triggers or other findings consistent with the clinical diagnosis of sleepwalking, but cannot determine if they were present on the night of the criminal incident.[17] Third, there are no reliable biomarkers for sleepwalking in the sleep study. Early studies reported that sleepwalking was often associated with frequent arousals from deep sleep as well as so-called hypersynchronous delta waves. The classic electroencephalograph (EEG) findings have been shown to have poor sensitivity and specificity for sleepwalking.

In the late 1960s these findings were further extended by Dr. Roger Broughton, who noted that sleepwalking and related disorders often appeared to follow a sudden arousal from deep sleep.[18] Since that time, sleepwalking along with sleep terrors and confusional arousals have been classified as Disorders of Arousal because of the fact that their pathophysiology is thought to be similar.

Legal Aspects of Automatisms

The traditional evaluation of automatisms was related not only to criminal responsibility, but also to public policy concerns about future dangerousness. A finding of insane automatism suggests that the defendant requires an indefinite hospital order because of the likelihood of dangerous behavior recurring. A finding of noninsane automatism suggests future danger is limited or nonexistent. The classic test—still in use in the United Kingdom—of whether future dangerousness exists is whether the behavior was (is) caused by an internal or external factor. An example of an automatism caused by an external factor is a sudden blow to the head. Because a second or third blow to the head was not thought to be likely, the risk of the automatisms recurring and endangering the public was thought to be very low. On the other hand, disorders that occurred as the result of internal factors—epilepsy, schizophrenia, sleepwalking—were thought to represent potential continuing danger to the public. Of course, these rules were established during a time period in which effective treatments did not exist.[19] The weakness and unfairness of this system was recognized even in the nineteenth century. The internal/external factor system could result in epilepsy being labeled as insanity as well as indefinite hospitalization in an insane asylum. The legal standing of sleepwalking as an insane automatism was established in the United Kingdom in 1991 in *R v. Burgess*. The court ruled that because the defendant was essentially unconscious, he could not form the necessary *mens rea*, and because sleepwalking was caused by an internal factor sleepwalking it was consistent with M'Naughten and qualified as insanity. However, not all courts in the United Kingdom continue view sleepwalking as an insane automatism, and there are recent examples of defendants acquitted and allowed to walk free with no punishment or court-ordered supervision. The Law Commission of the United Kingdom recently recommended abandoning the internal/external system as archaic and based on out-of-date science.[19]

In Canada, there has been a recent shift in the legal approach to sleepwalking as a defense. The 1985 Parks case had established that sleepwalking was to be considered a non-insane automatism.[13] The Supreme Court of Canada found that sleepwalking was not a "mental disease or defect," and because sleep was a normal state of consciousness, that sleepwalking could not be considered insanity. Thus, until 2012 all sleepwalking cases were tried as non-insane automatisms, and as such a finding might not result in any punishment or continuing supervision by the court or other government body. Mr. Parks was acquitted of murdering his mother-in-law and the attempted murder of his father-in-law.

The appeal of the more recent Luedecke case to the Ontario Supreme Court changed this completely.[20] Mr. Luedecke was arrested for sexual assault. And although he had been alcohol intoxicated at the time, his defense successfully argued that the alcohol had triggered an episode of sleepwalking and sexual behavior in sleep. The Crown Prosecution did not present a counterargument via its own expert, and Mr. Luedecke was found to have been in a state of non-insane automatism at the time of the sexual assault. He was acquitted and released without any required supervision. His acquittal and release led to a national uproar, and the Crown appealed the verdict. The Court of Appeals for Ontario did not allow a retrial, but did make several important changes to the law. First, they declared that a sleepwalking defense would heretofore be an insane automatism. The reasoning was that insanity is a legal term, not to be confused with medical/psychological terminology such as psychosis or schizophrenia. The purpose of insanity statutes is not just to determine if there was criminal intent, but also to protect the public from future dangerous behavior. Thus, sleepwalking was to be considered an insane automatism in the future with the burden of proof on the defense. If the court were to determine that the defendant was not criminally liable because of an insane automatism, the defendant would not criminally responsible on account of mental disorder (NCR-MD) and be remanded for a determination of dangerousness and disposition.

In recent times sleep medicine has become a full-fledged specialty. Forensic psychologists, psychiatrists, and others who have not specialized in sleep medicine may lack the knowledge and expertise to perform sleep medicine evaluations and expert testimony. The effect of evidence-based medicine has also had an effect on whether or not scientific evidence is considered to be currently reliable.

A good example of the effect of evidence-based medicine and its corresponding legal field of reliable scientific evidence is the relationship between alcohol and sleepwalking. In the last 10 years numerous criminal cases, especially in the United Kingdom and Canada, have offered the theory that the criminal actions of severely alcohol-intoxicated defendants should not be evaluated based on voluntary intoxication laws that would severely limit or exclude an alcohol-related defense.[21] Rather, they pointed to the fact that alcohol has appeared for many years on lists of potential triggers for sleepwalking. Thus, they advanced the theory that the criminal act did not result directly from alcohol intoxication, but rather that alcohol merely triggered sleepwalking, therefore allowing an automatism defense and the potential for an acquittal or a legal disposition that did not include prison. These lists never provided even a single scientific citation to support this alcohol-induced sleepwalking theory.

Evidence-based medicine has produced a number of scientific publications that point out the lack of reliable evidence supporting this theory. There has never been a sleep laboratory study in which alcohol was given to a clinically diagnosed sleepwalker under controlled conditions. There are no normative, sensitivity, or specificity data. More recently, studies employing retrospective questionnaire techniques have reported a small percentage of patients who believe prior episodes to have been related to alcohol.[22] However, these same patients have also reported amnesia for these same episodes, strongly suggesting that descriptions of prior episodes could not have originated with them. Recall bias and hearsay make these reports very unreliable. This has resulted in a change in how the major classification/diagnostic publications (DSM-5,[23] ICSD-3[24]) and major textbooks have approached this question.[25] The DSM-4 TR published in 2000 stated:

> Associated descriptive features and mental disorder: Internal stimuli (e.g., a distended bladder) or external stimuli (e.g., noises) can increase the likelihood of a sleepwalking episode as can psychosocial stressors and alcohol and sedative use. (p. 640)
>
> Differential Diagnosis: Sleepwalking may be induced by use of, or withdrawal from, substances or medications (e.g., alcohol, benzodiazepines, opiates, cocaine, nicotine, antipsychotics, tricyclic antidepressants, chloral hydrate). (p. 643)

However, the DSM-5 had removed all reference to alcohol as a trigger or risk factor for sleepwalking and instead inserted language to alert the diagnostician that alcoholic blackout should be considered.

> Risk and Prognostic Factors: Environmental. Sedative use, sleep deprivation, sleep-wake schedule disruptions, fatigue and physical or emotional stress increase the likelihood of episodes. Fever and sleep deprivation can produce an increased frequency of NREM sleep arousal disorders. (p. 401)
>
> Differential Diagnosis: Alcohol-induced blackouts. Alcohol-induced blackouts may be associated with extremely complex behaviors in the absence of other suggestions of intoxication. They do not involve loss of consciousness but rather reflect an isolated disruption of memory for events during a drinking episode. By history, these behaviors may be indistinguishable from those seen in NREM sleep arousal disorders. (p. 403)

The International Classification of Sleep Disorders (ICSD), 3rd ed., has removed all reference to alcohol as a trigger or risk factor for sleepwalking. Instead, it explicitly states sleepwalking should not be diagnosed in the presence of alcohol intoxication.

The ICSD is the only diagnostic and coding manual specially published for sleep disorders. Originally published in 1979, the second version of the ICSD was published in 2005, but included no scientific citations after 2000. In ICSD-2 under Confusional Arousals (p. 139), alcohol consumption is listed as a "precipitating" factor. Under Sleepwalking (p. 143) "Alcohol use and abuse are other factors" noted to be precipitators. However, ICSD-3, published in March of 2014, has eliminated all reference to alcohol as a trigger or risk factor for sleepwalking and related disorders.

> Alcohol has been identified in previous reports as a potential sleepwalking trigger. However, the amnesia associated with disorders of arousal makes these reports unreliable.

> More recent evidence-based reviews have found no compelling relationship between alcohol and disorders of arousal. (p. 234)
>
> Disorders of arousal should not be diagnosed in the presence of alcohol intoxication. The behavior of the alcohol-intoxicated individual may superficially resemble that of the sleepwalker. However, the sleepwalker is typically severely cognitively impaired, but with only limited motor impairment. The alcohol-intoxicated individual's level of cognitive functioning may be reduced, but not absent, whereas motor behavior is often severely impaired. In alcoholic blackouts, where anterograde amnesia is, by definition, the cardinal manifestation, it is important to note that outward motor behavior and cognitive function may not be impaired and may be perceived as normal. Thus, the importance of appreciating the neuroscience of alcoholic blackouts and its potential role in the explanation of unusual and bizarre nocturnal behaviors cannot be understated because these can mimic parasomnias. The former are exponentially more prevalent and thus should be given appropriate weight when attributing likely causation in cases with criminal allegations. (p. 237)

A common defense tactic in sleepwalking cases is to focus solely on whether or not alcohol could be a trigger for sleepwalking while essentially ignoring the exceptional strong scientific and forensic data showing that alcohol is linked to violence in general as well as to violent criminal acts and sexual assaults. On the scientific side, a recent PubMed search found no experimental studies of alcohol on the behavior of known sleepwalkers. However, almost 5000 experimental studies of the effects of alcohol on brain and behavior in humans were noted. This included 400 published studies of alcohol and sexual behavior as well as 105 studies of alcohol and violence. Forensic data from the United States and the United Kingdom report millions of episodes of alcohol-related violence and sexual assault every year.

Forensic experts and the courts should approach the published sleep medicine literature carefully. Recent advances in sleep medicine and sleep science may not immediately find their way into court as part of expert evidence.[26] New data or data that corrects, repudiates, or contradicts previously published data may not even find their way into clinically oriented books, book chapters, or review articles for many years after publication. Even articles that have been retracted continue to be cited for many years. Corrected articles have been reported to require 8 to 12 years before they are cited more often than the original articles. How often contradicted, corrected, repudiated, or retracted articles are cited as the basis for expert evidence in sleepwalking defense cases is unknown.

Many misconceptions regarding sleepwalking continue to be presented in court due either to the fact that the admitted expert is not really a sleep or sleepwalking expert, a failure by the experts to keep up the scientific literature, or a deliberate attempt to mold expert testimony to fit the defense or prosecution theories of the crime.

These are common misconceptions not only of forensic experts, but are likely to be thought of as common knowledge by the jury.

1. *Sleepwalkers are acting out their dreams.* It has been known for almost 50 years that sleepwalkers are not acting out their dreams. However, recent published research suggests that some sleepwalkers may recall frightening images associated with their walking.
2. *Sleepwalkers are enacting dreams related to prior psychological traumas.*
   This pseudo-Freudian theory has shown a lot of staying power even in the face of direct tests of clinically diagnosed sleepwalkers with psychological tests that show that sleepwalkers are no more prone to psychological disorders or trauma than normal controls.
3. *Sleepwalking is a kind of seizure.* The lay public may describe thrashing around in bed as a form of seizure, and seizure can occur concurrently with sleepwalking. However, for the overwhelming majority of sleepwalkers there are no abnormalities in the EEG or the brain.
4. *Alcohol can trigger sleepwalking.* As noted, there are no reliable scientific data to support this claim.
5. *Drugs can cause sleepwalking and variants of sleepwalking, such as sleep eating and sleep driving.* Complex and occasionally bizarre behaviors have been attributed to the effects of sedative hypnotics and antidepressants, but it is uncertain that these behaviors occur because of activation or deactivation of the same areas of the brain or nerve pathways responsible for sleepwalking.
6. *Sleepwalkers generally have anterograde amnesia for the episodes.* Alcohol intoxication may produce the same effects on memory.
7. *Sleepwalkers re-enact behaviors or intents from prior wakefulness.* In sleepwalkers, higher cognitive functions such as memory, planning, and social skills are essentially turned off. Thus, a true sleepwalker should not have access to memories or intents formed earlier while awake.
8. *Waking a sleepwalker in the middle of an episode can cause injury to the sleepwalker.* There is no evidence that attempting to awaken a sleepwalker will do any harm to him or her, but it may elicit defensive aggression and violence against the person trying to awaken the sleepwalker.
9. *Sleepwalkers are violent and seek out victims for revenge.* There is no evidence that sleepwalkers seek out and initiate violent behaviors. Alternately, in the overwhelming majority of cases of sleepwalking-related violence, the ultimate victim of violence comes to the sleepwalker and may block or grab him or her. Sleepwalkers cannot recognize faces.[27]
10. *Sleepwalkers have their eyes closed.* Sleepwalkers walk with eyes open. Sleepwalkers are reported to have eyes open. They appear able to navigate in familiar surrounding but frequent injury due to falls or bumping into furniture are reported.
11. *Sleepwalking episodes may wax and wane.* There is no evidence that sleepwalking episodes may wax and wane over long periods. All evidence suggesting that if a sleepwalking episode stops, sleepwalking may only resume again if the complete process is repeated—fall asleep, enter deep sleep, arousal is triggered. And then there is no guarantee that the same behaviors will recur.

12. *Sleepwalking episodes can last for hours.* The overwhelming majority of episodes of sleepwalking are reported to last seconds or minutes. Longer episodes are much rarer, although occasional episodes are reported to last 30 to 60 minutes.

Occasionally novel or unreliable science has been admitted by judges in sleepwalking defense cases. On several occasions this occurred when the prosecution did not present an expert witness of its own. The prosecution should be made aware that both judges and juries appear willing to consider a sleepwalking defense. Also, a successful cross-examination of an expert is not likely to be effective without the assistance of a knowledgeable sleep medicine expert.

Finally, the forensic expert in a sleepwalking defense trial should remember that the goal of an evaluation is to determine if the defendant was in a state of parasomnia during the episode, not that he or she currently—months or years later or in the past—had signs or symptoms suggestive of sleep walking or sleep sex.

References

1. Rosen v Ciba-Guigy Corp. In: Court of Appeals, 7th Circuit 1996.
2. Bonkalo A. (1974). Impulsive acts and confusional states during incomplete arousal from sleep: Crinimological and forensic implications. *Psychiat Quart, 48*, 400–409.
3. Ohayon MM, Mahowald MW, Dauvilliers Y, Krystal AD, & Leger D. (2012). Prevalence and comorbidity of nocturnal wandering in the U.S. adult general population. *Neurology, 78*, 1583–1589.
4. Petrain D. (2010). An English translation of John William Polidori's (1815) medical dissertation on Oneirodynia (somnambulism). *Eur Rom Rev, 21*, 775–788.
5. Ray I. (1838). *A treatise on the medical jurisprudence of insanity.* Boston: Charles C. Little and James Brown.
6. Aserinsky E, & Kleitman N. (1953). Regularly occurring periods of eye motility, and concomittant phenomena, during sleep. *Science, 118*, 273–274.
7. Hodes RDWC. (1963). *Abolition of electrically induced reflexes during rapid eye movement (REM) periods of sleep normal subject (preliminary report).* Brooklyn, NY: Association for the Psychophysiology of Sleep.
8. Jacobson AKA, Lehmann D, & Hoedemaker FS. (1964). Muscle tonus in human subjects during sleep and dreaming. *Exp Neurol, 10*, 418–424.
9. Oudiette D, Leu S, Pottier M, Buzare MA, Brion A, & Arnulf I. (2009). Dreamlike mentations during sleepwalking and sleep terrors in adults. *Sleep, 32*, 1621–1627.
10. Schenck CH, Bundlie SR, Ettinger MG, & Mahowald MW. (1986). Chronic behavioral disorders of human REM sleep: A new category of parasomnia. *Sleep, 9*, 293–308.
11. Jacobson A, Kales A, Lehmann D, & Zweizig J. (1965). Somnambulism: All-night electroencephalographic studies. *Science, 148*, 975–977.
12. Kales A, Jacobson A, Paulson MJ, Kales JD, & Walter RD. (1966). Somnambulism: Psychophysiologi cal correlates. I. All-night EEG studies. *Arch Gen Psychiatry, 14*, 586–594.
13. R. v Parks. 2 S.C.C.R. 871; 95 D.L.R. (4th) 27 (1992).
14. Arizona v Scott Falater (1999).
15. Mahowald MW, Schenck CH, & Cramer-Bornemann M. (2007). Finally—Sleep science for the courtroom. *Sleep Med Rev, 11*, 1–3.
16. Pressman MR. (2007). Factors that predispose, prime and precipitate NREM parasomnias in adults: Clinical and forensic implications. *Sleep Med Rev, 11*, 5–30.

17. Pressman MR. (2004). Hypersynchronous delta sleep EEG activity and sudden arousals from slow-wave sleep in adults without a history of parasomnias: Clinical and forensic implications. *Sleep, 27*, 706–710.
18. Broughton RJ. (1968). Sleep disorders: Disorders of arousal? Enuresis, somnambulism, and nightmares occur in confusional states of arousal, not in "dreaming sleep". *Science, 159*, 1070–1078.
19. Law Commission (UK). Criminal Liability: Insanity and Automatism Discussion Paper In; 2013. (http://lawcommission.justice.gov.uk/docs/insanity_discussion.pdf)
20. R. v. Luedecke (2008). ONCA 716 (CanLII), <http://canlii.ca/t/217d9>
21. Pressman MR, Mahowald MW, Schenck CH, & Bornemann MC. (2007). Alcohol-induced sleepwalking or confusional arousal as a defense to criminal behavior: A review of scientific evidence, methods and forensic considerations. *J Sleep Res, 16*, 198–212.
22. Lopez R, Jaussent I, Scholz S, Bayard S, Montplaisir J, & Dauvilliers Y. (2013). Functional impairment in adult sleepwalkers: A case-control study. *Sleep, 36*, 345–351.
23. American Psychiatric Association. (2000). *Diagnostic and statistical manual of mental disorders*, DSM-IV-TR (4th ed.). Washington, DC: American Psychiatric Association.
24. Medicine AAoS. (2014). *International classification of sleep disorders* (3rd ed.). Darien, IL: American Academy of Sleep Medicine.
25. Cramer Bornemann M, & Mahowald MW. Sleep forensics. In MH Kryger, C Roth, & WC Dement (Eds.), *Principles and practice of sleep medicine* (5th ed., pp. 725–733). Philadelphia: Elsevier Saunders.
26. Peterson GM. (2010). The effectiveness of the practice of correction and republication in the biomedical literature. *J Med Libr Assoc, 98*, 135–139.
27. Pressman MR. (2007). Disorders of arousal from sleep and violent behavior: The role of physical contact and proximity. *Sleep, 30*, 1039–1047.

22

Nobody Wins Without a Good Team

Kathleen Brown

The practice of forensic psychiatry, by its very definition, requires team work. Medical education moves students from a realm of one to one, patient and doctor, to a health care world of working with many other professionals. All physicians learn to work within a health care team comprising fellow physicians with specialized training, nurses, scientists, and many other professionals.

Psychiatrists who choose to work in a forensic capacity must work within the health care team and the criminal justice team. These two teams do not work with each other or against each other; rather, they exist in parallel universes. One team is incredibly cooperative, with everyone working together for the betterment of the patient. The other team is an adversarial one that aspires to find justice via rigorous debate. The dance between and among these two systems is one all forensic psychiatrists must learn. Some dance so admirably they are sought after by members of the criminal justice team. Good dancers have rhythm that can be used as an important vehicle for winning one side of an argument—the side of the defense or prosecution team hiring the psychiatrist.

Navigating two systems that share no historical bond to each other and no obvious connection to each other is challenging. Allied professionals who understand the difficulties and the rhythm make the life of the forensic psychiatrist easier and more productive. Allies also assist the forensic psychiatrist in maintaining central values such as patient health and safety and minimizing harm, while producing an objective, scientific, and useful opinion to the court. One of the best allies for forensic psychiatrists, the best dance partners, if you will, are nurses.

Forensic psychiatrists answer legal questions put forth by the criminal and civil justice systems. The questions put forth by the justice system to forensic psychiatrists vary greatly. The practice of forensic psychiatry requires devotion to meticulous document review, interviews, testing, report writing, and testifying in court. The practice also requires a large amount of admirable creativity, because no two cases are identical.

Psychiatrists moving in the world of forensic psychiatry cases do not leave behind their colleagues in the health care system. Forensic psychiatry requires team work and partnerships with the justice system and the health care system. Knowledge of both systems and the players within them is a requirement for successful practice of all forensic psychiatrists.

The nursing profession is an important part of both teams the forensic psychiatrist must navigate. Physicians who practice medicine in any specialty area cannot imagine a practice of medicine without nursing at its side. Nurses have worked beside physicians since Florence Nightingale, and although nursing practice has changed over the years, working with physicians has always been equally important to nursing as it is to medicine.

Nursing: Definitions and Psychiatric Mental Health Nursing

Nursing, by definition, is the protection, promotion, and optimization of health and abilities, prevention of illness and injury, alleviation of suffering through the diagnosis and treatment of human response, and advocacy in the care of individuals, families, communities, and populations.[1]

Psychiatric mental health nursing is a specialty within nursing. Psychiatric mental health registered nurses (PMHN) work with individuals, families, groups, and communities, assessing their mental health needs. The PMHN develops a nursing diagnosis and plan of care, implements the nursing process, and evaluates it for effectiveness.[1]

Psychiatric Mental Health Advanced Practice Registered Nurses (PMH-APRNs) offer primary care services to the psychiatric-mental health population. The PMH-APRNs assess, diagnose, and treat individuals and families with psychiatric disorders or the potential for such disorders using their full scope of therapeutic skills, including the prescription of medication and administration of psychotherapy.[1]

Through the APRN Consensus Model, all PMH-APRNs are academically prepared to provide mental health promotion and mental illness diagnosis and treatment across the life span. Areas of subspecialty include child and adolescent mental health nursing, gerontological-psychiatric nursing, forensics, or substance use disorders.[2]

Forensic psychiatrists work most closely with registered nurses who have chosen psychiatric mental health nursing as a specialty area and with advanced practice psychiatric mental health nurses who have chosen forensics as a subspecialty. Forensic nursing is a recognized specialty in nursing.[1] This specialty allows for application of nursing art and science to clinical legal situations. The nurse's level of education and practice experience greatly influences the role of the nurse on the health care team and the criminal justice team.

Forensic psychiatric mental health advanced practice nurses' most important practice skills are: listening skills, confidence, clinical knowledge, communication skills, nonjudgmental attitude, empathy, patience, knowledge of offending behavior, and ability to do multidisciplinary work.[3]

Research Support for Interdisciplinary Health Care Team Work

Nurses, physicians, and health care organizations must focus on patient safety as well as care quality and always ask the question, "What is best for our patients?"

Rapid advances in biomedical science, improved disease prevention and management, integration of new clinical care technologies, and shifts in care delivery to a broad array of clinical sites contribute to the rapidly increasing need for well-educated, experienced nurses on every health care team.

In 1999, the Institute of Medicine (IOM) issued a comprehensive report, *To Err Is Human: Building a Safer Health System*, summarizing problems of patient safety in the US health system.[4] One important recommendation was to create improved safety systems inside health care through implementation of safe practices at the delivery level, including interdisciplinary clinical practice among health professionals. Interdisciplinary practice or collaboration is defined as a joint decision-making and communication process among health care providers with the goal of satisfying the needs of the patient while respecting the unique abilities of each professional involved in the care.[5] Attributes of interdisciplinary collaboration include trust, knowledge, mutual respect, good communication, cooperation, coordination, shared responsibility, and optimism.[6]

Today's best integrated health delivery systems are evolving toward a model of care in which interdisciplinary teams of providers manage the care of complex patients. Studies of environments that support collaboration among physicians, nurses, and allied health professionals have shown evidence of improved outcomes for both acutely and chronically ill patients.[7]

Science and Technology

The shift to science and technology in medicine and nursing has reconfigured the health care team. Physicians and nurses continue to work together as important allies for their patients, but the practices of both disciplines are increasingly complex, requiring scientific assessment, diagnoses, and treatment, balancing the need for technical competence with the still-important traditional arts of nursing and medicine. Science and technology have driven the team to greater dependence on each other in order to provide the best care and treatment for patients, whether inpatients or outpatients. Skilled nurses are needed to achieve a balance of care, which preserves the humanity and dignity of patients, their relatives, and their caretakers.

The practice of psychiatry is not immune to the shift toward science and technology. The growing fields of genetics and neuroscience interface with forensic psychiatry, and the translation of neurological sciences can be important to answering select legal questions for the forensic psychiatrist.

Nursing in Criminal and Civil Justice Systems

Nurses who work in areas of health care that directly interface with the public interact with the health care team and additional team members. Law enforcement commonly interacts with nurses who work in urgent health care settings such as trauma units, emergency departments for adults or children, and psychiatric mental health emergency units. Patients often arrive in these units accompanied by law enforcement officers. A professional relationship develops with nursing and law enforcement as they work side by side in attempts to achieve and secure the safety of the person under their care. The overall mission of the nurse in urgent care situations is to work with the health care team providing the best possible care to each and every patient. The overall responsibility of law enforcement is public safety. While working with nurses, law enforcement officers will ensure safety for the entire health care team and their patients, while at the same time seeking evidence that may be used for purposes of arrest, thereby ensuring safety to the public at large.

The role of nurses working in urgent care situations in tandem with law enforcement officers often requires their explaining actions and findings to law enforcement as well as prosecutors and defense attorneys. Examples include child abuse cases, cases of child and adult sex crimes, automobile accidents that cause physical injury, shootings and stabbings, and injuries from domestic violence. If a patient with mental health issues is determined to require an evaluation in a psychiatric mental health inpatient unit because of threats of injury to self or others, law enforcement is often present to ensure the safety and security of the patient and the health care team.

Explanations given by nursing professionals may occur during or shortly after treatment, but most often explanations are given long after the acute event. Assistance may be in the form of explanations, can be in the form of reading and understanding health records, since it is not at all unusual for law enforcement officers, prosecutors, and defense attorneys to lack understanding of health records, which may contain important information relevant to legal investigations.

Law enforcement, prosecutors, and defense attorneys often need assistance understanding hospital policy and procedures such as transfers to psychiatric inpatient units and other units within the hospital system. Reasons for such procedures involved in transfer are important to law enforcement officers in order to ensure safety, security, and prevent loss of evidence.

Prosecutors or defense attorneys may contact nurses for information that may enhance investigation and/or assist in preparation for a trial. A nurse's level of education and years of experience influence and limit the explanations given. Nurses may be asked to explain anatomy and physiology, appropriate to the situation of nursing care, behavior related to trauma, or mental or physical illness. Nurses may testify for either the prosecution or defense in court with the purpose of explaining aspects of nursing science to a jury.

Forensic nursing is a recognized discipline within nursing, but it is not an educational degree in nursing. Nurses who wish to increase consultations with the legal system do so via continuing education experiences and courses at universities. Similar to the path of some forensic psychiatrists, nurses may attend law schools and may obtain a law degree. Nurses may seek educational information specific to one aspect of the law, such as sexual assault, domestic violence, elder abuse, child abuse, or behavior of victims and offenders.

Psychiatric mental health nurses with a bachelor's degree are qualified to work with patients with mental illness without further education and can put forth opinions in a legal realm about nursing care related to patients for whom they cared. Bachelor's degree nurses are licensed by the state to practice nursing and can testify to issues related to standard of care. Nurses who complete a masters in nursing within the specialty area of psychiatric mental health nursing can assess, diagnose, and treat patients with mental illness via a state nurse practitioner license. They can testify about patients they have cared for and can speak to the standard of care for psychiatric nurse practitioners. A very small population of nurses obtains a Ph.D. in nursing, which prepares the nurse for professional life in academia, including conducting research. They are often consulted by the legal system for opinions related to nursing research. Recently, nursing developed a doctor of nursing practice as a specialty area. How this new specialty area will inform legal systems is yet to be determined.

Nurses can directly interface with the court when a question is put forth by the justice system that can be answered via nursing science and appropriate level of education and practice. Advanced practice psychiatric mental health forensic nurses can and do provide the courts with scientific knowledge for explaining or clarifying a legal matter within the psychiatric or mental health field.

De-institutionalization and Re-institutionalization

Nursing has a long history of working in inpatient and outpatient settings with patients diagnosed with mental illness. Nurses and medicine as a team were an important part of the mental health care system that institutionalized and de-institutionalized the mentally ill.

The history of de-institutionalization falls into several stages as policies and objectives changed over time. The early focus was on moving individuals out of state public mental hospitals. In the 1990s, entire institutions began to close in significant numbers because of a greater emphasis on patients' rights such as access to housing and jobs rather than on long-term treatment, and on liberty rights to be treated in the least restrictive setting.

Many people with serious mental illness were moved from mental institutions to other institutional settings: nursing homes, single-room occupancy buildings, and board-and-care homes. Others went to live with families who were ill-equipped and poorly supported to meet their needs.[8]

De-institutionalization, the emptying of state mental hospitals, has been one of the most well-meaning but poorly planned social changes ever carried out in the United States. It was a product of overcrowding and deterioration of hospitals; new medications that significantly improved the symptoms of about half the patients; and a failure to understand that many of the sickest patients were not able to make informed decisions about their own need for medication. De-institutionalization drew enthusiastic support from fiscal conservatives interested primarily in saving funds by shutting state hospitals, as well as from civil rights advocates who believed that mental patients needed to be "liberated." De-institutionalization continues to take place, despite clear evidence that for many patients it has been a disaster.[9]

By the early 1970s, it was becoming evident, particularly in California, that the emptying of state mental hospitals resulted in a marked increase in the number of mentally ill individuals placed in jails and prisons. In 1972 Marc Abramson, a psychiatrist in San Mateo County, published a study reporting a 36% increase in mentally ill prisoners in the county jail and a 100% increase in mentally ill individuals judged to be incompetent to stand trial. He also quoted a state prison psychiatrist who said: "We are literally drowning in patients.... Many more men are being sent to prison who have serious mental problems."[10]

At midyear 2005, according to the Department of Justice, more than half of all prison and jail inmates had a mental health problem, including 705,600 inmates in state prisons, 78,800 in federal prisons, and 479,900 in local jails.

Just as forensic psychiatry developed as a result of societal needs for a specific medicolegal role, the specialty of forensic nursing developed as a result of societal needs and the needs of patients. Nurses took over roles, at the request of society, performed by less qualified personnel in the legal and criminal justice system. The public criticized the criminalization of the mentally ill and demanded better health care for mentally ill offenders.

Nurses who care for mentally ill patients have followed their patients from institutions and hospitals to communities to jails and prisons. Nurses followed the patients into each of these systems and successfully integrated themselves into health care teams and criminal justice teams in all of these venues.

Forensic nurses work with correctional psychiatrists in forensic mental health facilities, jails, and prisons. Within these facilities they work every day in a difficult environment that requires a contradictory mandate of therapy and custody. Security trumps therapy within these environments; they work as agents of care as well as agents of control. Within these environments, nurses are working with initiatives to reduce or eliminate seclusion as a practice, viewing it as contentious and harmful to patients with mental illness.

Case Examples of Nurses and Forensic Psychiatrists Working Together

1. A middle-aged inmate detained in jail reported to sick call one afternoon saying that he wanted to die. He said that he did not want to kill himself, but hoped his life would end soon. He was triaged and referred to a psychiatric nurse practitioner (NP). The NP evaluated the patient, called the treating psychiatrist, and determined that the risk for suicide

was low. The NP ordered the inmate be placed on suicide precautions. Suicide precautions were put into effect and an appointment was made for the inmate to visit with his treating psychiatrist the next morning.

The inmate committed suicide between security checks at approximately midnight, several hours after his evaluation, in his cell via hanging.

A forensic psychiatrist and an NP with a Ph.D. were asked to review relevant records and interview the personnel involved in the case. The forensic psychiatrist focused on the actions of the treating psychiatrist and on the system for suicide watch as well as on the personnel responsible for the watch.

The NP focused on the actions taken by the nurses, in particular the NP, the risk assessment tools in place, and the particular assessment performed for this particular patient/inmate.

The medical examiner ruled the death a suicide. The jail via the Department of Corrections settled the case with the family of the inmate.

2. An elderly woman lived with her son and daughter-in-law. She was nonambulatory, but not cognitively impaired. The woman was left in an upstairs bedroom, not fed, and not cared for. There was no phone in her room and no one living close by who might hear the calls of the elderly woman. The elderly woman perished. When the death was discovered, charges were brought against the son and daughter-in-law.

Several people testified for the prosecutor in the case, including a forensic psychiatrist and an NP with a Ph.D. The forensic psychiatrist focused on the suffering aspect of the case. The NP determined via record review from hospitals and home health care workers that the woman was not cognitively impaired at the time of transfer to the son's home. The NP also testified as to the availability of medical and nursing care surrounding the son's home that was not accessed.

3. A male prison inmate was raped repeatedly over time during a 6-year sentence. He reported the rapes via sick call to several nurses over the 6-year period. None of the nurses encouraged him to officially report the rapes, and none of the nurses recommended protective custody for the inmate.

The inmate developed colon and rectal abnormalities that were not diagnosed or treated by any health care provider in the prison system.

The inmate requested a transfer to another prison. His transfer was granted, and while at the second prison, he was able to obtain the interest of an attorney. The second prison diagnosed and treated the inmate, who was hospitalized for needed colon/rectal surgery.

An NP wrote a report related to this case stating the responsibilities of the nursing personnel at the first prison where the rapes took place, and stating the responsibilities of the prison system via the Prison Rape Elimination Act.

Internal medicine physicians wrote reports related to the colon/rectal injuries.

A forensic psychiatrist evaluated the inmate and wrote a report about his pain and suffering related to the chronic rapes and his mental deterioration related to the rapes and the lack of needed medical and surgical care.

A settlement was reached in favor of the inmate.

Conclusion

Together, nurses and forensic psychiatrists determine risk for violence, provide psychiatric assessment, make recommendations for treatment, and provide expert testimony. Together, nurses and forensic psychiatrists design mental health care plans for every patient while infusing the criminal justice system with neutral fact-based opinions. The challenge in doing this well is ever-present. Physician and nurse teams, working together, assure that each and every person is treated with a humanistic approach as well as a scientific one while consulting with both members of the health care team and members of the criminal justice team.

References

1. American Nurses Association www.nursingworld.org.
2. National Council of State Boards of Nursing https://www.ncsbn.org.
3. Mason T, Lovell A, & Coyle D. (2008). Forensic psychiatric nursing skills and competencies: Role dimensions. *J Psychiatric Mental Health Nurs, 15*, 118–130.
4. Institute of Medicine. (1999). *To err is human: Building a safer health system*. Washington, DC: Institute of Medicine.
5. Colluccio M, & McGuire P. (1983). Collaborative practice: Becoming a reality through primary nursing. *Nursing Admin Quart, 7*, 59–63.
6. Arcangelo V, Fitzgerald M, Carroll D, & David J. (1996). Collaborative care between nurse practitioners and physicians. *Primary Care: Clin Office Pract, 23*(1), 103–113.
7. Pew Center for Health Professionals. (1998). *Recreating health professional practice for a new century*. Washington, DC: Pew Center
8. Torrey EF. (1988). *Nowhere to go: The tragic odyssey of the homeless mentally ill*. New York: Harper & Row.
9. Koyanagi C, & Bazelton D. (2007). *Learning from history: Deinstitutionalization of people with mental illness as precursor to long-term care reform*. Washington, DC: Center for Mental Health Law.
10. Abramson MF. (1972). The criminalization of mentally disordered behavior: Possible side effect of a new mental health law. *Hosp Commun Psychiatry, 23*, 101–105.

23

Criminology and Forensic Psychiatry

Sharing a Discipline

William S. Laufer and Danielle M. Dorn

> Criminology is the body of knowledge regarding crime as a social phenomenon. It includes within its scope the process of making laws, of breaking laws, and of reacting toward the breaking of laws.... The objective of criminology is the development of a body of general and verified principles and of other types of knowledge regarding this process of law, crime, and treatment or prevention.[1] (p. 3)

Leading textbooks in criminology reflect an academic discipline with fairly fixed boundaries.[2,3] Chapters on how crime is measured are followed by an outline of the classical, positive, and neoclassical schools of criminological thought. Critical perspectives, including left and Marxist takes on the state, crime, and law, are given cursory attention. Biological, psychological, and sociological explanations of crime and criminality precede detailed legal descriptions of crimes. Finally, an overview of the criminal law sets the stage for a discussion of the various stages of the criminal justice system. If textbooks reflect a discipline's evolution, the word *stayed* seems to capture Criminology's steady but slow progress. It is both remarkable and telling that Sutherland's (1947) definition of criminology seems as current, enlightened, and informed of recent advances as it did when the first edition of his *Principles of Criminology* was published nearly a century ago.

Textbooks and timeless definitions, though, fail to capture how advances in the methods and approaches employed by criminologists mark the field's progress. From the increasing use of randomized controlled experiments to satisfy stringent evidence-based criteria, to the consideration of a crime's "place" and "context," the discipline is gaining a sophistication that, in some ways, extends it stayed boundaries.[4–7] Criminology is fast becoming a formidable social science.

Much of the same may be said of forensic psychiatry, acknowledging, of course, its more narrow scope, methods, and objectives, such as training, assessment, treatment, and public policy. Forensic psychiatry sits comfortably at an interface between psychiatry and the law where, with distinct subject matter boundaries, the kinds of questions asked are increasingly impressive. From developments in understanding mentally ill offenders; new ways of treating mental illness; to maturing public opinion about mental illness and mental health, this branch of psychiatry is tightly bounded but well-equipped to grapple with the most challenging of all questions.[8] How research from both fields translates into fair, just, and humane policy remains an unmet challenge.[9–11] Criminology and forensic psychiatry inherit many of the limitations and constraints from the very system they serve. At the same time, there does not appear to be a strong enough constituency in either to powerfully influence crime and mental health policy.

Criminology and forensic psychiatry also rely on many of the same methodological advances and opportunities to employ new scientific approaches. Both are concerned with the broad aims of justice, and wrestle with contentious decisions about who is deserving of criminal blame and who should be excused for reasons of mental illness. Both are concerned with the profound effects of correctional and mental health care institutionalization, the availability of treatment, the extent of mental illness in jails and correctional facilities, the prediction of violence in community and institutional settings, and the adversarial role of expert forensic testimony. Of course, both think about their contribution or possible contribution to the successive stages of the criminal process, including determinations of fitness to stand trial and competency to be punished.

In this chapter, we first explore how these allied disciplines are related, and why their relationship is complex and yet close. Second, we attempt to connect some of the leading thinking in criminology to the discipline of forensic psychiatry. Finally, the potential for a more activist and less provincial approach is outlined for both fields.

Sister Disciplines

There is remarkably little discussion in criminology about the field of forensic psychiatry. A review of leading criminology journals reveal very few references to this sister discipline or its journals. Perhaps this may be explained by the fact that both fields have a distinctly bounded subject matter, different training and degree requirements, generally separate outlets for scholarship, and a long intellectual history that—no matter how different from its modern incarnation—supports a strong and proud professional identity.

This is unfortunate because the history of criminology reveals a concentration of psychological and psychiatric determinists whom criminologists claim as their own. Without apologies, criminology takes ownership over psychological and psychiatric explanations of criminality. The psychology and psychiatry of criminal law also fits neatly into criminology. And advances in criminology, most particularly in the neurosciences and biology, are shared outside the field and branded "neurocriminology."[12,13] As Sutherland's definition suggests, criminologists tend to be moved by all forms of science that address the problem of crime and criminal behavior. There need not be a direct application or connection to criminal law or the criminal justice system.

This description of criminology may be enough to conclude that forensic psychiatry is in some important ways related to criminology, perhaps a distant cousin or neglected nephew. In the following, we suggest that the relationship is actually closer, in spite of all the noted differences.

Forensic Psychiatry

Oosterhuis and Loughnan (2014) offer a nuanced account of the history of forensic psychiatry by noting its many "...successions of innovations, advances and successes as well as breaks, detours, reversals, recurrences, and setbacks" (p. 2).[14] According to these authors, "Old views and practices endured while new ones were introduced, rejected, and reintroduced. The meanings of phrases such as 'unsound mind' and the concept of legal non-responsibility, and their consequences for mentally deranged defendants, has varied" (p. 2).[14] More important, the very nature of the inquiry into the accountability of human action—the central question of forensic psychiatry—melds principles, science, ethics, norms, and law that reflect profound social, political, and intellectual traditions. As with other fields of scientific inquiry, the progress of forensic psychiatry is neither linear nor entirely predictable.

Not so long ago, the field of forensic psychiatry was conceived quite narrowly. Selling (1949), for example, waxed poetically about how the practice of psychiatry in relation to courts was one of the oldest forms of psychiatry.[15] In recounting the history of forensic psychology, Bartol and Bartol (2005) observe that many notable figures in the field connect this branch of clinical psychology to a very limited clinical practice that concerns the specific questions raised by laws and the legal system.[16] A more modern and broad view sees both forensic psychiatry and psychology as split between a research function and a professional or clinical practice.[17] Bartol and Bartol (2005) cast this function and practice in terms of *production of knowledge* and *application* to criminal and civil justice system.

This modern or broad view was captured, in large part, by Jonas Robitscher (1972) many years earlier in his influential paper, "The New Face of Legal Psychiatry."[18] Robitscher distinguished old conceptions of psychiatrists confined to the custodial care of inpatients with more enlightened conceptions.[19] Forensic psychiatrists serve courts but are not so limited in function and discipline. Instead, Robitscher (1972) argues, "...the forensic psychiatrist has widened his role to include much more than the courtroom appearance. He uses his psychiatric background and his familiarity with law and the legislative process to deal with juvenile delinquency, aggression, violence, drugs, sexual standards, and a host of other problems that have psychiatric, legal, social, and even political and economic components" (p. 92).[18]

For Robitscher and Robert Sadoff, his successor at the University of Pennsylvania, forensic psychiatry is part of a larger scholarly conversation shared by law, psychiatry, psychology, sociology, social work, and other social and behavioral sciences. As such, leading forensic psychiatrists wrestle with how to capture, in one disciplinary label, the broadening of the discipline's boundaries and the vast "patient-society interaction." Robitscher, for instance, prefers to think of the discipline as "social-legal psychiatry."

There is little doubt that the principal architects of modern forensic psychiatry, such figures as Jonas Rappeport, Karl Menniger, Manfred Guttmacher, William Alanson White, A. Louis McGarry, Seymour Pollock, Bernard Diamond, Alan Stone, Gregory Zilboorg, Maier Tuchler, Irwin Perr, Stanley Portnow, and Robert Sadoff, would express different preferences. There is also little doubt that all would say that the field now has a broad subject matter boundary, a multidisciplinary reach, a distinct and identifiable literature, its own accreditation, unique ethical issues, and a vast number of connections to legal and societal institutions.[20,21]

Consistent with the notion that this field is defined, at least in part, by knowledge production, a host of forensic psychiatrists chronicle advances in substantive knowledge and scientific methods, from significant leaps in knowledge about the biology of criminal behavior to a cascade of research on the neurocorrelates of criminality. Witzel et al. (2008)[22] reflect on the potential for a paradigm shift from traditional models of forensic psychiatry to the emerging field of neuropsychiatry. This entails a move from the subjectivity of psychosocial evidence to the more objective biopsychosocial criteria, criteria reflected in brain–behavior relationships. Glenn, Raine, and Laufer (2011)[23] reflect on mounting neurological evidence that might explain differences in how psychopaths and non-psychopaths calculate risks. This leads to the question, Must criminal law accommodate new understandings of the brain? Dressing et al. (2008) do not go so far and, instead, offer concerns about the potential implications and applications of neurological evidence.[24–28] The broader question about what scientific evidence is appropriately entered into evidence is raised by Bernstein (1995).[29]

While science moves forward, pushing the boundaries of forensic psychiatry, some wrestle with the broad normative concerns that, in some ways, further define the field. Grounds (2004), for example, asks, "To what extent should forensic psychiatrists as a professional body be involved in issues of political controversy, particularly concerning legal standards and human rights?" (p. 192).[30] There are significant moral and political questions about the provision of mental health care to incarcerated populations, the execution of the mentally ill, and other vexing issues that would benefit from an engagement of the discipline, if not activism. We return to these questions in the final section of this chapter.

Not all of the most prominent forensic psychiatrists, though, see an expansive view of the field as an opportunity for engagement. Park Dietz, for example, is concerned with how the broadening of the discipline's boundaries invites a dilution of proficiency in certain core areas that threatens the value of forensic assessments. The solution is to scale back on the breadth of training and, instead, focus on core competencies in one or more of the following four distinct areas: criminal behavior, mental disability, forensic child psychiatry, and legal aspects of psychiatric practice.

The future of forensic psychiatry, according to Dietz, requires subspecializing in ways that allow for deep and specialized domains of knowledge. "The alternative vision of forensic psychiatry that I advocate," Dietz (1987) writes, "is focused on the branches and emphasizes depth over breadth. . ." (p. 217).[31] There has never been a forensic psychiatrist, Dietz argues, who has mastered all domains of disciplinary knowledge.

Dietz's cautionary tale about subspecialization considers the vast proliferation of research within the discipline; advances in relevant and sister disciplines; the difficulty of maintaining an expertise across a multidisciplinary field, and an increasing awareness that definitive scientific evidence should guide clinical practice. In this post *Daubert* period, forensic psychiatrists are held to very high standards—standards that require experimental evidence when and where reasonable and feasible.[32,33] Evidence-based practice is increasingly synonymous with scientific proof.[34] For example, producing evidence that forensic psychiatric rehabilitation works, and that measures of competency to stand trial are effective, are good illustrations of an evidence-based practice movement.[35,36] Efforts by the Campbell Collaboration to review programs for mentally ill offenders,[37] parent–infant psychotherapy for improving parental and infant mental health,[38] the effectiveness of forensic nurse examiners versus doctors for the forensic examination of rape and sexual assault complainants,[39] and the effects of parental imprisonment on child antisocial behavior and mental health[40] are also illustrative of a strong evidence-based trend in the field.

With such active knowledge production, a focus on evidence-based practices, and a unifying interest in crime and criminality, just how close is forensic psychiatry to criminology? A cursory review of the modern history of criminology suggests both complexity and closeness—and points of convergence and divergence.

Psychiatry and Criminology: It's a Complex but Close Relationship

Laub (2004) extends a life course metaphor to the history of modern criminology by looking at the three key periods and associated turning points.[41] The first phase (1900–1930) is defined by the multifactor approach. Laub writes about the atheoretical accumulation of descriptive data during this period. The second phase (1930–1960), called the Golden Age of Theory, gives credit to Merton, Sutherland, Cohen, Cloward and Ohlin, and other sociologists who crafted some of the most creative and long-standing structural and process theories of delinquency. Laub laments that there was not nearly as much systematic research as theory generation. The final phase (1960–2000), is characterized by extensive theory testing with increasingly sophisticated empirical methods. Here credit is due to Ron Akers, Travis Hirschi, Lawrence Cohen, Marcus Felson, Robert Sampson, and a small legion of others.[41]

There is an elaborate foundation for these three life course phases for those interested in a more complete history. Over the past 200 years, the pioneers of classical and positivist criminology devoted many lifetimes to the study of crime and criminality. The positive school has dominated, with biological determinists (e.g., Gall, Lombroso, Dugdale, Garofalo, Ferri, Hooten, Kretschmer, and Sheldon), psychological and psychiatric determinists (e.g., Ray, Maudsley, and Goddard), and sociological determinists (e.g., Quetelet, Comte, Guerry, Tarde, Durkheim, Goring, and the Gluecks). Of course, these determinists had to wrestle with the classical work of Beccaria and Bentham. The mix of disciplines and orientations from the eighteenth century onward is simply remarkable.

Forensic psychiatry may borrow much for other disciplines, but its focus has been and continues to be at the individual level. The same may not be said of criminology, in which, for example, there remains an active debate about the completeness of explanatory models of criminal behavior that disregard the variance explained by genetics, neuroscience, or at the other end of the spectrum, neighborhood or place. Criminological theory is offered and tested across and within levels.[42] At times, theory is subject to propositional and conceptual integration.[43] Some explanations are narrowly constructed and there are, of course, general theories of crime.[44]

The range of levels becomes apparent with even a cursory look at the contents of leading journals. In a recent issue of *Criminology* (May, 2014), the journal of the American Society of Criminology, articles included research on heart rate and impulsive sensation seeking; employment of ex-offenders and crime desistance; biosocial criminology in the postgenomic era; age effects and juvenile court sanctioning; and the effects of arresting a gang leader on criminal group embeddedness. It is revealing just how many disciplines and approaches are represented in a single issue of a criminology journal.

The normative orientation of the two fields differ, at times, as well. Criminologists represent multiple normative orientations, from desert-based principles to deterrence and peacemaking. Many are agnostic, preferring to maintain a dispassionate front. Others side with a positivist or neoclassical world view that reflects more profound justice orientations. By the very nature of their inquiry and role, forensic psychiatrists make determinations about the madness or badness of clients that bring about different forms of social control. Maintaining a treatment or welfare orientation for those who suffer from serious mental disease distinguishes forensic psychiatrists from their criminological counterparts.[45] This orientation and role also raise concerns about possible exploitation, the potential for compromised autonomy, and more general questions about the reach of the mental health care state.[46–51] Critical criminologists, like Turk (1967)[52] offered a harsh account of the "psychiatrization" of the criminal law some years ago—inspired by the much discussed work of Thomas Szasz. To be fair, critical criminologists offer somewhat comparable critiques of the criminal justice system.

How a field defines a crime and a criminal; the role that science plays in the production of knowledge; the place of evidence in decision making; the dominance of generalists by training, research, and clinical applications; and the constraints imposed by law and the criminal justice system, all combine to reveal additional points of convergence and divergence. This is what makes the relationship complex.

What makes forensic psychiatry and criminology increasingly close is captured by the idea that there is more to either field than the generation of disciplinary knowledge and the reliance on leading paradigms and methods. Criminology and forensic psychiatry both share a connection and commitment to justice systems—a commitment to use research in support of justice systems.[53,54] This is increasingly apparent in the leading journals (e.g., *Journal of the American Academy of Psychiatry and Law; Law and Human Behavior; American Journal of Forensic Psychology; Journal of Psychiatry and Law; Bulletin of the American Academy of Psychiatry and Law; British Journal of Psychiatry; American Journal of Psychiatry; and International Journal of Psychiatry and Law*).

In this sense, Bartol and Bartol's (2005)[55] conceptual division of forensic psychiatry and psychology into knowledge production and applications to justice systems captures something unique and special about these "sister" disciplines. Research on perceptions of procedural justice in mental health courts,[56] the recidivism of child sex abusers in Sweden,[57] gun restrictions for the seriously mentally ill,[58] blame attribution and guilt feelings in violent offenders,[59] and post traumatic stress disorder and substance use in male prisoners[60] appear in current forensic psychiatry and psychology journals. They would be equally at home in criminology and criminal justice journals.[61]

The domains of knowledge and focus on knowledge production bring the two fields together in subject matter, research focus, and relevance to systems of justice. It is, though, the commitment to making a system of justice more just, effective, and humane through research that enhances the relationship. It is the confluence of what moves research and practice. And, Appelbaum (1997) writes, "For forensic psychiatrists, the primary value of their work is to advance the interests of justice" (p. 234).[48]

In the next two sections, we explore how the body of knowledge and expression of principles of justice might be enhanced through a stronger relationship between these sister disciplines.

Criminological Musings

The presidential addresses of the American Society of Criminology and addresses of the Sutherland Award recipients (those recognized for outstanding contributions to theory or research in criminology) cover significant territory. Much of these criminological musings may not immediately connect with the standard fare of forensic psychiatry. They are, though, worthy of some consideration by psychiatrists. Not attending to the progress of criminological thinking for a field so aligned with the study of crime and criminality may be a missed opportunity.

In the most recent presidential address, Agnew (2014)[62] wonders why theories of crime and corresponding crime control policies make assumptions about the self-interested nature of offenders when mounting evidence from outside of criminology reveals that most people are both self-interested and socially concerned. According to Agnew, this may include "... caring about others, forming close ties to and cooperating with others, following certain moral intuitions, and conforming" (p. 1).[62]

What if social concern or some variants of social concern, like empathy, have direct, indirect, or mediating effects on criminal behavior? How could such evidence connect with psychiatric research on psychopathy or evidence of dysempathy in other psychiatric patients? According to Blair (2005),[63] empathy is tied to a variety of neurocognitive functions, each of which may be disrupted. "Such selective disruptions," Blair maintains, "are at the heart of specific psychiatric disorders: autism, psychopathy, childhood bipolar disorder, and intermittent explosive disorder. The continued elucidation of these forms of empathy dysfunction will one day make likely the successful treatment of these disorders" (p. 711).[63]

Garland's (2013) Sutherland address explores the impact of penal practices and policies in the United States with a call to "... attend more closely to the structure and operation of the penal state" (p. 1).[64] This address raises some familiar questions: How does the penal state connect to the therapeutic state? What does Garland's thesis say about Wexler and Winick's (1990) notion of therapeutic jurisprudence?[65] Or Braithwaite's (2002) consideration of restorative justice and therapeutic jurisprudence?[66]

The balance of recent addresses, marking the progression of criminological leadership, are equally thought-provoking and relevant. Peterson's (2010) call for greater attention to racial inequality by criminologists could just as easily served as a call in forensic psychiatry.[67,68] Hicks' (2004) call matches Peterson's: "As a field, forensic psychiatry should encourage research in the area of race and ethnicity, because it affects the validity of our opinions and complicates clinical care in the special populations with whom we work" (p. 30).[69]

Rosenfeld (2010) asks for greater attention to macro-level analyses of crime data, concerned that criminologists are too occupied by micro-level questions.[70] That shift in criminology might inspire its sister discipline to engage in more frequent systematic reviews and meta-analyses while, at the same time, looking more often at effect sizes from the analysis of larger, more representative datasets.[71]

Finally, in his ASC presidential address, Clear (2010) challenges an academic organization of criminologists to work toward "... building a broad and forward-looking evidentiary base for fundamental innovation in justice policy" (p. 1).[72] Clear reviews the shift in attitudes about evidence in criminal justice policy, and delights in a new evidence-based world. At the same time, he seeks an opportunity to raise "friendly" questions about the bridge between evidence and policy. "A part of my concern," Clear (2010) writes, "has to do with the nature of evidence in our work. Another part has to do with the nature of policy. And finally, I am concerned about the potential ramifications of the emergence of a kind of hegemony of "what works" (p. 4).[72]

Clear (2010) raises the need for successive positive evaluations of program or policies across different settings for evidence to be definitive; the fact that there are few truly randomized field trials; and a sense that "... on far too many policy questions, we do not have that sort of collection of studies" (p. 6).[72] He concludes that the "What Works" movement is "extraordinarily conservative," retrospective by its very design, and fails to lay a foundation for new and innovative strategic interventions.

Clear (2010) wants criminologists to rethink the kind of knowledge that constitutes evidence.[72] Controlled experiments should be one of a number of evidentiary methods, joined by the methods of qualitative research, policy studies, and natural experiments. Knowledge of all sorts—basic research—will contribute to "action-relevant evidence." To pair action only with consistent experimental evidence will "... shackle us from taking bold action when only bold action makes sense" (Clear, 2010, p. 14).[72] The balance of Clear's (2010) address details the kinds of policies that might be promoted from within the American Society of Criminology (ASC).

There are very reasonable arguments for and against the ASC and the American Academy of Psychiatry and the Law (AAPL) assuming and advocating strong policy positions. There are only good reasons, though, for forensic psychiatrists to know the positions taken by national organizations representing a sister discipline and, of course, for the ASC to know the same of the AAPL. After all, both the ASC and AAPL are united by commonly shared problems and challenges, questions raised about the same or parallel systems of justice, and profound normative concerns that wrap tightly around contested practices.

Collaboration and the End of Provincialism

Some issues of rights and justice cross-disciplines in ways that prompt and even encourage collaboration. One such issue, now raised regularly in the popular press, is how jails and prisons are the new mental health care asylums.[73] Data revealing the significant psychiatric morbidity among prison and jail inmates are, sadly, far from new. They are, indeed, nearly a century old.[74] In recent years, though, research from the Bureau of Justice Statistics shows significant, if not dramatic, growth in mentally ill offenders across the correctional enterprise in the United States.[75]

James and Glaze (2006), for example, reveal that 56% of state prison inmates acknowledge one or more mental health problem based on DSM IV criteria.[76] Forty-five percent of federal inmates and sixty-four percent of jail inmates reported the same. The Survey of Inmates in State and Federal Correctional Facilities, and the Survey of Inmates in Local Jails explore the symptoms in the past 12 months or since admission, and the reported disorders. More than 25% of state prison, federal prison, and local jail inmates report major depressive disorder symptoms and mania disorder symptoms. Notably, a systematic review and meta-analysis of multiple surveys of prisoners report comparable data.[77] And all of these data should be examined alongside Beck's (2001) report on the provision of mental health counseling and psychotropic medication in state and federal prisons.[78] Knowing how few of those in our custodial care receive needed treatment and counseling should engender action and change.

Fazel and Baillargeon (2011) and Gunn (2000) compare data from the United States with countries in Europe and elsewhere.[79,80] The data are far from good, but if you combine reports from the United Nations Office on Drugs and Crime and the World Health Organization with the regular failure to abide by prevailing United Nations Standards, the portrait is dire. There is an opportunity here for research, standards setting, and program development and evaluation—for forensic psychiatry and criminology. It requires a recognition both fields have strongly shared interests, norms and, at times, a moral imperative to act. Finally, it requires more than a provincial view of an American academic society or academy. The dismal treatment of the incarcerated mentally ill in the United States *and* around the world is an urgent human rights issue waiting for two sister disciplines to act.

References

1. Sutherland EH. (1947). *Principles of criminology*. Philadelphia: Lippincott.
2. Adler F, Mueller GOW, & Laufer WS. (2013). *Criminology*. New York: McGraw-Hill.
3. Siegel LJ. (2013). *Criminology*. Belmont, CA: Wadsworth.
4. Weisburd DL, Groff ER, & Yang SM. (2012). *The criminology of place: Street segments and our understanding of the crime problem*. New York: Oxford University Press.
5. Braga AA, & Weisburd D. (2010). *Policing problem places: Crime hot spots and effective prevention*. New York: Oxford University Press.

6. Boruch R, Weisburd D, & Berk R. (2010). Place randomized trials. In AR Piquero, & D Weisburd (Eds.), *Handbook of quantitative criminology* (pp. 481–502). New York: Springer.
7. Welsh BC, & Farrington DP. (2012). Science, politics, and crime prevention: Toward a new crime policy. *J Crim Just, 40*(2), 128–133.
8. Dietz PE. (1996). The quest for excellence in forensic psychiatry. *J Am Acad Psychiatry Law Online, 24*(2), 153–163.
9. Harsch S, Bergk JE, Steinert T, Keller F, & Jockusch U. (2006). Prevalence of mental disorders among sexual offenders in forensic psychiatry and prison. *Int J Law Psychiatry, 29*(5), 443–449.
10. Dolan M, & Smith C. (2001). Juvenile homicide offenders: 10 years' experience of an adolescent forensic psychiatry service. *J Forens Psychiatry, 12*(2), 313–329.
11. Vaillant GE. (1966). A twelve-year follow-up of New York narcotic addicts: I. The relation of treatment to outcome. *Am J Psychiatry, 122*(7), 727–737.
12. Raine A. (2013). *The anatomy of violence: The biological roots of crime*. New York: Random House.
13. Mednick SA, & Finello KM. (1983). Biological factors and crime: Implications for forensic psychiatry. *Int J Law Psychiatry, 6*(1), 1–15.
14. Oosterhuis H, & Loughnan A. (2014). Madness and crime: Historical perspectives on forensic psychiatry. *Int J Law Psychiatry, 37*(1), 1.
15. Selling LS. (1949). Forensic psychiatry. *J Crim Law Criminol, 39*, 606.
16. Bartol CR, & Bartol AM. (1999). History of forensic psychology. *Handbook Forens Psychol*, 3–23.
17. Grisso T. (1993). The differences between forensic psychiatry and forensic psychology. *J Am Acad Psychiatry Law Online, 21*(2), 133–145.
18. Robitscher BJ. (1972). The new face of legal psychiatry. *Amer J Psychiatry, 129*(3).
19. Pollack S. (1974). Forensic psychiatry: A specialty. *J Am Acad Psychiatry Law Online, 2*(1), 1–6.
20. Hamilton J. (1987). Violence and victims: the contribution of victimology to forensic psychiatry. *Lancet, 329*(8525), 147–150.
21. Prentice SE. (1995). A history of subspecialization in forensic psychiatry. *J Am Acad Psychiatry Law Online, 23*(2), 195–203.
22. Witzel J, Walter M, Bogerts B, & Northoff G. (2008). Neurophilosophical perspectives of neuroimaging in forensic psychiatry—giving way to a paradigm shift? *Behav Sci Law, 26*(1), 113–130.
23. Glenn AL, Raine A, & Laufer WS. (2011). Is it wrong to criminalize and punish psychopaths? *Emotion Rev, 3*(3), 302–304.
24. Dressing H, Sartorius A, & Meyer-Lindenberg A. (2008). Implications of fMRI and genetics for the law and the routine practice of forensic psychiatry. *Neurocase, 14*(1), 7–14.
25. Morse S. (2011). Avoiding irrational neurolaw exuberance: A plea for neuromodesty. *Law, Innovat Technol, 3*(2), 209–228.
26. Reeves D, Mills MJ, Billick SB, & Brodie JD. (2003). Limitations of brain imaging in forensic psychiatry. *J Am Acad Psychiatry Law, 31*, 89–96.
27. Rushing SE, & Langleben DD. (2011). Relative function: Nuclear brain imaging in United States courts. *J Psychiatry Law, 39*(4), 567–593.
28. Hayempour BJ, Rushing SE, & Alavi A. (2011). The role of neuroimaging in assessing neuropsychological deficits following traumatic brain injury. *J Psychiatry Law, 39*(4), 537.
29. Bernstein DE. (1995). The science of forensic psychiatry and psychology. *Psychiatry Psychol Law, 2*(1), 75–80.
30. Grounds A. (2004). Forensic psychiatry and political controversy. *J Am Acad Psychiatry Law Online, 32*(2), 192–196.
31. Dietz PE. (1987). The forensic psychiatrist of the future. *J Am Acad Psychiatry Law Online, 15*(3), 217–227.
32. Glancy GD, & Saini M. (2009). The confluence of evidence-based practice and Daubert within the fields of forensic psychiatry and the law. *J Am Acad Psychiatry Law Online, 37*(4), 438–441.
33. Schneider RD. (2009). Commentary: Evidence-based practice and forensic psychiatry. *J Am Acad Psychiatry Law Online, 37*(4), 503–508.

34. Glancy GD. (2008). Evidence-based practices applied to forensic psychiatry: Introduction to special issue. *Brief Treat Crisis Int*, *8*(1), 1.
35. Lindqvist P, & Skipworth J. (2000). Evidence-based rehabilitation in forensic psychiatry. *Br J Psychiatry*, *176*(4), 320–323.
36. Rogers R, & Johansson-Love J. (2009). Evaluating competency to stand trial with evidence-based practice. *J Am Acad Psychiatry Law Online*, *37*(4), 450–460.
37. Scott DA, McGilloway S, Dempster M, Browne F, & Donnelly M. (2013). Effectiveness of criminal justice liaison and diversion services for offenders with mental disorders: A review. *Psychiatr Serv*, *64*(9), 843–849.
38. Barlow J, Bennett C, & Midgley N. (2013). Parent-infant psychotherapy for the secondary and tertiary prevention of infant mental health problems: A systematic review. *The Campbell Collaboration*. Available at www.campbellcollaboration.org
39. Toon C, Gurusamy K. (2014). Forensic nurse examiners versus doctors for the forensic examination of rape and sexual assault complainants: A systematic review. *Campbell Systematic Reviews*, *5*, 1–56.
40. Murray J, Farrington D, Sekol I, & Olsen RF. (2009). Effects of parental imprisonment on child antisocial behaviour and mental health: A systematic review. *Campbell Systematic Reviews*, *4*, 1–105.
41. Laub JH. (2004). The life course of criminology in the United States: The American Society of Criminology 2003 presidential address. *Criminology*, *42*(1), 1–26.
42. Bernard TJ, & Snipes JB. (1996). Theoretical integration in criminology. *Crime Just*, *20*, 301–348.
43. Liska AE, Krohn MD, & Messner SF. (1989). Strategies and requisites for theoretical integration in the study of crime and deviance. *Theoretical Integration in the Study of Deviance and Crime: Problems and Prospects*, 1–19.
44. Hirschi T, & Gottfredson MR. (1993). Commentary: Testing the general theory of crime. *J Res Crime Delinq*, *30*(1), 47–54.
45. Adshead G, & Sarkar SP. (2005). Justice and welfare: Two ethical paradigms in forensic psychiatry. *Aust NZ J Psychiatry*, *39*(11–12), 1011–1017.
46. Halleck SL. (1974). Troubled view of current trends in forensic psychiatry. *Am J Psychiatry Law*, *2*, 135.
47. Stone AA. (1984). The ethical boundaries of forensic psychiatry: A view from the ivory tower. *J Am Acad Psychiatry Law Online*, *12*(3), 209–219.
48. Appelbaum PS. (1997). A theory of ethics for forensic psychiatry. *J Am Acad Psychiatry Law Online*, *25*(3), 233–247.
49. Appelbaum, PS. (1990). The parable of the forensic psychiatrist: Ethics and the problem of doing harm. *Int J Law Psychiatry*, *13*(4), 249–259.
50. Bonnie RJ. (2010). Howard Zonana and the transformation of forensic psychiatry. *J Am Acad Psychiatry Law Online*, *38*(4), 570–576.
51. Sadoff RL. (2011). *Ethical issues in forensic psychiatry: Minimizing harm*. New York: Wiley.
52. Turk AT. (1967). Psychiatry vs. the law—therefore? *Criminology*, *5*(3), 30–35.
53. Coid JW, Kahtan N, Gault S, & Jarman B. (2000). Ethnic differences in admissions to secure forensic psychiatry services. *Br J Psychiatry*, *177*(3), 241–247.
54. Coid J, Kahtan N, Cook A, Gault S, & Jarman B. (2001). Predicting admission rates to secure forensic psychiatry services. *Psychol Med*, *31*(3), 531–539.
55. Bartol, CR, & Bartol AM. (2005). *Criminal behavior: A psychosocial approach*. Pearson Prentice Hall, Upper Saddle River, New Jersey.
56. Canada KE, & Hiday VA. (2014). Procedural justice in mental health court: an investigation of the relation of perception of procedural justice to non-adherence and termination. *J Forens Psychiatry Psychol*, *25*(3), 321–340.
57. Nilsson T, Carlstedt A, Baudin C, Jakobsson C, Forsman A, & Anckarsäter H. (2014). Intra-and extra-familial child sexual abusers and recidivism in Sweden: a 10-to 15-year follow-up study. *J Forens Psychiatry Psychol*, *25*(3), 341–361.
58. Matejkowski J, Fairfax-Columbo J, Cullen SW, Marcus SC, & Solomon PL. (2014). Exploring the potential of stricter gun restrictions for people with serious mental illness to reduce homicide in the United States. *J Forens Psychiatry Psychol*, *25*(3), 362–369.

59. Johnsson M, Andersson B, Wallinius M, Hofvander B, Ståhlberg O, Anckarsäter H, & Radovic S. (2014). Blame attribution and guilt feelings in violent offenders. *J Forens Psychiatry Psychol, 25*(2), 212–223.
60. Sindicich N, Mills KL, Barrett EL, Indig D, Sunjic S, Sannibale C,... & Najavits LM. (2014). Offenders as victims: post-traumatic stress disorder and substance use disorder among male prisoners. *J Forens Psychiatry Psychol, 25*(1), 44–60.
61. Phillips MR, Wolf AS, & Coons DJ. (1988). Psychiatry and the criminal justice system: Testing the myths. *Am J Psychiatry, 145*(5), 605–610.
62. Agnew R. (2014). Social concern and crime: Moving beyond the assumption of simple self-interest. *Criminology, 52*(1), 1–32.
63. Blair RJR. (2005) Responding to the emotions of others: Dissociating forms of empathy through the study of typical and psychiatric populations. *Consciousness Cogn, 14*(4), 698–718.
64. Garland D. (2013). Penalty and the penal state. *Criminology, 51*(3), 475–517.
65. Wexler DB, & Winick BJ. (1990). Therapeutic jurisprudence as a new approach to mental health law policy analysis and research. *Univ Miami Law Rev, 45*, 979.
67. Peterson RD. (2012). The central place of race in crime and justice. *Criminology, 50*(2), 303–328.
68. Fernando S, Ndegwa D, & Wilson M. (2005). *Forensic psychiatry, race and culture*. New York: Routledge.
69. Hicks JW. (2004). Ethnicity, race, and forensic psychiatry: Are we color-blind? *J Am Acad Psychiatry Law Online, 32*(1), 21–33.
70. Rosenfeld R. (2011). The big picture. *Criminology, 49*(1), 1–26
71. Guy LS, Edens JF, Anthony C, & Douglas KS. (2005). Does psychopathy predict institutional misconduct among adults? A meta-analytic investigation. *J Consult Clin Psychol, 73*(6), 1056.
72. Clear TR. (2010). Policy and evidence: The challenge to the American Society of Crimnology. *Criminology, 48*(1), 1–25.
73. Konrad N. (2002). Prisons as new asylums. *Curr Opin Psychiatry, 15*(6), 583–587.
74. Glueck B. (1918). A study of 608 admissions to Sing Sing prison. *Mental Hygiene, 2*, 85–151.
75. Brink J. (2005). Epidemiology of mental illness in a correctional system. *Curr Opin Psychiatry, 18*(5), 536–541
76. James DJ, & Glaze LE. (2006). *Mental health problems of prison and jail inmates*. Washington, DC: US Department of Justice, Office of Justice Programs, Bureau of Justice Statistics.
77. Fazel S, & Danesh J. (2002). Serious mental disorder in 23 000 prisoners: A systematic review of 62 surveys. *Lancet, 359*, 545–550.
78. Beck AJ, & Maruschak LM. (2001). *Mental health treatment in state prisons, 2000*. Washington, DC: US Department of Justice, Office of Justice Programs, Bureau of Justice Statistics.
79. Fazel S, & Baillargeon J. (2011). The health of prisoners. *Lancet*, 377:9769, 956–965.
80. Gunn J. (2000). Future directions for treatment in forensic psychiatry. *Br J Psychiatry, 176*(4), 332–338.

SECTION SIX

Forensic Psychiatry and Legal Issues

24

Forensic Psychiatry and the Law

Litigation, Advocacy, Scholarship, and Teaching

Michael L. Perlin

I met Bob Sadoff on a snowy day in December 1971, and it changed my life.[1] I was a rookie public defender (PD) in Trenton, NJ, and I had been assigned to represent a young man (Raamon Jenkins), institutionalized in what was called the "Vroom Building," New Jersey's maximum security hospital for the "criminally insane." He had been charged with assaulting his treating psychiatrist. Not surprisingly, most of the psychiatrists whom I called, quickly declined the offer, but several said, "Contact Bob Sadoff. I bet he'd love to do the case." I didn't know who Bob was at the time, but when I researched him and found that he was president of the American Academy of Psychiatry and Law, I gulped. Why on earth would an expert as prominent as *this* want to come to the Trenton PD office to work on a case with me, who had been practicing law all of 4 months?

Heart in mouth, I called Bob, and introduced myself. He said, without hesitation, "Sure! Just make sure that the guards know that I'm coming so we don't kill half a day getting me access." I was floored. A few days later, Bob came to my office, and introduced himself. We chatted for a few minutes (I am sure about sports), and he said, "Let's get to work!" And we did.

The case turned into one of the ultimate shaggy-dog stories of my career. New Jersey was and is a *M'Naghten* state,[2–5] but, at this point in time (12 years before John Hinckley shot Ronald Reagan), it seemed certainly within the realm of possibility that the state supreme court could be persuaded to abandon it, and adopt, instead, the more liberal Model Penal Code/American Law Institute test—that the defendant "as a result of mental disease or defect, lacked substantial capacity to conform his conduct to the requirements of the law which he is alleged to have violated" (*United States v. Currens*, 1961),[6] which a decade earlier had been adopted by the third circuit for federal criminal trials.[7,8]

After Bob examined my client, he came back and said, "Do you want the good news or the bad news?"[9] Although I am generally an optimist, my few months as a criminal defense lawyer had already amply demonstrated that the bad news would eventually prevail, so I said, "Start with the bad." And Bob told me that my client did not meet the *M'Naghten* standard. Deflated, I asked, "So what's the good news?" To which Bob responded, "He *does* meet the American Law Institute (ALI) standard. Maybe you want to use this as a test case?" I thought about it for 12 seconds, and said, "Sure!" And we were off and running.

The trial came, and Bob got up to testify. And, after a detailed explanation of my client's actions, his motivations, his mental illness, and more, he explained to the judge (This was a bench trial; I might have been a rookie, but I realized that there was no way a jury could have grasped the nuances of this case) that my client did "lack substantial capacity to conform his conduct to the requirements of the law" (tracking the ALI test). At which point, the prosecutor jumped up and said, "Well, this is interesting, but it's not the law of New Jersey. And, in fact, Dr. Sadoff *did* prepare a report in this case in which the court might be interested." The judge looked at me, and said, "A report?" I said, "Yes, your honor. I was getting to that in a moment. I wanted to set the stage though, by putting on this testimony first." In his report, Bob concluded that my client was *not* insane under *M'Naghten* but would have been insane *if New Jersey were to adopt the ALI test.* It took the judge about 3 minutes to wish me luck on my appeal and find my client guilty.

This was not unexpected at all, and Bob and I agreed that this was the perfect test case to take to the New Jersey Supreme Court—I had clerked for the state appellate division the year before and that position had given me a lot of time to think about how the justices felt about the toughest criminal law and procedure issues—and that we had, all in all, a fairly good shot, in what would probably be a 4-3 decision. My client, unfortunately, thought the wheels of justice moved too slowly, and decided that he would be better off taking matters in his own hands, so, one day, when the laundry truck was leaving the jail, he hopped in somehow and took his leave, thus ending our chances of a test case appeal.[10]

This is not the kind of case one forgets, and it was the start of what has perhaps been the most remarkable professional relationship of my life. I worked closely with Bob on many, many cases over the years. He was a witness in many cases that I have litigated,[11,12] and has been the inspiration for others.[13]

We have taught together and presented on panels together,[14] we have shared the podium innumerable times at meetings of the American Academy of Psychiatry and Law (AAPL), the American Association of Law Schools, the American Psychiatric Association, the International Academy of Law and Mental Health, and other cross-professional organizations. He has served on monitoring committees of cases I have litigated.[15] We have made teaching tapes together,[16] have co-authored articles,[17,18] and I have written chapters in other books that he has edited.[19,20] I present regularly in his Practical Applications in Forensic Psychiatry Seminar series at the University of Pennsylvania Medical School.[21] Bob gave me my "national" start by inviting me to present at an American Academy of Psychiatry and Law meeting in 1975 (see Perlin, 1975). He has written about me in his books,[22] and I have written about him in my articles.[23,24] I have written introductory forewords to two of his books,[25,26] and I have participated in two *festschrifts* honoring Bob.[27,28]

I begin this chapter with these personal recollections because, in answering the question that was posed to me—to discuss the impact forensic psychiatry has had on my work and reciprocally the effect I have had on forensic psychiatry—I realized that so much of my answer flows from my relationship with Bob, a relationship that has touched on every aspect of my professional life.

I spent 13 years as a practicing lawyer and have now spent 30 as a law professor. Forensic psychiatry has had an impact on every aspect of my careers, in the context of litigation, advocacy, scholarship, and teaching. I hope that, both directly through my having taught forensic psychiatry fellows for many years, and less directly, through my scholarship—especially my foci on sanism and pretextuality and my incorporation of therapeutic jurisprudence in all aspects of my work, as discussed in the following—and my advocacy—especially my insistence that American mental health professionals learn about and incorporate international human rights principles and standards into their work—that I have had a modest effect on forensic psychiatric practice as well. Again, my work with Bob—my presentations at AAPL, my teaching in the fellowship programs, our co-authorships—form the core of that sphere of influence.

Litigation

I have spent much of the past 40 years seeking to persuade forensic psychiatrists that they could best influence the development of the law by working with plaintiffs' lawyers in test cases that challenge the way the civil commitment process is carried out, that challenge the conditions of confinement in public psychiatric facilities (including the prescriptive right to treatment and the proscriptive right to refuse treatment), that challenge the way that hospital release plans rarely meet any of the criteria of a true deinstitutionalization program, and by working with criminal defendants' lawyers in the full range of forensic issues, including competency to stand trial, responsibility determinations, sentencing, and the death penalty.[29]

At the same time, forensic psychiatry has influenced me by demonstrating to me—on multiple occasions—that there are significant limits as to what lawyers can do for a client if they fail to acknowledge the reality of the limitations, political influences, and funding pressures on forensic systems.

I believe that these influences have been—and continue to be—symbiotic. It is only if forensic psychiatrists continue to work with lawyers, who seek consciously to advance a social law reform agenda, and only if those lawyers continue to work with forensic psychiatrists who continue to ask questions—questions about forensic systems, about clients beyond the narrow legal inquiry that may be the only question before the court (e.g., is the defendant competent to stand trial?)—that the law often simply does not ask, that litigation in this area can become an effective tool for social change.[30]

Teaching: My Influence on Forensic Psychiatry

I began teaching in 1984. Almost immediately thereafter, students from the New York University (NYU) Forensic Fellowship program began to audit my mental disability law courses, and, from approximately 1986 to 2004, enrollment in and successful completion of one of my courses was a prerequisite for all NYU fellows. For many years, I was an adjunct professor of law and psychiatry at the University of Rochester Medical Center, and taught the forensic fellows affiliated with that program as well. For several years, I have done an annual lecture for the New York City Forensic Fellowship Consortium (attended by fellows in all the forensic programs in New York City and North/Central New Jersey). As noted, I present yearly at the Practical Applications in Forensic Psychiatry Seminar at the University of Pennsylvania Medical School, do grand rounds regularly at hospitals in New York, New Jersey, and elsewhere, and am a regular presenter at conferences and workshops offered by groups such as the American Academy of Psychiatry and Law, the American College of Forensic Psychiatry, and the World Psychiatric Association. Forensic psychiatrists from around the world have enrolled for many years in the masters program in mental disability law studies that I have directed at the New York Law School.

I think it is critical that psychiatrists understand the different perspectives of the legal system and how it is so different from the medical model taught in medical schools (even if the psychiatrist had had a course in "the law" in medical school that included case summaries or expository essays *about* cases). It is only by reading cases and by taking law courses or participating in legal seminars that psychiatrists in training can understand how the legal system works and why the questions posed by counsel and the courts may appear to be so discordant with the methodology in which they are versed.

Teaching: Forensic Psychiatry's Influence on Me

By working with forensic psychiatrists, teaching them, studying with them, sharing the seminar table with them, I have come to grasp the chasm in the ways that the pedagogy in law is different from the pedagogy in psychiatry, and to more fully understand how the two fields "work" and how we (lawyers *and* law professors) must learn from forensic psychiatry teachers the same ways that we hope they learn from us.

I believe that this training will expand the pedagogic and practical horizons of all involved, and will ultimately lead to a forensic system that is more consonant with legal requirements (especially, *constitutional* requirements), that is more humane, and, in the end, provides better care and treatment for patients.

Scholarship

Since the early 1990s, I have been writing regularly about how sanism and pretexuality have ravaged the legal system and poisoned mental disability law practice.[31] I define *sanism* as an irrational prejudice of the same quality and character of other irrational prejudices that cause (and are reflected in) prevailing social attitudes of racism, sexism, homophobia, and ethnic bigotry,[32] and define *pretextuality* as the ways in which courts accept, either implicitly or explicitly, testimonial dishonesty and engage similarly in dishonest and frequently meretricious decision making.[33] Since about the same time, I have begun to write about therapeutic jurisprudence, a model for assessing the impact of case law and legislation that recognizes that, as a therapeutic agent, the law can have therapeutic or antitherapeutic consequences.[34,35] The ultimate aim of therapeutic jurisprudence is to determine whether legal rules, procedures, and lawyer roles can or should be reshaped to enhance their therapeutic potential while not subordinating due process principles.[36–39] I have written about these approaches to the law in the *Bulletin of the Academy of Psychiatry and Law*,[40] the *American Journal of Forensic Psychiatry*,[41] and other publications that I believe are regularly read by forensic psychiatrists.[42–45] My hope is that, by publishing in such journals, I am able to reach out to forensic psychiatrists on their own turf so as to share some of what I think are the important aspects of understanding why and how the legal system treats persons with mental disabilities the way it does.

There is no question in my mind that scholarship is, and can be, a tool for social change.[46] By seeking to "unpack" how sanism and pretextuality can affect and infect the work of forensic psychiatrists, I seek to contribute to that social change. By reaching out to forensic psychiatrists in my work on therapeutic jurisprudence, I hope to sensitize this cohort to the contours of that discipline and to encourage them to apply those principles in their own writing. Not coincidentally, Bob Sadoff is one of the very few who has yet taken up that challenge.[47] other such writings by forensic psychiatrists include Glaser (2003) and Mossman (1996).[48,49]

Advocacy

Since the early 2000s, I have turned my attention to the intersection between mental disability law and international human rights law.[50–56] In recent years, I have presented papers, workshops and panels to groups of forensic psychiatrists in the United States, New Zealand, Austria, the Czech Republic, Australia, Turkey, Argentina, and elsewhere, seeking to emphasize how important it is that they understand this connection, begin to incorporate international human rights insights into their reports and evaluations, and emphasize that state psychiatry is still, in many nations, used as a tool through which to suppress political dissent.[57] Interestingly, most of the forensic psychiatrists I speak to abroad know about recent developments in this area of the law—specifically, the ratification of the United Nations Convention on the Rights of Persons with Disabilities[58]—but, domestically it is news to virtually everyone in my audiences. I hope to continue to share these insights with progressive forensic psychiatrists, in the hopes that, in the coming years, this will be as well known domestically as it is internationally.

Recently, I have written about the relationship between international human rights law and guardianship,[59] international human rights law and juvenile punishment,[60] international human rights law and mental health courts,[61] international human rights law and the treatment of patients in forensic facilities,[62] and international human rights law and the sexual autonomy of psychiatric patients.[63,64] Forensic psychiatrists should have something to say about each of these topics, and I hope that these pieces will lead to invigorated scholarship in that regard.

Conclusion

In this chapter, I have considered the relationship between forensic psychiatry and the law through four filters (litigation, teaching, scholarship, and advocacy) and one very unique lens—my relationship with Bob Sadoff. Bob and I have worked together for more than 40 years, and I continue to learn from him each time we meet, speak, or e-mail. I believe that his career is a template for forensic psychiatrists in each of these areas of social policy. His work continues to be an inspiration to all of us.

Acknowledgment

The author wishes to thank Katherine Davies for her excellent editing assistance.

References

1. Perlin ML. (2005). "May he stay forever young": Robert Sadoff and the history of mental health law. *J Am Acad Psychiatry*, 33, 236.
2. New Jersey had adopted the narrow, "right-from-wrong" *M'Naghten* test shortly after it was introduced in England, see *State v Spencer*, 21 *NJL*. 196, 204–05 (Oyer and Terminer 1846), and employed it consistently thereafter.
3. *State v. Coleman*, 46 *NJ* 16, 39, 214 *A*2d 393 (1965).
4. *State v Lucas*, 30 *NJ* 37, 72, 152 *A*2d 50 (1959).
5. *State v Maioni*, 78 *NJL* 339, 341–42, 74 *A*. 526 (E. & A.1909).
6. *United States v Currens*, 290 F2d 751 (3d Cir 1961).
7. Interestingly, at about the time of the *Jenkins* case, a NJ legislative commission had recommended that *M'Naghten* be discarded, and that the ALI test replace it. *Final Report. 1971, 96–97.* The Legislature eventually rejected this recommendation, and instead, codified *M'Naghten* in a 1978 global penal code revision. See NJ Stat Ann § 2C-4.1.
8. For a full discussion, see *State v Singleton*, 48 A3d 285, 295 (NJ 2012).
9. Personal communication with Robert L. Sadoff, MD.
10. The denouement? My client went to Texas, got a job working in a community mental health facility, and was found out years later only when he was given some sort of award, and his picture was in the local paper. A Trenton jail guard was, coincidentally, visiting family in that town at the time, saw his picture, and he was quickly extradited to serve his prison sentenc.... Bob discusses this case in a dialogue with Dr. Kenneth Weiss, in Weiss K, & Robert SL. (2012). From the journal of *Psychiatry & Law Archives*: Bernard L. Diamond, M.D. *J Psychiatry Law*, 40, 128–129.
11. Perlin ML. Mental Disability Law: Civil and Criminal. 2nd ed. 2002; 4(8A-6.3):88; discussing *State v Miller*, Indictment No. 1869-71 (NJ Mercer Cty. Ct. 1974).
12. Perlin ML. (1975). Psychiatric testimony in a criminal law setting. *Bull Am Acad Psychiatry Law*, 3(20), 1249.
13. Perlin ML. (2005). "May he stay forever young": Robert Sadoff and the history of mental health law. *J Am Acad Psychiatry*, 33, 236 (discussing *Dixon v Cahill*, Docket No. L.30977/y-71 P.W., NJ Super Ct.,

Law Div. 1973), final order reprinted in Perlin ML. Mental Disability Law: Civil and Criminal. 2nd ed. 2002; 4(§14-7):119-21; discussing *State v Miller*, Indictment No. 1869-71 (NJ Mercer Cty. Ct. 1974).

14. From 1979 to 1984, we taught together as members of the Faculty for Continuing Education in the Program in Psychiatry at the Institute of the Pennsylvania Hospital (Philadelphia).
15. Perlin ML. (2005). "May he stay forever young": Robert Sadoff and the history of mental health law. *J Am Acad Psychiatry*, 33, 243 (discussing the monitoring committee in *Doe v Klein*, Docket No. L-12088-74 PW, NJ Super Ct, Law Div 1977), In: Ment. Dis. L. Rep. 1977; 1:425 (Greystone Park Psychiatric Hospital case, Morris Plains, NJ).
16. The sample direct and cross examination that I include in my Treatise (p. 6 n. 5: Perlin, *supra* note 6. 2nd ed. 1998; 1(§2C-4.9): 338-53., is based on the Roland Rodney tape that Bob and I created in the late 1970s pursuant to a National Institute of Mental Health training project in conjunction with the Center for Studies in Social-Legal Psychiatry at the University of Pennsylvania Medical School (which Bob then directed). Bob also made a series of teaching tapes for me and with me ("The Case of Sharon Stevens"; "The Case of Darren Daniels") that I used in classes at New York Law School from 1990 to 2004.
17. Perlin ML, & Sadoff RL. (1982). Ethical issues in the representation of individuals in the commitment process. *Law Contemp Problems*, 45, 161.
18. Perlin ML, & Sadoff RL. (1978). The adversary system. In IL Kutash, SB Kutash, & LB Schlesinger (Eds.), *Violence: Perspectives on murder and aggression* (p. 394). San Francisco: Jossey-Bass.
19. Perlin ML. (1983). Recent developments in mental health law. *Psychiatry Clin North Am*, 6(4), 539–549.
20. Perlin ML. (2008). Competency to stand trial. In R Sadoff, F Dattillio (Eds.), *Crime and mental illness: A guide to courtroom practice* (p. 23). Mechanicsburg, PA: Pennsylvania Bar Institute.
21. Most recently, e.g., "The Death Penalty, International Human Rights Law, Mental Disability & Therapeutic Jurisprudence" (Feb. 26, 2013).
22. Sadoff RL. (2011). Ethical issues in forensic psychiatry: Minimizing harm. *BioMed Res Int*, 2014, p. 73.
23. Perlin ML. (2010). "They keep it all hid": The ghettoization of mental disability law and its implications for legal education. *St. Louis Univ Law J*, 54, 871.
24. Perlin ML. (2000). A law of healing. *Univ CT Law Rev*, 68, 417.
25. Perlin ML. (1992). Foreword: New directions in the legal regulation of the mental health professions. In R Simon, & RL Sadoff (Eds.), *Psychiatric malpractice: Cases and comments for clinicians* (p. ix). Washington, DC: American Psychiatric Press.
26. Perlin ML. (1982). Foreword. In RL Sadoff. *Legal issues in the care.*
27. Perlin ML. (2005). "May he stay forever young": Robert Sadoff and the history of mental health law. *J Am Acad Psychiatry*, 33, 236.
28. Perlin ML. (2012). "Justice's beautiful fact": Bob Sadoff and the redemptive promise of therapeutic jurisdprudence. *J Psychiatry Law*, 40, 265.
29. I consciously limit this to working with civil plaintiffs and criminal defendants, since my four decades of experience has taught me, sadly, that this is the only work that authentically leads to ameliorative developments in the law. Some may disagree.
30. Van Schaack B. (2004). With all deliberate speed: Civil human rights litigation as a tool for social change. *Vand Law Rev*, 57, 2338.
31. Perlin ML. (2000). *The hidden prejudice: Mental disability on trial.* Washington, DC: American Psychological Association.
32. Perlin ML. (1992). On "sanism." *SMU Law Rev*, 46, 374–375.
33. Perlin ML. (2009). "Simplify you, classify you": Stigma stereotypes and civil rights in disability classification systems. *Ga St Univ Law Rev*, 25, 621.
34. Perlin ML. (2009). "His brain has been mismanaged with great skill": How will jurors respond to neuroimaging testimony in insanity defense cases? *Akron Law Rev*, 42, 912.
35. Diesfeld K, & Freckelton I. (2006). Mental health law and therapeutic jurisprudence. In I Freckelton, & K Peterson (Eds.), *Disputes and dilemmas in health law* (p. 91). Sydney: Federation Press (providing a transnational perspective).

36. Perlin ML. (2008). "Everybody is making love/ or else expecting rain": Considering the sexual autonomy rights of persons institutionalized because of mental disability in forensic hospitals and in Asia. *Wash Law Rev*, 83(139), 510.
37. Perlin ML. (2008). "Baby, look inside your mirror": The legal profession's willful and sanist blindness to lawyers with mental disabilities. *Univ Pitt Law Rev*, 69, 591; (quoting, in part, Perlin, Disability on Trial, *supra* note xxx at 301) (discussing how TJ "might be a redemptive tool in efforts to combat sanism, as a means of 'strip[ping] bare the law's sanist façade' ").
38. Perlmutter BP. (2005). George's story: Voice and transformation through the teaching and practice of therapeutic jurisprudence in a law school child advocacy clinic. *St Thomas Law Rev*, 17(111), 599.
39. Freckelton I. (2008). Therapeutic jurisprudence misunderstood and misrepresented: The price and risks of influence. *T Jefferson Law Rev*, 30, 585–586.
40. Perlin ML. (1991). Morality and pretextuality, psychiatry and law: Of ordinary common sense, heuristic reasoning and cognitive dissonance. *Bull Am Acad Psychiatry Law*, 131.
41. See e.g., Perlin ML. (2005). Limited in sex, they dare: Attitudes toward issues of patient sexuality. *Amer J Forens Psychiatry*, 26, 25.
42. Perlin ML, et al. (2008). Psychiatric ethics and the rights of persons with mental disabilities in the community. *World Psychiatry*, 6, 33–34.
43. Perlin ML. (2013). "There must be some way out of here": Why the convention on the rights of persons with disabilities is potentially the best weapon in the fight against sanism. *Psychiatry Psychol Law*, 20, 426.
44. Perlin ML. (2012). "Too stubborn to ever be governed by enforced insanity": Some therapeutic jurisprudence dilemmas in the representation of criminal defendants in incompetency and insanity cases. *Intl J Law Psychiatry*, 33, 475
45. Payne A, et al. (1993). Sexual activity among psychiatric inpatients: International perspectives, *J Forens Psychiatry*, 4, 109.
46. Kukura L, & Mastman K. (2010). From page to practice: An introduction. *NY Univ Rev Law Soc Change*, 34, 428.
47. Sadoff RL. (1993). Therapeutic jurisprudence: A view from a forensic psychiatrist. *NY Law School J Hum Rts*, 10, 825.
48. Glaser B. (2003). Therapeutic jurisprudence: An ethical paradigm for therapists in sex offender treatment programs. *W Criminol Rev*, 4, 143.
49. Mossman D. (1996). Veterans affairs disability compensation: A case studying counter therapeutic jurisprudence. *Bull Am Cad J Psychiatry Law*, 24, 27.
50. Perlin ML. (2011). *International Human Rights and Mental Disability Law: When the Silenced are Heard*. Oxford, UK: Oxford University Press.
51. Perlin ML. (2013). "Yonder stands your orphan with gun": The international human rights and therapeutic jurisprudence implications of juvenile punishment schemes. *Texas Tech Law Rev*, 46, 301.
52. Perlin ML. (2013). Understanding the intersection between international human rights and mental disability law: The role of dignity. In B Arrigo, H Bersot (Eds.), *The Routledge handbook of international crime and justice studies* (p. 19). Abingdon, UK: Routledge.
53. Perlin ML, & Szeli E. (2012). Mental health law and human rights: Evolution and contemporary challenges: In M Dudley, et al. (Eds.), *Mental health and human rights: Vision, praxis and courage* (p. 98). New York: Oxford University Press.
54. Perlin ML. (2012). Promoting social change in Asian and the Pacific: The need for a disability rights tribunal to give life to the un convention on the rights of persons with disabilities. *Geo Wash Intl Law Rev*, 44, 1.
55. Perlin ML. (2011). "Abandoned love": The impact of Wyatt v. Stickney on the intersection between international human rights and domestic mental disability law. *Law Psychol Rev*, 35, 121.
56. Perlin ML. (2011). "Abandonded love": The impact of Wyatt v. Stickney on the intersection between international human rights and domestic mental disability law. *Law Psychol Rev*, 35, 121.
57. Most recently, in January 2014, at the request of the American Bar Association's Center on Human Rights' Justice Defenders Program, I have filed a declaration with the High Court of Kazakhstan in

the case of *Zinaida Mukhortova v. Republic of Kazakhstan*, a case involving the involuntary psychiatric commitment of a newspaper reporter/attorney who was institutionalized because she (quoting from the moving papers) "gave interviews to the media and started to write complaints to different bodies to 'restore justice'" in Kazakhstan. Perlin ML. (2006). International human rights and comparative mental disability law: The role of institutional psychiatry in the suppression of political dissent. *Israel Law Rev*, 39, 69.

58. See G.A. Res. 61/106, U.N. Doc. A/RES/61/106 (Jan. 24, 2007).
59. Perlin ML. (2013). "Striking for the guardians and protectors of the mind": The convention of the rights of persons with disabilities and the future of guardianship law. *Penn St Law Rev*, 1159.
60. Perlin ML. (2013). "Yonder stands your orphan with gun": The international human rights and therapeutic jurisprudence implications of juvenile punishment schemes. *Tex Tech Law Rev*, 46, 301.
61. Perlin ML. (2013). "The judge, he cast his robe aside": Mental health courts, dignity and due process. *J Ment Health Law Policy*, 3, 1.
62. Perlin ML, & Schriver MR. (2013). "You that hide behind walls": The relationship between the convention on persons with disabilities and the convention against torture and the treatment of institutionalized forensic patients. In: American University Center on Humanitarian Law (Ed.) *Torture and ill-treatment in health-care settings: A compilation*. Washington, DC: American University Center on Humanitarian Law.
63. Perlin ML, & Lynch AJ. (2014). "Love is just a four-letter word": Sexuality, international human rights and therapeutic jurisprudence. *Can J Comp Contemp Law*, in press.
64. Perlin ML, & Lynch AJ. (2014). "All his sexless patients": Persons with mental disabilities and the competence to have sex. *Wash Law Rev*, 89, 257–300.

25

Forensic Psychiatry

A View From a Trial Lawyer and a Judge

Hon. Robert J. Matthews

This chapter presents cases in which an attorney who is now a judge collaborated with forensic psychiatrists to develop defenses and to aid in disposition. Lawyers are often confronted with unusual scenarios in which it is necessary to obtain proper professional assistance. It is often difficult for the attorney to determine which cases require forensic intervention. The three examples given involve criminal law, products liability/medical misadventure, and family law.

Forensic Psychiatry in Criminal Cases

In the early 1970s I represented a client accused of committing a horrible crime: a firebombing that resulted in the deaths of four innocent children and their mother. My client vehemently denied guilt despite the fact that he was present at the scene and signed an eight-page confession. The district attorney also advised me that he had failed an inadmissible lie detector test. I always asked my clients if they did the crime for which they had been charged. This man told me he did not and I believed him despite the circumstantial evidence against him.

How could a young man with a tested IQ of 55 have convinced me that he was innocent? I continued to ask, Why would he do this and deny it? Why would I believe him? Why did his sixth grade teacher in his special education class testify that his former student could not have given an eight-page written statement? He had testified that the defendant with the limited intellectual capacity that he had was not capable of putting together such a complete story with minute details. He also said that his former student could not continually lie and remember the details of his previous denials.

Clearly, the police and prosecutor emphasized the importance of the results of the lie detector and the "confession." I was more focused on his denial of guilt and my belief that he did not do the crime. It was then that I referred the matter to a forensic psychiatrist, who stressed the limited intellect of the defendant and the complexity of both the questions of the original polygrapher and the detailed responses in his written statement. He suggested we give my client simple questions in the second polygraph, such as "Did you know there was a firebombing?" "Did you do it?" "Do you know who did it?" rather than the more complex questions I had proposed initially that he could not understand. He passed the "simpler questioned" polygraph, but was convicted by a jury, who of course did not hear about either lie detector test. The "confession" was suppressed, but an eyewitness was most convincing.

On post-trial motions, the eyewitness recanted, and the actual criminals confessed. It was later revealed that the police and the district attorney withheld exculpatory evidence from the court and the defense. A federal jury convicted the guilty parties and my client was exonerated.

Without the assistance of the forensic psychiatrist, my client would have been sentenced to prison. I had my belief in his innocence but little else with which to work. Belief in a client might result in self-satisfaction, but not a total exposition of the truth. The multidisciplinary approach provides the essential bases for effective collaboration when needed, especially when lives, families, and societal interests are at risk.

Forensic Psychiatry in Civil Cases

Can forensic psychiatry assist the attorney in civil legal cases, especially when medical misadventure is claimed? Several years ago, I was consulted by "Claire" (not her real name) who was in great discomfort from severe urinary obstruction. Tests were ordered, including an X-ray using contrast material containing iodine. She was known to be allergic to certain shellfish and seafood. During the procedure, Claire experienced a cardiac arrest. Although prompt treatment was provided, Claire developed an amnesia for the previous 10 years of her life. She did not recognize her husband nor their three children. She had been married previously and had three children with her first husband, all of whom she did recognize. She was disoriented to time and her current situation. Her urinary condition improved after treatment, but her confusion and amnesia persisted.

Claire also developed other symptoms, including amenorrhea, loss of body hair, headaches, distress, and other confusing symptoms. She did not recognize many of her close friends; her memory loss was quite frightening.

Both of Claire's biological parents died within 3 months of each other about a year prior to her cardiac arrest. During her anaphylactic reaction and cardiac arrest, she described a "near death" experience, reporting that she saw a bright white light at the end of a long tube. During one of these experiences, she said she saw her mother, who told her "Claire, go back, it is not your time." A second time she reported seeing her father who told her the same thing. Claire complied and recalls feeling she was not dead and began a slow recovery, but with the absence of memory for the past 10 years.

Claire's husband, Charles, was very patient and understanding and outwardly he appeared to handle things rather well. However, he was concerned for Claire and the children, who were confused by her lack of memory. He took Claire to an attorney who did little to help resolve the matter. Thus, Claire was referred to me. I was confronted with a vexing problem. The statute of limitations was about to expire in less than a month. I immediately called a forensic psychiatrist for help. His words of comfort were most welcome: "I believe I can help your client." I filed the lawsuit; the statute of limitations was tolled.

Claire's multiple symptomatology resulted in unusual treatment. The forensic psychiatrist gave the opinion that Claire suffered from Conversion Reaction (DSM III was in use at the time) and recommended hypnotherapy by a psychologist-dentist who used hypnosis for pain management and taught at various medical and dental schools. The treatment, which was video/audio taped consisted of 5½ hours, during which Claire engaged in automatic writing. She could not speak openly about the depths of her repressed feelings. In a very relaxed mood she disclosed a memory of a brutal rape to which she was subjected several years previously.

While preparing to enter her place of employment one night, five men grabbed her in the parking area and serially and savagely raped her. She told no one and completed her work shift. She suppressed the horror of that experience and held it all in until the trauma of the cardiac arrest and "near death" experiences. She was a vulnerable woman who had been the victim of a brutal attack and believed she was strong enough to handle the stress alone. She was wrong and paid the price.

Hypnotherapy and forensic psychiatry cured Claire of most of her symptoms. She regained her memory and improved in her medical symptoms.

I conducted a legal study for admissibility for what we lawyers refer to in the Law of Evidence as "memory refreshed." It was my opinion that the testimony of the forensic psychiatrist and the hypnotherapist would be admissible in court. I was wrong! The judge ruled that he would not allow the testimony, nor to have the videotape shown to the jury because he believed that there was too much speculation about "refreshed memory." Without this evidence, which formed the legal basis for the damages portion of the lawsuit, the case could not be won. We did not pursue the lawsuit, but forensic psychiatry won as Claire was cured of her symptoms. Claire and Charles renewed their lives together. Justice, from a lawyer's view, did not prevail, but the client was well served.

Forensic experts excel in their ability to meticulously analyze all known facts and work closely with the attorney in helping to resolve an issue. This collaboration may ultimately save a life, lead to a cure of a medical/psychological injury or disorder, prove or disprove a theory, or assist in the settlement of a dispute. The appropriate dispensation of justice often is the result of the collaborative efforts of the medical profession and the trial lawyer. Such efforts ultimately serve the needs of society.

Forensic Psychiatry in Family Law

How does forensic psychiatry assist a judge in dysfunctional child custody disputes? It is not uncommon to hear the saying: "In criminal court, we frequently encounter the worst people at their best, whereas in family court, we experience the best people at their worst." Tension, animosity, and open hostility are frequent in family disputes. Even though we jurists utilize every skill we have available, we cannot handle many of these acrimonious family matters alone. Can forensic psychiatry offer any benefits to the jurist, the children, or the family?

Absolutely, *yes*. Unfortunately, more often than not, funds are not available for such services. Insurance usually does not cover such costs. Nevertheless, the court must try to help these families. The children are the victims of such dysfunctional families and the damage may go on for generations. It is difficult for a judge in such situations to render a valid decision without forensic assistance. The judge must decide what is in "the best interest of the children" and often realizes that an in-depth forensic custody evaluation and report could be of significant assistance in rendering a proper decision.

Many parents and/or caregivers do not realize they have a condition aggravating the custody situation or that they may be causing the problem. Issues such as alienation, attachment, a lack of parenting skills, or psychological disorders may pose significant problems for the judge. Mental health assessment or forensic psychiatric examinations are extremely helpful to the judge in exposing the causes of the problems and finding reasonable solutions. Most state laws require a complete and extensive analysis of multiple relevant factors before a judge entering a final custody order. However, the judge cannot rely solely on the findings, opinions, or recommendations of a forensic team. It is the judge who must consider all relevant factors in justifying the order, not infrequently via an extensively written opinion for review by the parents and/or a higher court of law, if an appeal ensues.

Case Example

Barbara and Norman were married and produced three beautiful daughters. The marriage fell on hard times, resulting in Norman leaving, moving to another state, and filing for divorce. Barbara had a personality problem and could not handle the rejection by Norman. She vowed to get even with him by getting full custody of the children. Norman would regret his actions, especially marrying another woman. She would take the children from him as punishment. Norman did not agree and the decision fell to the judge. After a 12-hour trial, Barbara was awarded primary physical custody and Norman, partial physical custody on alternating weekends and other times as agreed on the interim order.

However, Barbara was not complying with the Order, the girls' grades were suffering, they were frequently late for school, and had too many absences. The children were referred to a court psychologist who opined that Barbara had a diagnosis of Bipolar II Disorder and Borderline Personality Features. Both parents had life circumstance difficulties, but Norman had no DSM diagnosis. The battles continued, with Barbara insisting on sole physical and legal custody. To her dismay, Norman was having a wonderful relationship with "her" girls.

A second trial was held. The children were not doing well in Barbara's care. In addition, Barbara had assaulted Norman's wife, the new stepmother, and was facing criminal charges for assault. Other unusual events occurred as well. A second mental health evaluation was conducted and the results were not favorable to Barbara's case. Norman was awarded primary physical custody with legal custody being shared by both parents.

After a request by Barbara for reconsideration, the family was referred for an in-depth forensic psychiatric custody evaluation. The children benefited greatly from this evaluation as they developed a closeness with members of the forensic team and began to realize that they were the victims in this battle between their parents. They did not wish to hurt their mother or father, so they made choices in their best interest with flexibility in their parental contacts. The oldest child eventually went with her mother to help care for her.

The result to date is that two of the daughters living with their father are excelling in their education and are socially active in school and after-school activities. The court has little information about the oldest daughter, who is near emancipation and is attached to her mother. The judge has encouraged the two younger girls to have as much physical access and electronic access with Barbara as they desire. Barbara asked the court for partial custody of her two younger daughters for their birthdays. I refused, but allowed mother to greet her daughters and wish them happy birthdays. Barbara cried and hugged each daughter, but they did not reciprocate. That moment revealed that the efforts of the forensic psychiatric team were worth the effort. These young women were affirmed and empowered.

Through cooperative efforts of law and mental health professionals, lives have been altered and children have found security and protection. Results are in "the best interests of the children." A judge is just as much a human being as the evaluating psychiatrist or psychologist, with varied life experiences, education, feelings, biases, beliefs, and opinions. Yet, we professionals, utilizing the cooperative interdisciplinary approach, as demonstrated in this book, realize that we must rely upon the "wholeness of our professional training" and experience in order to render a reasoned opinion or decision. The impact of a nasty custody dispute in court can have a devastating effect on a child. Working together, we can greatly alleviate potential damage to these precious children.

I have faith in the future of our professions: that we shall continue to honor our commitment to health, physically, morally, ethically, and professionally.

26

The Growing Intersection of Forensic Psychiatry and Federal Criminal Defense

NiaLena Caravasos

As federal law has undergone a metamorphosis in recent years regarding sentencing proceedings, the roles of the expert forensic psychiatrist and psychologist as well as the treating forensic psychiatrist have also evolved and become even more relevant.

The Sentencing Reform Act was a federal statute enacted as part of the Comprehensive Crime Control Act of 1984 with the stated goal of increasing consistency in federal sentencing. It established the United States Sentencing Commission as well as a rigid methodology to be undertaken every time a federal defendant was sentenced. Although the stated goal of increasing consistency in sentences handed down nationwide for similar crimes seemed on its face to be a worthy one, the rigid methodology resulted not only in eliminating much of the judiciary's discretion, but also in leaving little room for meaningful consideration of defendants' unique characteristics and circumstances contributing to their offenses. Over the next 20 years, the judiciary as well as various organizations advocating for defendants' rights slowly but surely began to voice discontent. As the years passed, the grumblings became stronger and change finally occurred.

These changes have also resulted in giving life to a much more expansive role of forensic psychiatry in the advocacy on behalf of a client in a federal criminal setting. Examples include, but are not limited to: (1) assessing and exploring a client's mental health challenges along with certain aspects of his or her life circumstances that may have played a role in the motivation for the commission of the crime; (2) facilitating an opportunity for clients to engage in treatment and therapy and/or self-rehabilitation that may then be translated into powerful arguments at the time of sentencing; and (3) assisting lawyers in evaluating the true motivations of a client by identifying a client who is truly suffering from a mental health challenge versus a client who may simply be engaging in manipulation tactics.

Before 2005, the federal sentencing guidelines were mandatory. As such, the opportunity for any federal judge to deviate from the mandatory guideline range in imposing a sentence was truly limited to extraordinary exceptions recognized by the United States Sentencing Commission. Consequently, unless a defendant's circumstances fit squarely into one of those extraordinarily limited exceptions, the hands of the federal judge were tied by the mandatory nature of the sentencing guidelines. Circa 2005, all of that changed.

In *United States v. Booker*, 543 U.S. 220 (2005), the United States Supreme Court invalidated the portion of the Sentencing Reform Act (18 U.S.C. §3553 (b)(1)) that previously made the sentencing guidelines mandatory. Even though sentencing courts must nevertheless still consider the federal sentencing guidelines, they must also consider all of the other factors set forth in §3553(a). Indeed, following *Booker*, the United States Court of Appeals for the Third Circuit outlined a three-step approach for sentencing courts. First, district courts must begin by correctly calculating the applicable sentencing guideline range, just as courts did before *Booker*. Second, sentencing courts must still rule on departure motions and determine, through the sentencing guidelines' calculus, the case-specific applicable sentencing guideline range. Although the sentencing guidelines are the starting point, they are by no means the only consideration. In fact, federal law is clear that the guidelines are no more controlling of the final sentencing decision than any of the other multiple factors that must be considered under §3553(a) as a whole. *United States v. Grier*, 475 F.3d 556, 571 (3rd Cir. 2007) ("the Sentencing Reform Act mandates that the district court "consider" the factors of 18 U.S.C. §3553(a)"); *United States v. Gunter*, 462 F.3d 237, 247 (3rd Cir. 2006).

In addition to listing the various sentencing considerations in sub-parts (a)(1) through (7), §3553(a) contains a preliminary directive that states that "[t]he court shall impose a sentence sufficient, but not greater than necessary, to comply with the purposes set forth in paragraph 2 of this sub-section." Generally referred to as the "parsimony provision," the Court stated in *Kimbrough v. United States*, 128 S.Ct. 558 (2007) that this provision is "overarching" in nature:

> The statute, as modified by *Booker*, contains an *overarching* provision instructing district courts to "impose a sentence sufficient, but not greater than necessary" to accomplish the goals of sentencing, including "to reflect the seriousness of the offense," "to promote respect for the law," "to provide just punishment for the offense," "to afford adequate deterrence to criminal conduct," and "to protect the public from further crimes of the defendant." Id. at 570 (emphasis added).

This language clearly suggests that the parsimony provision now functions as a lens through which all sentences must be evaluated at both the district and appellate court levels.

As the First Circuit noted in *United States v. Rodriguez*, 527 F. 3d 221 (1st Cir. 2008), *Kimbrough* indicates the following:

> [S]ection 3553(a) is more than a laundry list of discrete sentencing factors; it is, rather, a tapestry of factors, through which runs the thread of an overarching principle. That tenet (sometimes referred to as the parsimony principle), instructs district courts to impose a sentence sufficient, but not greater than necessary to accomplish the goals of sentencing. This overarching principle necessarily informs a sentencing court's consideration of the entire constellation of section 3553(a) factors, including the need to avoid unwarranted disparity. Similarly, judicial interpretation of section 3553(a) should be guided by the broadly worded goals of sentencing spelled out in section 3553(a)(2), to which *Kimbrough* pays homage.
>
> In the final analysis, then, the gloss supplied by *Kimbrough* signifies that a district court should not evaluate a request for a variant sentence piecemeal, examining each section 3553(a) factor in isolation, but should instead consider all the relevant factors as a group and strive to construct a sentence that is minimally sufficient to achieve the broad goals of sentencing. This inquiry should be guided by, but not made unflinchingly subservient to, the concerns expressed by the statute's various sub-parts. Id. at 228 (internal quotations and citations omitted); see also United States v. Foreman, 436 F.3d 638, 644 n.1 (6th Cir. 2006) ("...a district court's mandate is to impose 'a sentence sufficient, but not greater than necessary, to comply with the purposes' of section 3553(a)(2)"); United States v. Martinez-Barragan, 545 F.3d 894, 904 (10th Cir. 2008) ("When crafting a sentence, the district court must be guided by the 'parsimony principle'").

This metamorphosis in the law has truly served to transform the landscape of how a good federal criminal practitioner approaches a case and a client. Before *Booker*, the issues regarding a sentencing proceeding were not really contemplated and, even if contemplated, were certainly not dealt with before reaching that point in a case. Because the hands of the judiciary were tied to a very large extent, there was really no reason to focus on a sentencing proceeding at an earlier point in the timeline of the case. Very little could be done to change the course of destiny of a convicted defendant in any meaningful sense and, therefore, the primary focus of counsel was to try to defeat the charges at a trial or, alternatively, to try to reach the best possible plea agreement. As a result, more defendants went to trial because they had no other viable options, given the fact that this was usually perceived as the only realistic (or unrealistic) option by which they had to proceed, unless they were willing and able to cooperate with the government.

Fast-forwarding to the post-*Booker* era, a good lawyer with care and foresight begins to contemplate the sentencing of his or her client at the onset of the case, along with cultivating the legal aspects and phases of the case before sentencing (assuming that a conviction results). This foresight and forward thinking is especially critical in federal cases, which for the most part necessitate a long time to develop because of their inherent complexity and seriousness and often multiple defendants. The development of a federal case can typically run 1 year and perhaps even much longer, depending on the nature and circumstances of the case. Consequently, it is critical for counsel to spend the time at the onset of the case in order to really get to know the client as much as possible and to try to identify issues that are fertile and that can potentially be cultivated going forward. In doing so, it is especially important for a lawyer to be mindful of the ultimate goals of sentencing, as perceived by the federal courts and as delineated earlier in this chapter, and to try to figure out what endeavors during the development of the case may address those ultimate sentencing goals and ultimately serve to benefit the client. For these reasons, sophisticated federal criminal lawyers have found the opportunity in their practices to cultivate a growing intersection between the federal criminal law and forensic psychiatry.

Ali

One key example of a criminal case in which it was glaringly obvious that forensic psychiatry would and should play a critical role in helping the client, either at trial or sentencing or both, was during the federal criminal prosecution of a man in his thirties identified by the pseudonym of Ali.

When counsel first met Ali, it was under very precarious circumstances. His brother had contacted counsel in reference to potential representation for Ali, who had just been indicted by a federal grand jury. Unbeknown to his brother, Ali had been so devastated and ashamed by his arrest and the ultimate effect that he perceived it would have on his family that he had attempted suicide more than once while in lockup at the Federal Detention Center. When counsel first met him in the federal prison, he begged her not to tell his family about the suicide attempts because he did not want to worry them. Counsel had no choice but to agree to keep his secret, as it was a client confidence that must be held inviolate and there existed no overriding compelling need to disclose it. However, this presented quite a bit of challenge for counsel and put into play her credibility with his family because they could not understand why she wanted to hold off before making her request for pretrial release. It was clear to counsel that no federal judge in his or her right mind would even consider allowing Ali out on bail until and unless his mental health were stabilized and arrangements were put in place to ensure continued mental health treatment upon release. Of course, the fact that the government (mis)perceived Ali, an Arab American, as being tangentially connected to someone involved with terrorism added a whole new dimension of problems to the case and to the immediate issue of counsel's efforts to secure bail.

Nevertheless, counsel's first immediate challenge was to find a way to connect on a human level with Ali quickly and profoundly so that he would trust her, so that his anxiety level would decrease and he would hopefully no longer have an immediate suicidal urge, and so that she could try and help him stabilize to the point at which the focus could shift to putting into place the necessary arguments and safeguards that would allow a judge to comfortably entertain the thought of pretrial release. Although Ali was initially distrustful of counsel because of his own inherent paranoid tendencies, his perception ultimately changed through the course of time and counsel's persistent efforts to demonstrate to Ali that she was indeed worthy of his trust. Counsel also tried very hard to work as much as possible with the chief clinical psychologist in the Federal Detention Center because she knew that her ultimate recommendation would carry great weight with the judge regarding whether Ali presented any continuing risk to himself. All of this took a month, but counsel was finally able to secure Ali's pretrial release, along with a plan for continuing mental health treatment. Ali was in such a fragile mental state that counsel firmly believes to this day that he would literally not have survived if he had been forced to remain incarcerated during the pretrial phase of the case.

The federal indictment against Ali charged him with various offenses, including conspiracy to traffic internationally in counterfeit goods, conspiracy to make false statements to government officials in order to acquire a fake social security card, and conspiracy to commit passport fraud. A conspiracy is defined as an agreement between two or more people to commit an illegal act or a legal act in an illegal manner. In order to sustain a conspiracy charge, there has to be a finding of at least one overt act (e.g., conversation alone is insufficient to sustain a finding of conspiracy) that was performed in furtherance of the conspiracy. However, the illegal act need not have actually been committed in order to sustain a conspiracy charge. Among the key pieces of evidence in Ali's case were an enormous amount of conversations generated from wiretap surveillance and consensual recordings by an undercover agent. Ali's role in those conversations (in which he referred to himself by an alias name) constituted a critical factor, but not only in his indictment and the charges that were brought against him. The dissection of those wiretap conversations, along with the forensic psychological and psychiatric analyses that ensued, ultimately contributed greatly toward counsel's ability to secure a dismissal of the most serious charges, in Ali's ability to understand the genesis of his behavior and to begin to repair and transform himself, and in counsel's ability to secure a severely mitigated sentence for the one charge that remained.

When Ali arrived for his psychiatric evaluation by forensic psychiatrist Dr. S. (real name not used) and his subsequent psychological evaluation with forensic psychologist Dr. D. (real name not used), he was literally shaking like a leaf from the stress and anxiety of the situation. Indeed, although the probing analysis ultimately provided an enormous and life-altering benefit to both Ali's psychological healing and counsel's ability to best represent him in his case, the initial impact of the intense probing was so traumatic for Ali that it resulted in him pulling away from any discussion, or at least not any meaningful discussion, of his case for a period of months because he simply could not deal with thinking about it and became debilitated. Thankfully, he was fortunate enough to have his brother, who served as the backbone of his support system and as the person who would also communicate with counsel during the time period in which Ali was, figuratively speaking, in absentia.

Through the intense forensic analysis came the discovery that Ali was considered as the black sheep in his family and often felt lost and neglected at home because of the large number of children. Not only was he the recipient of physical and psychological abuse, primarily by his father, but also he engaged in constant arguing with his parents because he often felt unable to freely express his views. Additionally, Ali's father frequently drank an enormous amount of alcohol in order to cope with the family problems and his inability to financially provide for such a large family. He would often beat Ali while in a drunken state and had even knocked his teeth out at one point. In addition to feeling victimized by the physical and psychological abuse at home, Ali also felt that he was prejudiced in school and in his neighborhood because he was an Arab and also because of distasteful and cruel jokes associated with his real name (not disclosed herein), which thereby translated into behavioral problems and other difficulties at school and while growing up. Despite the turmoil, Ali managed to graduate high school and begin taking college courses. However, the physical exhaustion of maintaining a full-time job and a full-time college course load, coupled with the emotional toll of being a teenager and being thrust into the role of trying to be the sole provider for his parents and numerous siblings, forced him to drop out of college in order to support his family.

Although he managed to support his family successfully for a period of time, the devastation of 9/11 affected his business sales because most of the stores that he dealt with were in Manhattan. As his business profits began to decline and eventually were extinguished, Ali fell into what he believes was a major depression and ended up borrowing money from a loan shark in order to pay his mounting debts. Regrettably, not only had the trade shows dried up along with his ability to afford the rent at his store, but also his father (whom he had brought to help out in an effort to get him out of the house) began to alienate some of the other employees as well as some of the customers with his attitude, thereby contributing in large part to the eventual loss of the business.

In order to escape his growing debt to the loan shark that he was unable to pay, Ali attempted to free himself from his troubles by traveling to South America, where he began working and also became engaged. Unfortunately, he was not only shunned by his fiancée's father, who could not accept the fact that Ali was Arab, but also his fiancée miscarried their child. Ali became so extremely depressed between the loss of the child and the problems that they faced that he engaged in his first suicide attempt. The loss of his unborn child threw him into turmoil because this brought back a very painful childhood memory of a time when he suffered the loss of his baby brother, a loss about which he felt tremendous guilt and that he proceeded to carry with him throughout his life. When Ali's younger brother was born, the baby began receiving more of the family's attention, after which point Ali felt jealous of him and would often wish that his brother would die. The baby boy, who was less than 1 year old at the time, then became terribly ill from an immunization shot and passed away. As a result, Ali became consumed with guilt and carried that devastating guilt with him into adulthood. Since then, Ali tried to adopt his brother's name in some sense to keep his brother alive in his own mind and also because it served to help him shed some of the ridicule that he had received from others because of his own embarrassing given name.

Although Ali physically survived his first suicide attempt in South America, he did not surpass the losses that he had sustained thus far in his life. Returning to New York City, he tried to secure employment but was barely getting by. A couple of years later, in his effort to make connections for further business opportunities, Ali ended up getting involved with someone who was dealing in stolen merchandise and eventually got caught up in pretending to be someone important.

As revealed by the forensic examinations, Ali came to realize that having people believe that he was a major player in this field made him feel good about himself at a time when he had nothing else going for him except very low self-esteem. Ali then engaged in numerous lies just to impress a particular man in the hope that it would benefit him in the long run since he had been told that this man could get him a false social security number and driver's license to use for identification. Despite the fact that the government believed that Ali was involved in some major fraud scheme and was therefore in need of official paperwork to support an alternate identity, the truth is that he simply needed both items in order to re-establish his credit score that had imploded over the years.

Indeed, he jumped at the glimmer of hope that he saw for a new life without thinking of the consequences, as all he could visualize was the possibility of finally having a new prospect at life again since he was no longer really able to use his own name to start a business or get a social security card because he had been in bankruptcy and had creditors. Unfortunately, the man to whom Ali was lying in order to impress turned out to be an undercover federal agent. Nevertheless, the truth of the matter is that a number of the lies that he told were tremendous exaggerations of his criminal conduct. Also unbeknown to the federal government at the time of indictment was the fact that the alias name that was being used by Ali during the wiretapped conversations (and that the government mistakenly interpreted as some covert effort to hide his true identity for nefarious reasons) was really just the name of his deceased baby brother.

The results of the psychological testing revealed Ali to be a man with not only a severe level of anxiety and depression along with a bipolar variant, but also one with an extremely low sense of self-worth and poor self-esteem that had been ongoing for quite a long time. With regard to his personality dynamics, Ali had a very disdainful view of himself and the world around him and indeed often regretted being born. Moreover, there was also an indication that Ali not only suffered from some traumatic stress as a result of being abused during his childhood, but also that he may have been suffering a reoccurrence of traumatization as a result of the arrest that occurred in his federal case. Although this alone was not sufficient to create a condition of traumatic stress, it certainly did exacerbate the trauma of his earlier life that had been marked by the psychological and physical abuse by his father as well as the death of his baby brother.

Clinically, Ali's profile indicated a severely paranoid personality makeup with some almost borderline psychotic characteristics, as he was constantly struggling with hostile, tense, and agitated feelings, particularly when he felt that he was being trapped or threatened. Moreover, he was prone toward acting-out as a major defense mechanism with poor impulse control and defective judgment and forethought, and he was also severely depressed and anxious and very prone toward feeling misunderstood, unappreciated, and unfairly treated by others. He was also strongly prone to project his angry feelings and aggressive impulses onto others and tended to overreact not only to anger in others, but also especially to events that he saw as confirming of his own projections.

With regard to Ali's conduct that resulted in his federal arrest, the forensic evaluations and analyses further found clear indication that his weak ego functioning and poor sense of self-perception and self-worth contributed to him making up lies and exaggerating his involvement in illegal activity with his cohorts in order to make himself feel important. This was particularly significant since the individuals to whom he was lying seemed to represent some form of authority, which gave more impetus for him to impress them. Ali always wanted to be something special and, unfortunately, this was an avenue where he felt he could make a mark for himself and at least be somebody. Unfortunately, his blind need interfered with his use of reason and judgment, and he became embroiled in a scheme that was much more elaborate than he was aware. The reality, though, was that Ali was by no means a mastermind and was clearly someone who was vulnerable and got swept up in a situation that was beyond his control.

As a criminal defense attorney, it is always extremely significant and potentially extremely helpful to be able to craft out of logic and reason an alternative theory/explanation to the government's evidence. The fact that the forensic evaluations and analyses conducted by Drs. S. and D. were able to substantiate counsel's own alternative theory regarding Ali's behavior and his mindset was truly priceless and, without exaggeration, life-saving in his case. Armed with these forensic weapons, counsel was then able to marry the findings with her own evaluation and reasoned interpretations of the wiretapped conversations in order to demonstrate and convince the government of the fact that there was a very reasonable and actually quite likely alternative theory to their evidence, and that embracing this alternative theory, which was supported by forensic psychological and psychiatric evaluation and findings, necessarily and equitably would result in a dismissal of the most serious charges against Ali.

Obviously, counsel could have gone to trial on this alternative theory. Instead, counsel chose to aggressively explore with the government and pursue the option of a non-trial disposition (by embarking upon a path of using the ammunition that counsel had gathered to convince the government that the dismissal of most charges was warranted) because she believed that was in her client's best interest since the forensic evaluations had also revealed (unbeknown to the government, of course) that Ali's mental health was so fragile that he most likely would not be able to successfully survive the stress and ordeal of a trial. It was literally a race against the clock to help Ali at a time when it mattered most and could really make the most difference in his life. Without the benefit of the forensic ammunition that had been given to her, counsel would have never known that the clock was ticking so quickly, nor would she have had the tools necessary to find her way out of the labyrinth.

Of course, a reputable and ethical lawyer will never look for a psychiatric or psychological finding that is not born out of the evidence and that does not legitimately exist. Although there do exist those "hired guns" who are known in the industry for always providing a helpful opinion to a particular side, their opinion in reality holds no real value for just that very reason. Ultimately, a good lawyer will seek the opinion of someone who is totally and completely above reproach and who is viewed that way by all sides (i.e., the defense, the prosecution, and the judiciary). Indeed, in the case of Ali, counsel was only able to rely on the forensic findings to such a degree because she knew that the reputations of Drs. S. and D. were such that no one would ever question the integrity of their findings.

In addition to providing counsel with the necessary tools and critical insight in order to be able to best help Ali in his federal case and in his life, the forensic evaluations and analyses also helped counsel to really understand the deficiencies and challenges that Ali was struggling with from a psychiatric and psychological perspective. That critical insight was key in helping counsel to reinforce Ali's strengths and to address his deficiencies in a manner so as to give him the confidence to be able to go forward in the most productive way. Moreover, the insight along with the medication and psychotherapy in which Ali was engaging in separately really helped him to understand and begin to conquer his demons. After working his way through the pain, Ali was able to slowly learn how to believe in himself again. He re-enrolled in college and focused on achieving high grades, he worked very hard in therapy so that he could grow as a person and stabilize himself, he began to volunteer for an international organization that was aiding people in Africa, and he really began to soar.

As a result of the forensic analysis and findings, counsel was also able to instinctively understand the issues driving Ali's enormously low self-esteem as well as what might help to reverse that. Consequently, because counsel fiercely believed in Ali as well as his ability to ultimately succeed, counsel was inspired to "Name A Star" after him and in honor of his baby brother who had died. It was counsel's way of letting Ali know that she believed his star was rising and that by making something of his life and excelling, he would not only be able to proudly carry on, but also that he would be able to honor his baby brother's memory in the process. Ali was incredibly moved at this small gesture, primarily because no one had ever before done anything like that for him. He was so excited that he even shared the coordinates of his star with his college astronomy class so that they could help him locate it in the night sky.

Interestingly enough, this simple act of kindness was able to strike such a meaningful chord within Ali that it inspired him to truly want to excel in his studies, his therapy, and his life. At sentencing, the judge not only rewarded him and counsel's efforts by giving him a probationary sentence, but also the judge complimented him in open court and told him how truly impressed she was by everything that he had achieved during his transformation. Were it not for the incredible insight and sage advice of Drs. S. and D., none of this would have been possible.

In addition to the traditional route of securing a forensic expert for evaluation of the client defendant and analysis of the issues at play, the changes described in the preceding in the federal sentencing guidelines have allowed for the opportunity to really cultivate in a creative way the use of treating forensic psychiatrists, whom are very few and far between. Although forensic psychiatrists who also maintain a practice of treating patients are indeed a rare breed, they offer a unique set of skills that can be very creatively used to a defendant's benefit by a good federal practitioner who is thinking outside the box.

This is especially true under the scenario in which the defendant is a first-time offender who is accepting responsibility (and may even be cooperating with the federal government). The reason for this is because most defendants who are accepting responsibility and are first-time offenders do not have the kind of psychological makeup that would require additional expert forensic evaluation and analysis independent of treatment with a forensically trained professional. Rather, they usually tend to be individuals who have otherwise lived law-abiding, productive lives but yet harbor unresolved issues from the past that have somehow become intertwined with their current psychological makeup and have resulted in playing a key role as to what went wrong in their lives that contributed to them finding themselves at the doorstep of the federal criminal justice system.

Additionally, because these defendants may even be cooperating with the federal government in an effort to make amends for their wrongdoings in the hope of obtaining some leniency at sentencing, they are more likely to be the type of individuals who would be amenable to the kind of introspective analysis and transformation in which therapy and treatment would be most beneficial.

Gill

An illuminating example of a criminal case in which a psychiatrist who possessed not only a forensic background but who also maintained a cadre of patients requiring psychotherapy was able to play a critical role in both helping the client as well as the case was during the federal criminal prosecution of a another man also in his thirties and identified by the pseudonym of Gill.

When counsel first met Gill and he came to her office for the purpose of retaining her to represent him, he had already made the decision that he wanted to accept responsibility for his wrongdoings and begin cooperating with the federal government. He wanted very much to make amends for his leadership role in a very large criminal tax scheme. Consequently, he successfully embarked upon that path, a path that actually took more than 4 years to fully develop. The ensuing time proved extremely difficult for Gill because he was really struggling in his efforts to understand (so that counsel could then also understand) why someone like him who had an advanced degree from a good university had become so embroiled in a high-level white collar criminal case.

Counsel realized that Gill needed some professional assistance in order to begin to understand and work through his issues and, thus, she encouraged him to seek psychiatric/psychological counseling. He was relatively open to counsel's suggestion, but finances were his primary concern, as he was only holding down part-time employment and also had family responsibilities. Consequently, after putting counsel off for quite some time, he eventually sought out someone who was covered by his health insurance, which ended up being a licensed social worker. Counsel was not at all optimistic about how this would work out, but she did not want to put more financial pressure on him and therefore decided to allow him to give it a try. This effort lasted for close to 1 year. It was a disaster by all accounts. First and foremost, as counsel had predicted, the social worker really did not have the skills and insight necessary to recognize the client's issues and effectively help him work through them. Additionally, she (like many in the field who do not have advanced training and education and who also are not forensically trained) had a fear of and aversion to lawyers and was therefore unwilling to communicate with counsel in any meaningful manner. The therapist's total unwillingness to communicate with counsel, along with her inability to accurately assess and deal with the client's issues in psychotherapy, was pretty much the beginning of the end regarding her sessions with Gill.

Although the goals of treatment do not necessarily always mirror the goals of the legal case, they are nevertheless often closely related. It is therefore critical for counsel to have ongoing insight as to the progress being made during therapy in order to make certain that the various significant issues are being properly addressed. That way, counsel can later dissect the findings and attempt to use them in the most powerful way to help the client in his legal quandary. For the client's sake, counsel tried and tried to communicate with her over a period of months to no avail. Counsel finally told Gill in no uncertain terms that the social worker was not working out and that he had to allow counsel to refer him to an appropriately trained person who would be able to properly identify his issues as well as appropriately communicate with counsel. He continued to resist because he did not want to hurt the social worker's feelings and primarily because of financing concerns. Only when he developed suicidal ideations did he finally acquiesce and follow counsel's advice. Counsel's advice led him to the doorstep of treating forensic psychiatrist Dr. R. (real name not used). After he had begun treating with Dr. R. for only a few months, Gill acknowledged to counsel that he could not believe that he had resisted her promptings so greatly and that he had waited so very long to get the help that he now realized for himself he really needed.

When Gill first presented to Dr. R., he held himself out with his tough guy exterior. Even though he was hurting terribly inside and crying out for help, he was engaged in his own internal struggle about whether to allow himself to feel the pain in order to be able to accept the help. Dr. R. was very patient but stern with him, and he slowly began to open up and admit that he needed help. Progressively, he was able to stabilize his anxiety with medication and make tremendous strides in his own thought processes.

As a result of her forensic assessment as well as her treatment, Dr. R. was able to recognize the fact that Gill's very chaotic background, in both the distant and recent past, impacted his decision-making abilities, both generally as well as in his federal case, in a negative manner. As it turns out, not only had Gill been very close to his great-grandmother, who died when he was young, but also he had been very close to his sister, who died only a few years later. It was only a couple of years afterward that even more trauma ensued, with the death of Gill's brother and the murder of his nephew. Actually, there were so many deaths around the same time while Gill was growing up that he used to play "funeral" with his toy action figures and began missing school regularly because of depression that went untreated.

As it turned out, Dr. R. was able to conclude that at the time of the events having to do with the federal criminal tax scheme for which he was indicted, Gill was under the type of duress that caused him to repeat his childhood experience of having very close members of his family die or experience life-threatening illness. Indeed, his mother had suffered a stroke that she survived but needed his assistance, whereas his father developed cancer and required treatment. Additionally, Gill's grandmother, with whom he was extremely close and who helped raise him, died suddenly of a stroke at almost the same time. In her forensic analysis, Dr. R. found that although anyone could feel stressed by this situation, since it so closely paralleled the losses he experienced in youth, he had a recurrence of his overwhelmed feelings and impaired judgment.

Indeed, Dr. R. found not only that Gill had experienced post traumatic stress disorder (PTSD) as an adolescent, but also that he was vulnerable to the same emotional problems as an adult when he tried to deal with the severe illnesses of his parents and the death of a beloved grandmother, who was like a parent to him. Regarding his actions that led to the criminal tax indictment, the forensic findings concluded that Gill had a foreshortened sense of his own future, was impulsive, and wanted to provide a better material life for his family and show his sons that he was a good father, unlike his own father.

Consequently, although there was no legally justifiable theory to excuse Gill's criminal conduct, the forensic findings nevertheless did support the proposition that there was at least a medical explanation for his behavior. Through therapy, Gill was not only able to acknowledge that the short-term gain of his criminal actions was not worth the consequences, but also he was able to demonstrate genuine remorse in his sessions and also through volunteer work and cooperating with the authorities. By the time of sentencing, Gill had self-rehabilitated to the degree that counsel was able to successfully argue that the goals of sentencing had already been satisfied in large part in reference to him regarding promotion of respect for the law, just punishment, the need for deterrence, protection of society, and so on, thereby reducing his sentencing exposure from a period of several years to only several months incarceration.

Unlike most clients like Ali and Gill, who are truly seeking the best possible representation and outcome for themselves, there also exist those criminal defendants who are simply looking to game the system and their lawyers as much as possible. When such a scenario exists, it is critical that the lawyer realize it and endeavor not only to protect the client and advocate as best as possible on his or her behalf, but also to protect himself or herself from the client and inevitable repercussions that may follow as part of the client's "gaming" efforts.

Steve

One such example, in which a client was looking to manipulate his lawyer by calling into question his own mental stability, is the federal criminal prosecution of a man in his twenties identified by the pseudonym of Steve.

Steve was federally indicted and charged with conspiracy to possess with the intent to distribute multi-kilo quantities of cocaine as well as several distribution counts, along with various charges involving the possession of firearms by a convicted felon and also in furtherance of a drug trafficking offense. The evidence against Steve involved not only the seizure of drugs and guns and large amounts of cash in his place of residence, but also several hundred wiretapped conversations involving him and numerous co-conspirators, buyers, and suppliers. After evaluating the bulk of the evidence against Steve and listening to the majority of the phone conversations, counsel clearly saw the bleakness of Steve's chances of success at trial and urged him to seriously consider allowing her to explore the option of a possible non-trial disposition that would hopefully spare Steve from spending the rest of his life in prison.

Steve refused to consider exploring any such options and instead assured counsel that he would not spend the rest of his life in prison. When counsel pressed him on what he meant by this, given the evidence against him and the certainty of a conviction if not on all of the counts then on enough of them to secure an extraordinarily lengthy lifelong sentence, Steve acknowledged the reality of his case but emphasized that he would not be spending the rest of his life in prison. When counsel verbalized her suspicion that he was suggesting he would commit suicide if convicted, Steve acknowledged that this is what he was suggesting. When counsel expressed great distress and dismay over this realization, Steve urged her not to worry about it. Although most criminal defense attorneys would not have worried about it and would simply have disregarded it and proceeded with the case, counsel for Steve felt quite differently about the matter. By her estimation, there were various ethical obligations as well as practical factors at issue.

The first issue had to do with Steve's mental stability and competency to proceed with the case versus the possibility that he was simply trying to "game" his lawyer by proceeding under some ill-conceived notion that counsel could win the case for him if she were motivated enough to do so. The second issue had to do with counsel protecting herself from future liability if Steve did indeed commit suicide following a conviction and counsel had not done anything to try to prevent this when the matter was brought to her attention. The third issue had to do with the fact that counsel believed that Steve was engaging in a manipulation game and therefore felt the need to call him on it in an effort to shift the power dynamics and protect her reputation as well as gain control of the attorney–client relationship. Consequently, counsel advised the judge that there existed an issue of grave concern upon which she could not elaborate further without revealing a client confidence but that had to be addressed before counsel could proceed with the case. Counsel then proceeded to seek the assistance of forensic psychiatrist Dr. W. (real name not used) for the purpose of evaluating Steve.

Although initially Steve was unwilling to be evaluated, counsel advised him in no uncertain terms that she would not be willing to continue representing him unless he allowed and participated in the evaluation. Steve desired for counsel to continue representing him and therefore acquiesced to the request. Dr. W. was then able to meet with Steve and counsel together and also separately with Steve in order to evaluate him and render his opinion not only about his mental competency, but also about his true motivations. By engaging Dr. W. in this regard, counsel was able to meet her ethical obligations, ensure that Steve was mentally fit to proceed with his case and participate in his defense, and protect herself from any future liability in the event that Steve ultimately did commit suicide.

Ultimately, though, counsel's suspicions (which had been reinforced by Dr. W.'s opinion) about Steve's agenda were ultimately proved correct. When this first effort at manipulation failed, Steve subsequently continued his quest and even tried to use counsel's good name in order to further game the system and potentially endanger the lives of third parties. In the end, counsel's interests in protecting her hard-earned reputation and well-known integrity took precedence over Steve's interest in having a zealous advocate, and counsel ultimately moved to withdraw from any further representation of him.

Conclusion

Although traditionally the role of forensic psychiatry/psychology in a criminal case was far more constrained and limited to the typical evaluations mostly for competency and less often for sanity, the evolution of federal criminal law now allows the role of the forensic psychiatrist/psychologist to be as expansive as a creative and forward-thinking lawyer will allow. Perhaps this is a result of the law's growing recognition and appreciation for mental health forensic matters. Perhaps, on the other hand, it is more likely a result of the explosion of federal inmates who can no longer be adequately housed by the existing prison system, thereby allowing for arguments that may result in the imposition of a sentence sufficient but not greater than necessary to meet the goals of sentencing. Either way, whether the law has evolved because of insight or reality or some combination of those factors, it nevertheless has evolved so now is the time to maximize the positive effects of that evolution.

Truth be told, many federal judges are not eager to incarcerate a defendant for a lengthy period of time if they do not have to and, therefore, truly welcome some real insight about the defendant and his or her life and circumstances and difficulties and motivations that contributed to the commission of the offense. That way, a jurist can meaningfully dissect the entire panorama of information presented by the defense as well as the government in an effort to impose the most appropriate (and often least restrictive) sentence. Although a lawyer may believe and represent this or that about a particular client, such representations often carry little weight and have minimal impact unless they are backed up with true insight and analysis and solid findings and recommendations by an appropriately trained professional. In counsel's humble opinion, it is without question that the use of forensic psychiatric consultations and evaluations along with the collaborative efforts of the forensic expert and the attorney have immensely benefited not only defendants but also the administration of justice as a whole. To put it bluntly, counsel would not have been able to save the lives and futures of many of her clients were it not for the forensic psychiatrists and forensic psychologists with whom she has had the pleasure and honor to work over the past several years.

27

Forensic Psychiatry in Law Enforcement

A Practitioner's Perspective

George Cronin*

The Police and the Mentally Ill

The police are responsible for the safety and welfare of the community they serve. They are empowered by law to bring a solution or resolution to any problem upon which they are called. In some communities, particularly rural areas, the police are the first and only resource to handle urgent problems.[1] These problems may be violations of law, but more commonly, the police are called to bring order. We trust they will respond when we call no matter the day or time, and latently we acknowledge police will use whatever force is required.[2,3] It is within this framework that police assume authority when responding to problems.

The police officer in the field responds to a variety of situations, among which is dealing with the mentally ill. The police prioritize their response to where a violation of law is discovered.[3] The police receive extensive training in preparation for these situations and their actions are dictated by statute and procedural law. But the majority of time the police are engaged in activities related to keeping the peace or problem solving. In performing these activities the police have a great deal of discretion in finding solutions beyond an arrest. When exercising discretion the police find some guidance in their department policy or training, but most follow the rules of common practice. In most cases the police officer's interaction with the mentally ill is highly discretionary. However, with every interaction

*The views presented in this chapter are those of George Cronin, Ph.D. and do not necessarily represent the views of the Pennsylvania State Police.

the police officer always must be aware of the liability associated with excessive use of force, wrongful arrest, or failure to act.[3,4]

During the 1950s there was an ideological change in the treatment of the diagnosed mentally ill. Deinstitutionalization, for purposes of this paper, is defined as the transfer of the mentally ill from hospitals. The catalyst for this change was the public perception of warehousing of the mentally ill in deteriorating hospitals, the development of new medications, and major reductions in spending by the states, shifting the financial burden to the federal government. These changes dramatically reduced funding for mental health services and states created more restrictive rules for involuntary mental health commitments.[5,6] Conceptually, the plan was for community based services to assume care for the diagnosed mentally ill, but that did not materialize. Instead there was a sudden and steady increase in the numbers of mentally ill without proper treatment plans or supervision in the community, particularly in urban areas.

With the increased numbers of mentally ill in the community has come an increased demand on the police as the number of contacts between the mentally ill and the police increase.[7] In Pennsylvania, the Pennsylvania State Police (PSP), primarily a rural police agency, report from 2012 to 2013, there were 6400 contacts with the mentally ill.[8] In 2000, The New York City Police estimated they respond to about 18,000 calls for emotionally disturbed persons every year.[9] The literature indicates that the number of calls for police service across all police agencies regarding the mentally ill are ever-increasing.[7]

Largely from personal experience and anecdotal accounts from other officers, the police perceive the mentally ill as unpredictable and dangerous. Although it is not the function of the police to make psychiatric diagnoses, the police do have competency in diagnosing dangerous situations and dangerous persons, and measure their response according to their assessment.[10] With increased contact between the police and the mentally ill, there has been an increase in violent and tragic events. Torrey et al. report an increase in justifiable homicides as a result of an attack on the police.[7] The following case studies illustrate the dangerousness and the potential for tragedy when the police and mentally ill come into contact.

In the case of *Broadwater v. Fow*, PSP troopers were dispatched to serve involuntary commitment papers on a mentally disturbed person. After some resistance, the subject was handcuffed and placed in a patrol car. The subject continued to actively resist and was beaten. A trooper was arrested but later acquitted by a criminal jury; civil proceedings have been initiated.[11]

In the case of *Wingard v. PA State Police*, a young man suffered from a number of medical conditions, including depression. His girlfriend found him to be confused and disoriented; she called 911, and the PSP arrived. The verbal interaction escalated to the point where the troopers used force to handcuff the subject and he was tasered. The subject later died because of positional asphyxia.[12]

In the case of *Schorr v. Borough of Lemoyne*, Schorr suffered from bipolar disorder. With a court order, two police officers went to Schorr's apartment with a court order and took him to a hospital where he was placed in a "high security" room to wait for an evaluation. When a crisis intervention worker entered the room, Schorr pushed past the worker and escaped from custody. Schorr was located at his apartment. Two police officers were again dispatched to take him back into custody and to the hospital. A violent confrontation ensued and Schorr was shot and killed by one of the officers.[13]

The literature informs us that mental illness is not a predictor of violence, and that most interactions between the mentally ill and the police are successfully resolved without violence.[14] But for those interactions that end tragically the consequences are severe, realized not only by the subject and officers involved, but by families, community, and the police organizations. They include the loss of life, the loss of a loved one, loss of reputation, and confidence in the police among community members. Civil judgments awarded as a result of excessive force, unlawful death, and violations of the Americans with Disabilities Act can severely impact the individual officers and their organization.[15,16] Mishandled incidents have cost chiefs and elected officials their careers.[7,9]

The Role of Police Discretion and the Mentally Ill

The police come into contact with the mentally ill in one of three ways. One is through the service of a lawful warrant issued directing the police to locate, detain, and deliver the subject to the appropriate facility or location such as the court and/or psychiatric facility. These warrants may be issued by a court as part of a civil commitment process or as a result of the violation of probation, parole, or other formal supervision ordered by the court. A second way is responding to a call from a citizen regarding the behavior of someone suspected of being mentally ill. Third, the police may encounter a mentally ill person during the course of their duties. Most contacts between the police and the mentally ill occur through chance encounter or in response to a citizen complaint.[10]

It is not a violation of the law to be mentally ill; therefore, for the police, these encounters are considered disturbances or problems. However, often co-occurring with mental illness are substance abuse issues or behaviors that disturb the peace and security of the community, which amount to minor violations of the law.[17–19] Depending on the circumstances, the police will exercise their substantial discretionary powers in resolving the matter; most often without input from psychiatrists or other mental health experts. The police officers can decide to execute an arrest, pursue an involuntary hospitalization, find an informal settlement on the spot, or take no action. However, in cases of felony crimes, mental condition does not mitigate the offense and offenders are usually arrested and committed to jail.[20]

The police have a de facto role when encountering the mentally ill; most police officers do not operate under clear guidelines, legal or organizational, when interacting with the mentally ill absent a serious criminal violation. Police generally receive little or no training regarding psychiatry, mental illness, symptoms, or de-escalation techniques. Officers learn how to deal with the mentally ill through contacts in the field and interactions with other police officers. The officer's own attitudes, experiences, and assumptions play a significant role in determining outcomes, such as whether the mental health or criminal justice system can best meet the needs of a particular mentally ill individual.[10,21]

Several factors are in play when a police officer makes a dispositional decision. When a police officer is assigned to the field, performance is usually measured by the number of arrests made in combination with the number of calls handled. Police strive to minimize time spent on activities not related to arrest. Time committed to a problem is time away from providing protection and service to areas of responsibility. For the police officer in the field, making an arrest that includes booking and jail, and pursuing an involuntary hospitalization of the mentally ill, are among the most time-consuming activities. The latter activity does not benefit the officer's performance evaluation and while away from his beat, places those within his community at risk.

When considering dispositional options police officers are faced with the stringent standards for an involuntary commitment. The criteria for an involuntary commitment in Pennsylvania follow the model for other states. The guiding criterion for involuntary commitment is whether the mentally ill subject is a clear and present danger to himself and others; the standard of proof is reasonable belief. The law provides that a clear and present danger is defined as follows:

1. Conduct occurring within the previous 30 days in which the person has inflicted or attempted to inflict serious bodily harm on another, and there is a reasonable probability that such conduct will be repeated.
2. The subject is unable to care for himself or herself such that the subject is at risk of death or serious bodily injury.
3. The subject is suicidal, that the person has made threats to commit suicide and has committed acts that are in furtherance of the threat to commit suicide.
4. The subject has engaged in self-mutilation.[22]

The rules provide authorization for police officers to take a subject into custody and transport to the nearest appropriate facility, typically the emergency room of the local hospital. The subject should be examined by a physician who then determines if the subject should be treated further; if so, then the physician has the authority to order the subject's confinement at a place for treatment. If the physician feels the subject does not require treatment, the subject is to be released and returned to a place of his choosing.[22]

For most police officers the process of an involuntary commitment is tedious and frustrating because of several factors: (1) unreliable or inconsistent acceptance rates by hospital staff, (2) the substantial time commitment waiting for the hospital staff to arrive at a disposition, (3) if the hospital rejects the commitment the officer must still deal with the problem, and (4) the organizational pressure to avoid being out of service for extended periods of time. Consequently, police officers generally will not exercise their discretion and take a subject for involuntary examination unless they believe failure to do so will result in serious problems.[10,21]

These factors are widespread. The most recent census of state and local law enforcement agencies finds that of the 17,985 agencies, most employ fewer than 10 officers, and most police agencies serve populations of less than 50,000. This means that if there is 24-hour coverage, there is often one officer on duty for his jurisdiction. Similarly, most police agencies cover rural areas where officers are responsible for a large geographic area.[23] In rural areas transporting and processing a mentally ill subject at the appropriate treatment facility can take an extraordinary amount of time.[24] Time spent by a police officer has an organizational impact as well. Overtime costs can stress a smaller department's budget. An officer who is handling a response to a mentally ill subject becomes unavailable for other tasks and effectively transfers other responsibilities to other officers.

The aforementioned attributes are the foundation for dispositional decisions by police officers and often result in the arrest of the mentally ill. Scholars report psychologically disturbed individuals were more likely to be arrested than nondisturbed persons for similar crimes. Scholars also report that police officers choose to arrest and incarcerate those they perceive require mental health services believing these persons were more likely to receive treatment in jail than in the mental health system. This dispositional choice ensured that these individuals did not immediately return to the community.[21,25–28] However, arrest is a short-term solution that does not address the etiology of the illness and co-occurring disorders. Research shows that mentally ill persons once arrested are very likely to recidivate. One example cited is of a mentally ill female who was arrested more than 200 times before being admitted to a psychiatric hospital.[5]

The cycle of arrest, incarceration, re-entry, and arrest has been labeled "criminalization of the mentally ill" and has been observed since the 1970s. The result has been increasing numbers of mentally ill persons in jails and prisons, accounting for as much as 20% of the inmate population. Scholars note that prisons and jails are not the appropriate place for the treatment of the mentally ill.[5,28–30] Unless a mentally ill person commits a murder or other grave offense, he or she is released back to the community and is likely to re-enter the cycle of arrest, incarceration, re-entry, inadequate treatment, and re-arrest.[6,28]

Crisis Intervention Teams

The law enforcement, mental health communities, and scholars recognize the inadequacies of the "street corner psychiatrist approach" in which the police officer is the sole arbiter of how best to manage the mentally ill.[10] The safety of the community and community members is the concern of the police; mental illness is a medical condition.

Concerns of diagnosis, management, and treatment are concerns for the medical community. In the 1980s law enforcement recognized the importance of partnership building among entities outside law enforcement in problem solving.[31] In the Los Angeles area beginning in the late 1980s, the law enforcement and mental health communities developed co-responder teams that pair law enforcement officers with mental health professionals to respond to scenes involving a person in mental health crisis. The goal of this approach was to divert disturbed persons from the criminal justice system into the mental health treatment system.[32]

In 1988, the Memphis Police Department joined in partnership with the Memphis Chapter of the National Alliance on Mental Illness (NAMI), mental health providers, and two local universities (the University of Memphis and the University of Tennessee) in the creation of Crisis Intervention Teams (CITs).[33] The model provides for the creation of a specialized unit of police officers specifically trained to recognize mental illness, de-escalation techniques, and diversion to the appropriate services. The team is also populated with non–law enforcement mental health specialists and facilities that deal specifically with persons the police have detained. This arrangement has helped reduce the demand on police coverage by dispatching the CIT to calls involving the mentally ill. It has reduced the bureaucracy and long wait times that usually frustrate police officers and lead them to arrest, rather than hospitalize mentally ill individuals. The CIT model is evolving with input from mental health professionals with the goal of diverting the mentally ill from the cycle of arrest, incarceration, and re-arrest as well as defusing situations without the necessity of lethal force.[34] Although there is agreement among leaders in the criminal justice and mental health fields in calling for the adoption of the CIT model, replication of the CIT model across the many police agencies in the United States has been slow.[32,35]

Implementation of a CIT program is problematic for many police agencies. The training protocol calls for 40 hours of training for the police officer. Most police departments do not have sufficient manpower to accommodate this training schedule. Once an officer is trained, most departments do not have the budget to support dispatching the CIT officer on every call. Sustaining a CIT program can be problematic because of attrition. The CIT-trained officers may be promoted, transferred, or retired and must be replaced. Similarly, mental health specialists may be lost through attrition. With the loss of key personnel often comes a loss of initiative to sustain the program.

The CIT model is urban based; most police departments are in rural areas where distances create a barrier to the development of partnerships with the appropriate facilities and mental health agencies. The original CIT model calls for dispatching a mental health specialist to the scene of an incident. For most police agencies distances prohibit a timely response by a third party. Some police departments will not assume the liability for the possible harm that could come to civilians. From a tactical perspective, the introduction of civilians into potentially dangerous situations with a mentally disturbed person is an error that unnecessarily increases the level of risk to all involved.

For the model to work there must be sustained high-level agreement and cooperation across agencies to support training and partnerships. Funding is a concern and a potential impediment to implementation of the CIT model, not only from the law enforcement perspective but from the treatment providers as well.[36]

Although the CIT concept is popular, there are no empirical data to support effectiveness and limited data to support its perceived effectiveness. There is no accurate census of how many CIT programs exist, and scholars report that implementation of a CIT varies so much across jurisdictions, it is problematic to evaluate.[35]

There is almost no disagreement among practitioners and scholars concerning the importance of diverting the mentally ill from the criminal justice system. The concept of a team approach in responding to and resolving situations involving the mentally ill has the greatest utility. The CIT model's greatest success is in changing perceptions of how such collaboration may work.[37] The CIT model is criticized for its emphasis on creating a core group of specially trained police officers and reduced emphasis on partnership building with personnel such as emergency room doctors and psychiatrists.[35]

James Fyfe, a scholar and expert in police practices, calls for training all first responding police officers in techniques and strategies for dealing with the mentally ill. He minimizes the need for a group of police specialists in this area of policing. He finds no support for the argument that a police specialist can or should perform better than the generalist police officer. Fyfe argues that the techniques and strategies for dealing with the mentally ill are relatively simple and can be mastered by the officers who inevitably will be the first contact with the mentally disturbed subject. Such an approach is sustainable and may be the impetus for a culture change among police officers regarding the disposition of the mentally ill.[9]

Integration of Psychiatry and Law Enforcement

The diagnosis, management, and treatment of the mentally ill is the domain of psychiatry. One of the goals of forensic psychiatry is to effectively interface with the criminal justice system and to provide ethical, quality, and timely professional expert services. It is a best practice for the law enforcement to collaborate with psychiatrists when interacting with the mentally ill.

A significant development in this area is telemedicine and its application to psychiatry. This technology has great potential for collaboration among the police and mental health experts. Telepsychiatry is currently being used in court-ordered treatment programs, court-supervised re-entry programs, and other outpatient treatment programs.[38] Emergency telepsychiatry has the potential to bring the expertise of the psychiatrist to the police at the earliest stages of intervention with the mentally ill.

As the name suggests, emergency telepsychiatry is usually delivered by videoconference or sometimes by telephone. With technology, a videoconference with a psychiatric expert could be delivered using a handheld device. This effectively brings the expertise of the psychiatrist to the police, and perhaps patient, in real-time at the scene and/or the hospital without requiring the personal presence of the psychiatrist. Telepsychiatry significantly expands a doctor's service area.[38–41]

Factors in the dispositional decision process for police include difficulties encountered at area hospitals and in rural areas access to the appropriate experts and facilities. Research shows that 40% of hospitals have difficulty maintaining adequate psychiatric coverage to meet patient demand in the emergency room. Emergency telepsychiatry is an effective alternative to the shortage of psychiatric doctors and timely medical evaluations.[38] This technology appears to be particularly well-suited to servicing rural areas and overcoming the geographical barriers to consultation.[38,40,41]

It is well established that interacting with the mentally ill can be dangerous for the subject and the police. The best way to prevent an unfavorable outcome is proper preparation.[9] This technology can introduce the forensic psychiatrist into the planning stage in preparation for contact with a mentally disturbed subject. Risk assessments, medical record reviews, and strategies for dealing with the mentally ill are more effectively performed by a forensic psychiatrist than law enforcement.[34]

Discussion

Policy changes in the treatment of the mentally ill have led to increased contacts with the police. The police are mandated to respond to and deal with the mentally ill.[9,10] Because policing is a discretionary business, the police can exercise several options when interacting with the mentally ill to include referral to the medical community or arrest. Historically, there has been incongruence between the goals of law enforcement and the policy of the medical community regarding the handling of the mentally ill. This leads the police to choose arrest, conveying the responsibility for management of the disturbed subject to the criminal justice system. This has proved to be an ineffective means of dealing with the mentally ill, addressing their etiology, or providing treatment. In this environment, the mentally ill enter a cycle of arrest, incarceration, re-entry, and re-arrest. Mental illness is the domain of psychiatry. The medical model offers the best opportunity for the mentally ill to manage their condition and peacefully re-integrate into the community. Inclusion of mental health experts in the law enforcement response is the best practice. With the advent of new technologies come new opportunities to effect this change and improve outcomes.

References

1. Lamb HR, Weinberger LE, & DeCuir WJ. (2002). The police and mental health. *Psychiatr Serv, 53*(10), 1266–1271.
2. Bittner E. (1967). The police on skid-row: A study of peace keeping. *Am Sociol Rev, 32*(5), 699–715.
3. Bittner E. (1974). Florence Nightingale in pursuit of Willie Sutton: A theory of the police. In H Jacobs (Ed.), *The potential for reform of criminal justice* (pp. 17–43). Beverly Hills: Sage.
4. Green TM. (1997). Police as frontline mental health workers: The decision to arrest or refer to mental health agencies. *Int J Law Psychiatry, 20*(4), 469–486.
5. Torrey EF, Kennard AD, Eslinger D, Lamb R, & Pavle J. (2010). *More mentally ill persons are in jails and prisons than hospitals: A survey of the states.* Arlington, VA: Treatent Advocacy Center.
6. Markowitz FE. (2011). Mental illness, crime, and violence: Risk, context, and social control. *Aggress Violent Beh, 16*(1), 36–44.
7. Torrey EF, Kennard AD, Eslinger DF, Biasotti MC, & Fuller DA. (2013). *Number of justifiable homicides by law enforcement officers and by circumstance, 1980–2008.* Arlington, VA: The Treatment Advocacy Center and National Sheriffs' Association.
8. Pennslyvania State Police. Automated Incident Memo System—Request Assistance Mental Health Act 2012–2013.
9. Fyfe J. (2000). Policing the emotionally disturbed. *J Amer Acad Psychiatry Law Online, 28*(3), 345–347.
10. Bittner E. (1967). Police Discretion in emergency apprehension of mentally ill persons. *Social Problems, 14*(3), 278–292.
11. *Broadwater v. Fow*, 945 F. Supp. 2d 574 945 F. Supp. 2d 574 (M.D. Pa. 2013) (United States District Court for the Middle District of Pennsylvania 2013).
12. *Wingard v. Pa. State Police*, 2013 U.S. Dist. Lexis 97800 2013 U.S. Dist. Lexis 97800 (W.D. Pa. June 21, 2013) (United States District Court for the Western District of Pennsylvania 2013).
13. *Schorr v. Borough of Lemoyne*, 243 F. Supp. 2d 232 243 F. Supp. 2d 232 (M.D. Pa. 2003) (United States District Court for the Middle District of Pennsylvania 2003).

14. Appelbaum PS. (2013). Public safety, mental disorders, and guns. *JAMA Psychiatry, 70*(6), 565–566.
15. Brodin RE. (2005). Remedying a particularized form of discrimination: Why disabled plaintiffs can and should bring claims for police misconduct under the Americans with Disabilities Act. *Univ PA Law Rev, 154*(1), 157–200.
16. Alpert GP, & Smith WC. (1994). How reasonable is the reasonable man? Police and excessive force. *J Crim Law Criminol, 85*(2), 481–501.
17. Yoon J, Domino ME, Norton EC, Cuddeback GS, & Morrissey JP. (2013). The impact of changes in psychiatric bed supply on jail use by persons with severe mental illness. *J Ment Health Policy Econ*, 16(2), 81–92.
18. Lurigio AJ. (2013). Criminalization of the mentally ill exploring causes and current evidence in the United States. *Criminologist Off Newslett Amer Soc Criminol, 38*(6), 10.
19. Brink RH, Broer J, Tholen AJ, Winthorst WH, Visser E, & Wiersma D. (2012). Role of the police in linking individuals experiencing mental health crises with mental health services. *BMC Psychiatry, 12*(171), 1–7.
20. Cooper VG, Mclearen AM, & Zapf PA. (2004). Dispositional decisions with the mentally ill: Police perceptions and characteristics. *Police Quart, 7*(3), 295–310.
21. Patch PC, & Arrigo BA. (1999). Police officer attitudes and use of discretion in situations involving the mentally ill: The need to narrow the focus. *Int J Law Psychiatry, 22*(1), 23–35.
22. Mental Health Procedures Act (July 9, 1976).
23. Reaves BA. (2011). *Census of state and local law enforcement agencies, 2008*. U.S. Department of Justice, Office of Justice Programs, Bureau of Justice Statistics.
24. Skubby D, Bonfine N, Novisky M, Munetz MR, & Ritter C. (2013). Crisis intervention team (CIT) programs in rural communities: A focus group study. *Commun Mental Health J*, 49(6), 756–764.
25. Teplin LA, Pruett NS. (1992). Police as streetcorner psychiatrist: Managing the mentally ill. *Int J Law Psychiatry, 15*(2), 139–156.
26. Menzies RJ. (1987). Psychiatrists in blue: Police apprehension of mental disorder and dangerousness. *Criminology, 25*(3), 429–453.
27. Robertson G. (1988). Arrest patterns among mentally disordered offenders. *Br J Psychiatry, 153*(3), 313–316.
28. Chappell D, & O'Brien A. (2014). Police responses to persons with a mental illness: International perspectives. *Int J Law Psychiatry, 37*(4), 321–426.
29. Abramson MF. (1972). Criminalization of mentally disordered behavior—Possible side effect of a new mental health law. *Hosp Commun Psychiatry, 23*(4), 101–105.
30. Shah SA. (1989). Mental disorder and the criminal-justice system—Some overarching issues. *Int J Law Psychiatry, 12*(2–3), 231–244.
31. Goldstein H. (1987). Toward community-oriented policing potential, basic requirements, and threshold questions. *Crime Delinquency, 33*(1), 6–30.
32. Reuland M, Draper L, & Norton B. (2013). Developing a statewide approach to specialized policing response (SPR) programme implementation. In D Chappell (Ed.), *Policing and the mentally ill: International perspectives* (pp. 3–17). Boca Raton, FL: CRC Press.
33. Major Robert Vaughn, Memphis police department. Crisis intervention team: The "Memphis Model." http://www.memphispolice.org/Crisis Intervention.htm. Accessed March 10, 2014.
34. Augustin D, & Fagan TJ. (2011). Roles for mental health professionals in critical law enforcement incidents: An overview. *Psychol Serv, 8*(3), 166–177.
35. Cross AB, Mulvey EP, Schubert CA, et al. (2014). An agenda for advancing research on crisis intervention teams for mental health emergencies. *Psychiatr Serv, 65*(4), 530–536.
36. Pinals DA. (2014). Forensic services, public mental health policy, and financing: Charting the course ahead. *J Amer Acad Psychiatry Law Online, 42*(1), 7–19.
37. Morabito MS, Watson A, & Draine J. (2013). Police officer acceptance of new innovation: The case of crisis intervention teams. *Policing: Int J Police Strategies Manage, 36*(2), 421–436.
38. Yellowlees P, Burke MM, Marks SL, Hilty DM, & Shore JH. (2008). Emergency telepsychiatry. *J Telemed Telecare, 14*(6), 277–281.

39. Fortney JC, Pyne JM, Mouden SB, et al. (2013). Practice-based versus telemedicine-based collaborative care for depression in rural federally qualified health centers: A pragmatic randomized comparative effectiveness trial. *Amer J Psychiatry, 170*, 414–425.
40. Hilty DM, Yellowlees PM, Ferrer DC, et al. (2013). The effectiveness of telemental health: A 2013 review. *Telemed e-Health*, 19(6), 444–454.
41. Seidel RW, & Kilgus MD. (2014). Agreement between telepsychiatry assessment and face-to-face assessment for emergency department psychiatry patients. *J Telemed Telecare*, *20*(2), 59–62.

SECTION SEVEN

Future Directions

28

Linking Brain and Behavioral Measures in the Medical-Legal Context

Ruben C. Gur and Oren M. Gur

Based on experiences over the past several decades consulting and testifying in criminal cases in which questions arose about the relationship between brain function and behavior, we describe the process of applying neuroscience expertise in a medical-legal context. Beginning with a brief historical overview of the context surrounding the evolution of behavioral neuroscience to the point of becoming relevant to courts, we next present a brief history of how we became involved in court cases, offering neuroscience-based expertise in mitigation of capital offenses. After describing the process established for analyzing brain and behavioral measures, and providing illustrative examples from cases, we conclude by forecasting an expanding role for neuroscience in the judiciary moving forward.

Discovering the Relevance of the Brain to Behavior

It is noteworthy that the role of the brain in regulating behavior is a relatively recent discovery in the history of civilization. The ancient Greeks, for example, believed that courage arose from the heart, reason the head, and "base qualities" the stomach.[1] It was not until the thirteenth century that Albertus Magnus concluded that behavior was controlled by the brain, except he (and others) thought that the action was in the three ventricles[1]: the first processed the five senses, passing images to the middle reasoning and thoughtful ventricle, before being remembered in the final ventricle.[2] It was not until René Descartes that the idea was articulated that the seat of the "soul" was in brain tissue.[3,4] However, for Descartes, who was familiar with brain anatomy, it was incomprehensible that the soul be located in two "separate organs," the cerebral hemispheres. He therefore concluded that the pineal gland, one brain structure that does not have two hemispheres, must be the seat of the soul. Phrenology, much maligned and ridiculed already by the nineteenth century, nonetheless is a discipline that further influenced scientific thinking about brain and behavior. Lacking the tools to investigate the brain itself, phrenologists studied the head and attempted to correlate the size and shape of different portions with human "faculties."[5] For example, large foreheads were said to be associated with intellectual abilities. This methodology was not accepted by the mainstream of science or supported by empirical research, and the whole idea of localizing behavioral domains in brain regions became tarnished.[5] Unfortunately, perhaps, the dismissal of phrenology has led to a negative attitude regarding any efforts to localize cognitive "faculties" in specific brain regions.

The Seven Words of Monsieur Lelong

With that background, a French neurosurgeon, Pierre Paul Broca (1824–1880), reasoned that the criticism against phrenologists may relate to their failure to study important human faculties and link them to direct evidence of brain integrity. He argued that, of all human faculties, speech is both unique and of major importance, and should have a localizable brain structure to support it. Proceeding to search for a patient whose speech abilities were compromised, but who was otherwise not demented, he encountered Monsieur Lelong, an elderly gentleman who suffered a sudden onset of speech loss. By the time he was examined by Broca and his staff, Lelong used only seven words: "yes," "no," "one," "two," "three," "Lelong," and "*toujour*," the French word for "always." However, Broca was able to demonstrate that the patient understood speech, and applied his limited vocabulary appropriately. Thus, he used "one" for the number "one," "two" for the number "two," and "three" for any number larger than two; "yes" for affirmation, "no" for negation, and "*toujour*" for everything else. Having documented this patient's deficits, Broca was able, upon Mr. Lelong's death, to perform an autopsy that revealed a large lesion in the third frontal convolution of the left hemisphere. The publication of his findings in 1861 presaged the field of neuropsychology (Broca, 1861).[5a]

Clinical-Pathological Correlation Method

Subsequent neuroscientists have followed Broca's paradigm, which became established as the clinical-pathological correlation method. Thereafter, Wernicke (1970) documented that lesions more posterior to Broca's area were associated with relatively preserved speech output, but diminished capacity to comprehend speech.[6] Other such investigators, such as John Hughlings Jackson (1932),[7] reported that lesions in the right hemisphere produced deficits in spatial abilities. Links between brain abnormalities and behavioral aberrations also have been established in emotional behavior. Babinski (1914)[8] reported a series of patients ($N = 16$) with significant brain damage who were characterized behaviorally by denial of symptoms ("*anosognosie*"), and even unusual jollity about having these symptoms ("*anosodisaphorie*"). Notably, all these patients had major lesions in the right hemisphere. The British neurosurgeon Wilson described a patient who laughed incessantly, to the point of not being able to eat (1924).[9] Wilson had to overcome the danger of dehydration by sitting at the patient's bedside and yawning deliberately, which induced the patient to yawn long enough for the nurse to feed him. This patient's lesion too was in the left hemisphere. Subsequent studies have indicated that right hemispheric lesions were associated with positive symptoms of jocular affect, whereas left hemispheric lesions were associated with release of negative affect.[10] Thus, both cognitive and emotional processing are disrupted in patients with brain lesions, and different behavioral domains are affected depending on the location and nature of brain damage. Importantly, brain lesions can produce both negative symptoms (e.g., behaviors such as fluent speech or memory that patients can no longer perform at normative levels) and positive symptoms (e.g., new behaviors, such as aggressive or depressed mood) that may emerge because of damage to regions that inhibit or regulate such behaviors.

Brain Stimulation

Demonstrations of very specific regional control of behavior by the brain came about in the middle of the twentieth century, when the Canadian neurosurgeon Roger Penfield began publishing his studies of brain stimulation.[11-13] Penfield performed surgery on patients with temporal lobe epilepsy and, because the patients were awake, he could observe the effects of stimulating different brain regions on behavior. He found that stimulating a specific region in the back of the frontal lobe would cause patients to lift their contralateral arm; stimulating an adjacent region would cause patients to lift their contralateral index finger. Methodically mapping the motor system in this way, Penfield discovered a "homunculus" along the fissure that separates the frontal lobe from the parietal lobe. The entire human body was represented, and each limb (e.g., individual fingers) could be activated by an electrical pulse administered to specific contralateral locations of the brain. A parallel homunculus was demonstrated in the parietal side of the same fissure, where stimulation would lead to sensations from corresponding body parts. Of relevance to the medical-legal context, during Penfield's procedures, when patients were asked why they moved their arm or finger, or why they started or stopped talking, they usually reported a subjective feeling that this was their wish. Patients invariably perceived actions induced by electrical stimulation as being under their voluntary control.

Psychometric Methods

Progress in neurological evidence linking behavioral domains to regional brain function was paralleled by progress in psychometric methodology, allowing for reliable measurement of behavioral performance. For example, to measure verbal output fluency, psychologists have developed standardized tests in which a subject is given a limited amount of time to produce as many words as possible that start with a certain letter. Applying such a test in neurological patients proved sensitive to the presence of left fronto-temporal lesions. Similarly, tests of memory proved sensitive to temporal-limbic anomalies, and tests of concept formation and set-shifting sensitive to frontal lobe damage. Research and clinical work using this methodology helped solidify the field of neuropsychology, and it is now a recognized subspecialty of the American Board of Professional Psychology (ABPP). Neuropsychology has become the discipline that links behavioral domains to the functioning of brain systems.

Neuroimaging

Progress in neuropsychology has accelerated exponentially with the advent of neuroimaging. In the late 1970s and early 1980s, several methods became available for safely and reliably measuring brain function and structure in humans. Among the first methods was the Xenon-133 clearance technique, which demonstrated that cerebral blood flow increases during cognitive activity compared with a resting ("default mode") state,[14] and that it increases more to the left hemisphere for a verbal-reasoning task and to the right hemisphere for a spatial task.[15] This methodology was augmented by positron emission tomography (PET), which allowed measurement of both cerebral blood flow and metabolism with three-dimensional resolution. Spatial resolution was low (~1.5 cm) at the beginning but reaches 3 to 4 mm^3 with modern devices. The introduction of magnetic resonance imaging (MRI) has vastly enhanced the scope and pace of research linking brain systems to behavior. Because it is noninvasive and does not expose research participants to ionizing radiation, MRI studies can be done in babies and children, which is not possible with the isotopic methods. Furthermore, advanced MRI methodology can generate multimodal information on the brain, with exquisite spatial resolution. Magnetic resonance imaging affords reliable volumetric data that can be segmented into brain compartments (gray matter, white matter, cerebrospinal fluid), and MRI sequences are available that provide information on white matter connectivity through diffusion tensor imaging (DTI), regional cerebral perfusion with arterial spin-labeling methods, and resting state connectivity and response to neurobehavioral probes with blood oxygenation level dependent (BOLD) measures. Application of these methodologies has generated more precise models of brain system involvement in regulating behavior. For example, functional MRI (fMRI) studies have shown activation of the frontal system when participants were deliberating ethical dilemmas.[16] Such studies have also demonstrated the developmental trajectories of different brain systems and showed, for example, that frontal lobe regions related to executive function do not mature until early in the third decade of life.[17–19] Such data have relevance to criminal culpability of adolescents and of individuals with frontal lobe damage. The field is rapidly evolving, and multimodal integration will pave the way for heretofore unimagined mechanistic insights; a potential hazard for the neuroscientist involved in expert testimony is that data, although more precise and reliable, will become increasingly more difficult to understand, and therefore, explain.

Initial Involvement in Medical-Legal Consultation

A neuroscientist can become involved in medical-legal cases in several ways: some do research on issues that a lawyer thinks are germane to particular types of cases (e.g., death penalty), others study relevant topics more directly (e.g., brain development, bias). In the early-1990s, the first author (RCG) was involved in research that harnessed the evolving neuroimaging technology to understand the neural substrates of behavior, gaining experience working with clinical populations and applying budding neuroimaging methods in diagnosis and treatment planning. In one case, RCG testified:

> The first PET scanner I worked with was called PET three. It was technically the third PET scanner that was ever built. And when MRI came on the scene[,] because of my background and work in imaging in relation to behavior[,] I was involved with that work literally from the outset (transcript of record at 104, *U.S. v. Montgomery* (W.D.Mo. 2007)). No. 05CR06002 (or No. 05-6002-01-CR-SJ-GAF).[20]

This research was both basic, involving healthy populations, and clinical, with neurological (stroke, seizure disorders, tumors, head injuries, movement disorders, dementias) and psychiatric patients (primarily psychosis, mood, and conduct disorders). The resultant normative PET database—the largest in the country at the time—was known to Dr. Frank Wood, a neuropsychologist who was also involved in neuroimaging at what was then called Bowman Grey School of Medicine (now Wake Forest). Dr. Wood wanted to check values he obtained from a recent medical-legal PET study he performed, and asked whether they could be compared against our normative PET database.[21,22] Most regional-to-whole-brain values supplied by Dr. Wood were well within the expected range of the controls. However, the measured value for the amygdala was several standard deviations below the control group from the sample. The next day, the first author was on a plane to Ocala, Florida, and the following day testified in a death penalty case in the Fifth Judicial Circuit.

Robert "Bobbie" Joe Long (aka the "classified ad rapist") was a serial rapist and murderer in Florida in the early 1980s who received 28 sentences of life and, on July 25, 1986, a death sentence.[23] He started his crime spree while still wearing bandages after a motorcycle accident that resulted in a severe head injury with coma. After, on appeal, the Florida Supreme Court remanded the case back to the trial court, in 1994[24] the issue of the hypometabolism in PET scans came up during the sentencing phase.[25] The transition from the academic arena to the legal realm was greeted by an opposing expert, Dr. Leon Prockop, chairman of the Department of Neurology at the University of South Florida, who "admitted that Drs. Raquel and Ruben Gur are leading experts in the country on PET research and interpretation. (R. 1603-04)."[24]

For RCG, the first time testifying as a neuroscience expert in court was memorable, providing opportunities to observe the "patient" in spite of the short notice. During the trial the defendant had to be kept in a separate room because he would get upset easily and begin screaming out of control, threatening the judge and his lawyers. He could still be heard occasionally screaming from the remote room. Upon examining the defendant during a break in the trial, RCG noted that Mr. Long displayed other signs of frontal lobe damage, including disinhibition and tactlessness.[I] Although subsequently sentenced to death, as a mitigating factor the judge listed that "Long's ability to conform his conduct to the requirements of law

I. For example, while measuring his cranial circumference, Mr. Long gyrated his hips while commenting "anything else you want to measure, Doc?"

was substantially impaired."[24] After that, involvement continued in cases in which neuropsychology and neuroimaging expertise was sought.

A decade later, Marc Bookman, Esq., from the homicide unit of the Defender Association of Philadelphia,[II] contacted RCG and requested an affidavit summarizing the literature on brain development and its implications for legal culpability. Brain development was a major research interest for RCG, and much of the literature reviewed in the affidavit was in the process of being cited in a forthcoming technical manuscript.[18] The affidavit was used to help support ineligibility for the death penalty of juveniles, because the research showed that indices of brain maturation in regions related to legal culpability did not reach their apex until around age 22. The affidavit eventually became part of an amicus brief to the Supreme Court of the United States, in *Roper v. Simmons* (2005):[26] the case that resulted in the decision to ban the execution of individuals who are under the age of 18 when they commit crimes for which the prosecution might otherwise seek the death penalty.[25]

In summary, initial involvement began organically, neither pursued nor advertised, and has remained that way for several years. In the first case involving PET, Dr. Wood and RCG happened to serve on an NIMH Study Section together, and became familiar with each other's current research, including the growing PET database RCG was collecting. In the second case, a homicide lawyer in a unit of the local public defenders office,[III] who had defended many young people charged with murder, had an idea after looking into research on brain maturation, and decided to contact one of the people doing the research "in his backyard." However, referrals continued to stream in, as the methodology became more widely known and standardized, and colleagues were recruited to perform part of the analysis for which they already had a "pipeline" and medical-legal cases could join the queue. For example, Dr. Andrew Newberg, a nuclear medicine physician who performs and analyzes PET scans routinely, processed the PET scans, whereas Dr. Christos Davatzikos, a nationally renowned image analysis expert, processed the MRI data. With participation of postdoctoral students and support staff at the University of Pennsylvania—especially in recent years from Stace Moore, Michael Keutmann, Sherry Wang, and the late Raymond Hill—we established a "Neuroforensics Service" at Penn, using the reimbursements to further research into brain processes pertinent to violent behavior. Since 2007, with the assistance of the second author, a systematic process has been developed to respond to requests for assessment of behavior, brain structure, and function. The following section illustrates the elements of a typical case.

II. Mr. Bookman now directs the Atlantic Center for Capital Representation (ACCR).

III. Empirical research based on data drawn from a sample of "3,412 defendants charged with murder (18 Pa C.S. § 2502, 2011) in municipal court between 1994 and 2005" has shown that public defenders in Philadelphia are more effective for their clients than private appointed counsel in homicide cases.[26a] "Compared to private appointed counsel, [Philadelphia] public defenders reduce the murder conviction rate by 19%. They reduce the probability that their clients receive a life sentence by 62%. Public defenders reduce overall expected time served in prison by 24%. This suggests that defense counsel makes an enormous difference in the outcome of cases."[26a]

Handling a Typical Case Involving Neuroimaging

Over the years, a standard procedure has been developed for obtaining and analyzing behavioral (neuropsychological), structural (MRI), and functional (PET) neuroimaging data for both civil and criminal cases in which linkage was needed between behavior and brain function. The first step is to determine whether neuroimaging records exist electronically—today it would typically be in the Digital Imaging and Communications in Medicine (DICOM) format. If available, neuroimaging (i.e., MRI and PET) records are requested and reviewed by respective experts (see Figure 28.1) to determine whether they are of appropriate quality for a "comparison analysis."[27,IV] When prior neuroimaging is not available, efforts are made as necessary to guide legal teams in how to locate appropriate facilities, consult with medical doctors on which MRI and PET specifications to request, and, once imaging has been conducted, analyze the data that is received at Penn.

Although neuroscience techniques are the focus of our effort, they are usually not the only material we rely on, and often other records are more readily available for immediate review (i.e., while awaiting results of neuroimaging). In most cases this work is done in the context of an in-depth evaluation by another clinician, neuropsychologist, or neuropsychiatrist, who integrates our analysis with the history and their own clinical interviews to render a diagnosis. However, when a diagnosis is requested, RCG will complement BI, MRI, and PET modalities by conducting personal clinical evaluations and administering a Computerized Neurocognitive Battery (CNB). The CNB is a compilation of tasks that have been used in functional neuroimaging studies that have documented which regions are recruited in order to perform them.[28–30] They have been adapted for large-scale genomic studies for use as biomarkers ("endophenotypes") of behavior related to brain systems.[V] The

IV. Regarding "Comparison Analysis," Blume and Paavola (2011) write: "The traditional mode of neuroimaging analysis has been a visual review of the scan films by a radiologist or a neurologist. This method creates a number of problems related to subjectivity, bias, and error[.]"[27] Because the films or scans are generated from underlying numeric data, the computer literally "paints" the scan by scaling these numbers on a gray or color scale. Each "dot" on the scan represents a three-dimensional pixel, or "voxel," with known width, breadth, and height—"slice thickness" (e.g., 1 mm × 1 mm × 1 mm)—and a number associated with it. Methods have been developed for quantitatively analyzing these data to obtain precise measures of brain structure and function. Such data are obtained from healthy individuals, and these provide "normative" information that can help detect "abnormal" brains. Quantitative analysis allows for the application of validated computer algorithms to analyze data generated during an imaging study. Neuroradiologists are well trained to detect most abnormalities that can be lethal, such as tumors, strokes, malformations, MS lesions, and blood collections. This is because such lesions are focal and have unique tissue characteristics and therefore can be visualized. However, damage that is more diffuse, such as that caused by traumatic brain injuries or environmental exposure, is not visible even to the most well-trained eye. There is accumulating evidence that scans of patients with mild traumatic brain injury (TBI) that were read as "normal" by neuroradiologists had tissue loss clearly documented by volumetric analysis.[27a] "Quantitative analysis results in a more precise—and, it is hoped, more accurate—determination of whether the brain is structurally and functionally normal. Furthermore, quantitative analysis can permit a comparison of an individual client's brain to a database of brains with known abnormalities (such as schizophrenia)."[27,27b]

V. The battery has been translated to multiple languages and administered more than 200,000 times in studies around the world.

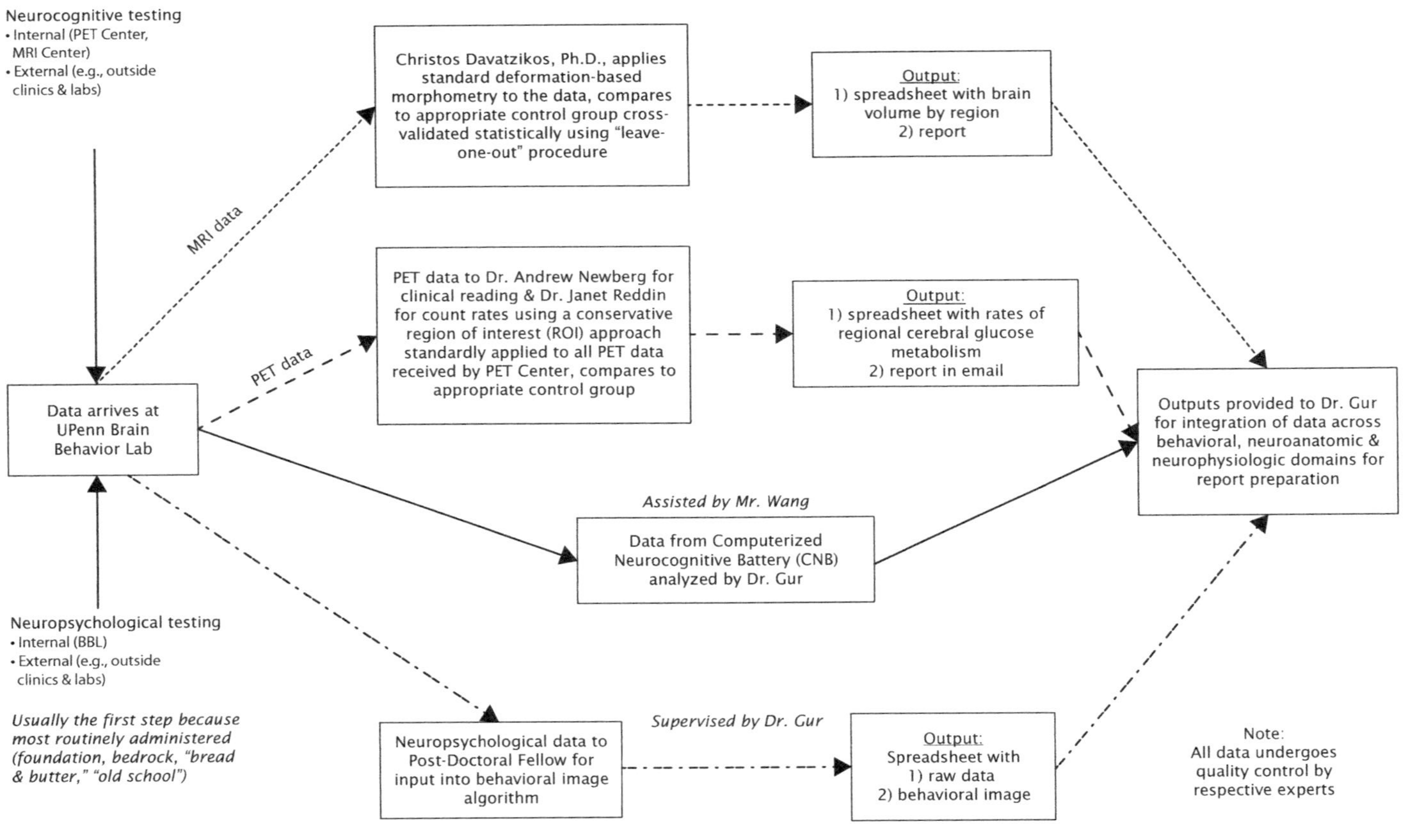

FIGURE 28.1 A schematic illustration of medical-legal data flow.

CNB permits more rigorous characterization of brain systems involved in the patient's specific deficits.

In cases in which a complete diagnostic work-up is requested, additional records are reviewed when available, such as social, medical, educational, military, criminal justice, and other "official statistics" generated by agencies,[31] including information pertaining to the immediate offense and litigation. Sometimes records are not always known to be relevant, and the sheer volume (and illegibility) can make searching for pertinent details cumbersome—even compared with neuroimaging. Record review can be timely and not cost-effective when done by neuroimaging experts, and in our experience is best done by a mitigation specialist already involved with the case, an assistant or aspiring criminologist instructed on what to look for (e.g., head injuries, substance use, alcohol use by mother, inconsistent school performance, time in public housing with lead paint).[VI] Last, reports and the testimony of other experts who assess the client are usually made available as the case unfolds, and feedback solicited as necessary, particularly when neuroimaging becomes an important issue.

Preparing a Report of Findings[VII]

Reports can be issued at different phases (as requested by the legal team), and multiple reports are often written for the same case, reflecting the emergent nature of information gleaned from the multifaceted approach to linking brain function, structure, and behavior. For example, an initial report might be issued based on information available prior to conducting neuroimaging (i.e., based on records and a "behavioral image" [BI] constructed from results of neuropsychological testing). The initial report might suggest that neuroimaging seems appropriate, given what is known,[VIII] and indicate what additional information is needed and how it can be obtained. If the BI suggests brain damage, then structural neuroimaging (MRI) and functional neuroimaging (PET) can be recommended. Because most clients in capital cases are unable to travel to Penn for scanning, this stage may involve communication with a scanning facility adjacent to the prison or sanctioned by the court.

VI. Although not all cases are as apparent as Robert Joe Long's motorcycle accident, many individuals referred for assessment have quite troubled pasts. For example, in one case, the authors traveled to California to assess an individual who huffed solvents from an early age, was regularly raped by older youths after being placed in foster care, experienced a range of other traumas, and then went on to kidnap and murder as an adult. As a child, another California client was forced by his (alcoholic) father to get into fistfights with his peers, while the father would take bets on the outcome. These early head traumas may have played a role in his misidentification of innocent passers-by as rival gang affiliates based on the color of their shirts and his impulsive response that resulted in their death.

VII. Reports may become public domain as part of the legal record; a recent *Wired* article includes a behavioral image,[31a] an example of its dissemination in media.

VIII. Neuroimaging might not be advisable in every case. Sometimes, it is clear from history and neuropsychological testing that there is brain damage, and there is no need for further proof. In other cases, legal considerations may influence the decision (e.g., cost, risk of negative findings, local factors). It is also worth noting that although our methodology is quite sensitive to the presence of brain damage, in some situations there may be evidence of organic damage that will not be revealed in a PET or MRI (e.g., very diffuse effects of TBI, small local cerebral areas of encephalomalacia).

Initially, it required travel to the site to assure that the correct sequences were executed and the data properly stored, but today most centers administer the essential sequences for valid quantitation and can store results in DICOM format. Once the results of MRI and PET become available, a second report would follow, which might also include results of the CNB and clinical assessment. The dates and locations of all assessments and names of other experts involved are included in the reports.

Reports usually begin with a summary of background information culled from record review, and an overview of the forthcoming analysis. The BI follows, where an algorithm[32–35] is applied to results of neuropsychological evaluations performed with the client to provide a quantitative analysis of cognitive performance as it relates to regional cortical functioning. This BI algorithm can help to further establish the localization of brain damage based on the neuropsychological test scores. The process for this schematic representation of clinical data has been clinically reliable and stable in defining and localizing affected areas of neurological impairment. The image is a true topographic display of the neuropsychological data in reference to the dysfunctional areas and severity of impairment implicated by the performance.

Applied to one specific capital defendant, the algorithm has produced the BI shown in Figure 28.2. The image depicts three views of a defendant's brain from the left (*top left panel*), the right (*lower left panel*) and the top (*right panel*, with the front of the brain oriented

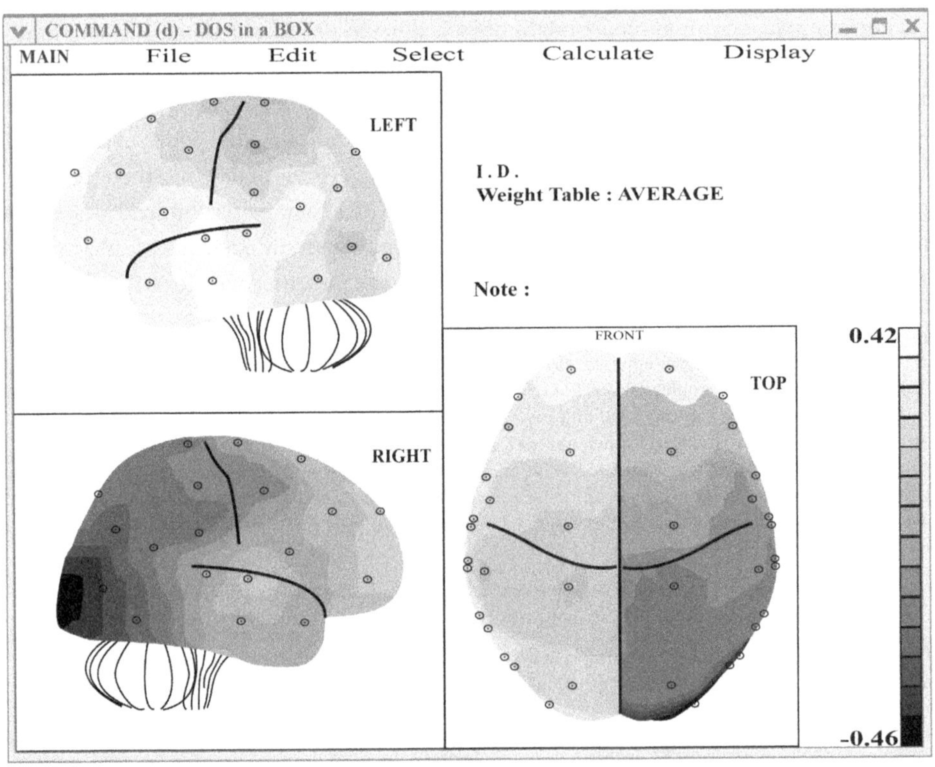

FIGURE 28.2 Behavioral image of performance.

toward the top of the panel). The scale in the lower right of the image represents functional capacity relative to the most intact ability. In the BI shown in Figure 28.2, there is moderate diffuse neuropsychological impairment. Most pronounced is impairment in the right hemisphere, starting at posterior regions and extending anteriorly to superior parietal and supramarginal gyrus and less pronounced in frontal regions.

Next, volumetric structural analysis of MRI are presented based on quantitative analysis and examination via delineation of regions of interest (ROI) assisted by a semi-automated template-warping algorithm applied by the developer of the algorithm, Christos Davatzikos.[36] Regions showing a reduction in volume of at least 1.5 standard deviations (SDs) below normal, and their corresponding contralateral structures, are displayed in Figure 28.3. These results show that the overall volume of the defendant's brain are in the normal range, except for reduced volume in the frontal lobe bilaterally, parietal lobes mostly on the right, and the limbic system on the left. Examining smaller regions, reduced in size are volumes of the frontal pole bilaterally, right anterior and posterior frontal orbital regions, precentral gyrus bilaterally, left postcentral, right superior parietal lobule, right supramarginal gyrus, right precuneus, left superior occipital, left middle occipital, left anterior cingulate, entorhinal area bilaterally, left hippocampus, parahippocampal formation bilaterally, anterior insula bilaterally, and the posterior internal capsule bilaterally. Also notable is an enlarged right ventricle.

Results of PET establish the regional distribution of cerebral glucose metabolic activity using fluorine-18 labeled deoxyglucose (FDG). Andrew Newberg provides a clinical reading of the technical quality of the scan in a report, which includes images of the PET

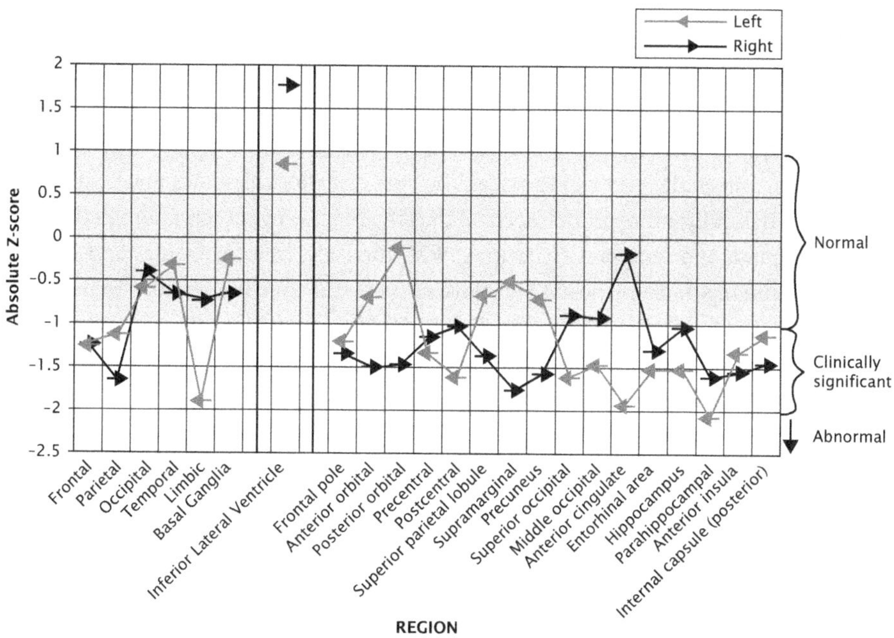

FIGURE 28.3 Volumetric analysis of magnetic resonance imaging. Volumes are expressed as absolute z-scores (standard deviations from the mean) relative to healthy individuals.

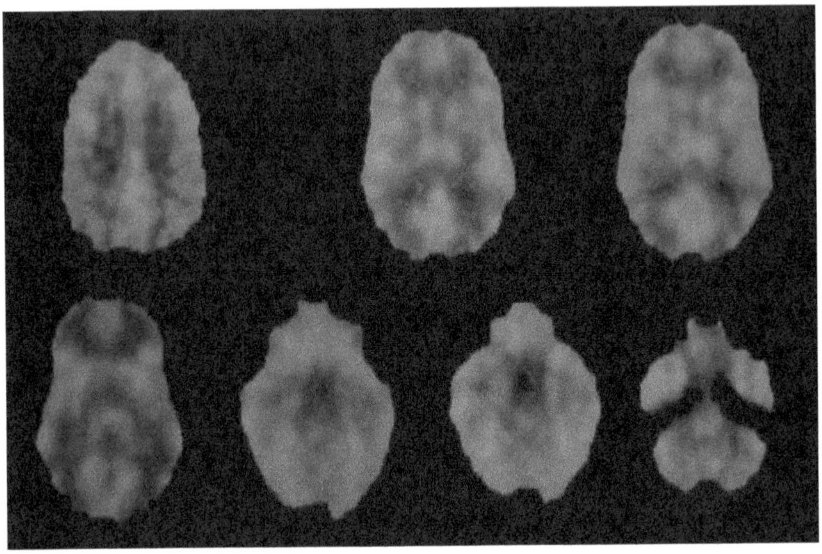

FIGURE 28.4 Positron emission tomography images of the brain.

scans (see Figure 28.4). The PET study is subjected to a quantitative analysis using a standard ROI approach.[21,22] The quantitative analysis of cerebral metabolic rates relative to the whole brain (Figure 28.5) supports Dr. Newberg's clinical reading and points to more specific sets of regions that show abnormal glucose uptake. For example, in Figure 28.4 the analysis indicated relative decreases in nine regions (see key for region abbreviations in Figure 28.5): left DM, TP, right PH, HI, AM, right IN, C1, C2, and right LM (when hemisphere not indicated, it is bilateral). Eighteen areas show relative increases in metabolism: right SF, right DL, MF, IF, left SM, SP, AG, PC, OM, OL, LI, OT, MT, right OF, left UN, CP, TH, and left HY. These results indicate a pattern of hypoactivation in limbic structures, most notably the hippocampus, amygdala, and right insula. The corpus callosum shows markedly reduced metabolism bilaterally, more pronounced on the left. There is hyperactivation in the frontal, parietal, occipital, and temporal structures, with the right inferior frontal and bilaterally superior parietal region being near 4 SD above normal. The hypometabolism in the anterior corpus callosum is quite abnormal, exceeding 3 SD below normal bilaterally, and on the left, nearing 5 SD below average. Also conspicuous is the strong hypermetabolism in the thalamus, exceeding 3 SD above normal bilaterally.

Computerized neurocognitive battery testing is used to further establish behavioral manifestations of regional brain dysfunction. The computerized battery was validated through functional neuroimaging[28–30,37] and established as sensitive to the existence of a major neuropsychiatric disorder.[38] It is scored by automated procedures and yields measures of accuracy and speed on several major neuropsychological domains. These include: Executive: Abstraction and mental flexibility (ABF); attention (ATT); working, memory (WME); Episodic memory: verbal, spatial and facial memory (VME, SME, and FME, respectively); Complex reasoning: language (LAN); Social cognition: spatial

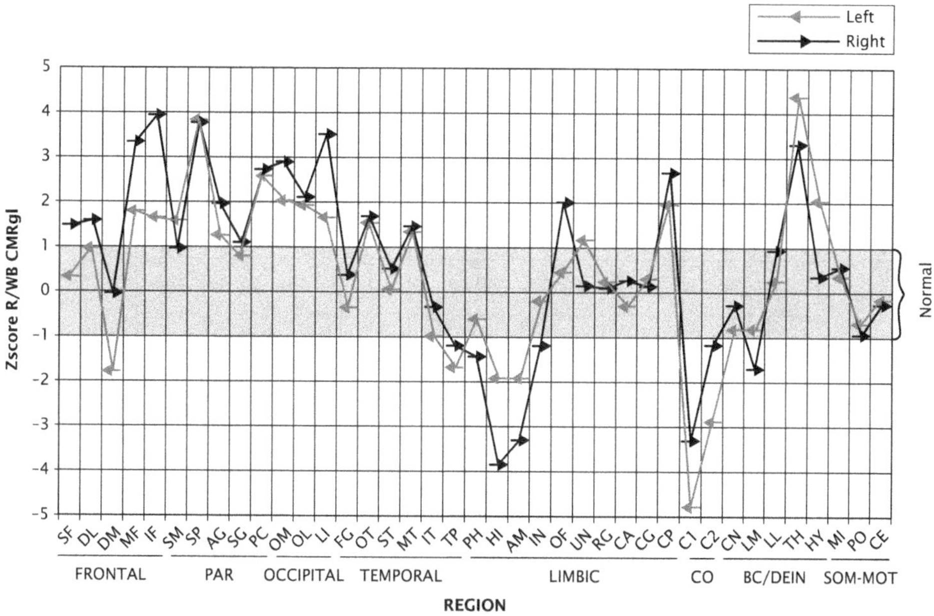

SF = Superior Frontal; DL = Dorsal Prefrontal - Lateral; DM = Dorsal Prefrontal - Medial; MF = Mid-Frontal; IF = Inferior Frontal; SM = Sensorimotor; SP = Superior Parietal; AG = Angular Gyrus; SG = Supramarginal Gyrus; PC = Precuneus; OM = Occipital cortex, Medial; OL = Occipital cortex, Lateral; LI = Lingual Gyrus; FG = Fusiform Gyrus; OT = Occipital Temporal; ST = Superior Temporal; MT = Mid-Temporal; IT = Inferior Temporal; TP = Temporal Pole; PH = Parahippocampal Gyrus; HI = Hippocampus; AM = Amygdala; IN = Insula; OF = Orbital Frontal; UN = Uncus; RG = Rectal Gyrus; CA = Cingulate Gyrus - Anterior; CG = Cingulate Gyrus - genu; CP = Cingulate Gyrus - Posterior; C1 = Corpus Callosum - Anterior; C2 = Corpus Callosum - Posterior; CN = Caudate Nucleus; LM = Lenticular - Medial (Globus Pallidus); LL = Lenticular - Lateral (Putamen); TH = Thalamus; HY = Hypothalamus; MI = Midbrain; PO = Pons; CE = Cerebellum.

FIGURE 28.5 Positron emission tomography region-whole brain ratio (R/WB) results for cerebral metabolic rates for glucose (CMRgl) in a client. Results are expressed as z-scores relative to a comparison group of healthy people.

processing (SPA); emotion processing (EMO); and sensorimotor speed of information processing (SM). The results of the testing are summarized in Figure 28.6.

Results show that the subject performed both accurately and with normal speed on several domains including ATT, WME, and LAN. However, his performance was severely slow in the verbal memory and spatial processing tasks, and moderately impaired in abstraction and mental flexibility and facial memory. He also performed poorly in the spatial processing domain despite taking a long time to complete the tasks. He was also abnormally slow for spatial memory, emotion identification, and sensorimotor processing speed.

Reports conclude with a summary of the results of neuropsychological and computerized neurocognitive testing, as well as structural and functional imaging, highlighting convergent areas of brain impairment and their meaning. Ascertaining the etiology of abnormalities can be difficult, requiring clinical evaluation and integration with historical information that was not recorded with the present circumstances in mind. Opinions expressed with regard to the neuroimaging findings have to meet standards of scientific validity.

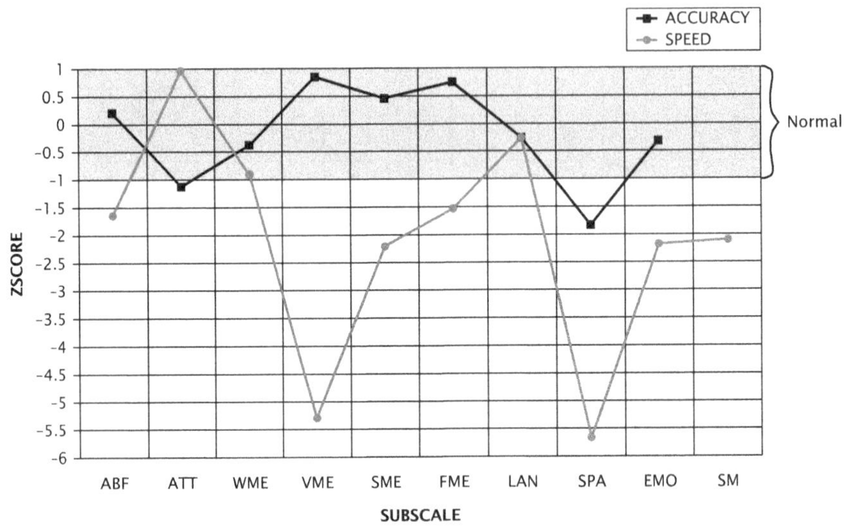

FIGURE 28.6 Performance of a client on computerized neurocognitive testing expressed as z-scores (standard deviations from the mean) relative to healthy people age 41 to 55.

Conclusion: "My Amygdala Did It" versus Reality

A response to neuroscience applications in capital cases ubiquitous among the lay public, and even in some academic and legal circles, is that such testimony offers an excuse for violence by deflecting responsibility from the person to a brain structure. Such an attitude has been articulated by Stephen Morse, a professor of Law and Psychiatry at the University of Pennsylvania, who noted "Brains don't kill people. People kill people."[39] As is hopefully evident from the preceding text, the brain controls behavior, and behavior informs culpability. Therefore, Morse's characterization is at best a caricature of the nature of neuroscience involvement in the court. First, in most cases, neuroscience evidence is presented during sentencing as a mitigating factor. Here, neuroscience is presented as one of myriad possible mitigating circumstances post-conviction, which may include testimonials from school friends, teachers, and family. If someone's kindergarten teacher can offer relevant testimony, how could a neuroscience expert documenting brain dysfunction not be germane?

Second, from the standpoint of neuroscience, Morse's statement is either tautological, or dualistic, and hence flawed. Because behavior is considered by neuroscientists to be the product of brain processing, and killing is a behavior, the statement—"Brains don't kill people. People kill people."—makes as much sense as its opposite: "People don't kill people. Brains kill people." Neuroscience offers a level of explanation for behavior, which is inherent to the question of culpability and mitigation.

Notwithstanding these paradoxical objections, it is likely that neuroscience will continue to play a role in jurisprudence, and that its inclusion will only increase. The field is becoming more accessible to other experts and the public, and its ability to shed light on more subtle aspects of human behavior is evolving rapidly. Technologies have herein been described that could contribute not only to improved sensitivity for detection of brain abnormalities, but also information that can speak directly to fact-finding, such as methods for lie detection.[40–42] Although currently the polygraph is not accepted in court,[43–45] there is reason to believe that fMRI vastly outperforms polygraphy (unpublished data) because it does not rely on the subject's autonomic response to lies, which may be attenuated in someone who is not anxious about lying. Instead, it keys on the extra step required by the brain to divert a veridical response. This methodology is likely to encounte r even greater resistance, but eventually it could become useful to the extent that it is reliable and valid. Although explaining neuroscience methods can become increasingly challenging, involving the explication of complex analytical techniques, tools for illustrating the relevant features of the data are also more prevalent. Contrary to assertions that such illustrations are designed to mislead or confuse the jury,[46,47] they are typically the products of standardized rigorous data processing, and their link to specific brain systems can be elucidated by a knowledgeable expert. Those interested in the intersection of neuroscience and the law can look forward to interesting times ahead.

References

1. Finger S. (1994). *Origins of neuroscience: A history of explorations into brain function.* New York: Oxford University Press.
2. Spencer F. (1997). Germany. In F Spencer (Ed.), *History of physical anthropology: An encyclopedia.* New York: Garland.
3. Descartes R. (1649). *The passions of the soul* [in French].
4. Descartes R. (1664). *Treatise of man* [in French].
5. Rafter N. (2008). *The criminal brain: Understanding biological theories of crime.* New York: NYU Press.

5a. Broca P. (1861). Remarques sur le siege de la faculte du langage articule, suivies d'une observation d'aphemie (perte de la parole) [Remarks on the seat of the faculty of articulated language, following an observation of Aphemia (loss of speech)]. *BUN Sot Anat, 6*, 330–357.

6. Wernicke C. (1970). The Aphasic Symptom-complex: A Psychological Study on an Anatomical Basis. *Arch Neurol, 22*, 280–282.
7. Jackson JH. (1932). On affections of speech from diseases of the brain. In J Taylor (Ed.), *Selected writings of John Hughlings Jackson* (vol. II, pp. 155–204). London: Hodder and Stoughton.
8. Babinski J. (1914) Contribution a l'etude des troubles mentaux dans l'hemiplegie organique cerebrale (anosognosie) [Contribution to the study of mental disorders in organic cerebral hemiplegia (anosognosia)]. *Rw Neural (Paris), 27*, 845–848.
9. Wilson SAK. (1924). Some problems in neurology, II: Pathological laughing and crying. *J Neurol Psychopathol, 16*, 299.
10. Sackeim HA, Greenberg MS, Weiman AL, Gur RC, Hungerbuhler JP, & Geschwind N. (1982). Hemispheric asymmetry in the expression of positive and negative emotions: Neurological evidence. *Arch Neurol, 39*, 210–218.
11. Penfield W. (1952). Memory mechanisms. *AMA Arch Neurol Psychiatry, 67*, 178–198.
12. Penfield W. (1975). *The mystery of the mind: A critical study of consciousness and the human brain.* Princeton, NJ: Princeton University Press.
13. Jasper H, & Penfield W. (1954). *Epilepsy and the functional anatomy of the human brain* (2nd ed.). Boston: Little, Brown and Co.
14. Gusnard DA, & Raichle ME. (2001). Searching for a baseline: Functional imaging and the resting human brain. *Nat Rev Neurosci, 2*, 685–694.

15. Gur RC, & Reivich M. (1980). Cognitive task effects on hemispheric blood flow in humans: Evidence for individual differences in hemispheric activation. *Brain Lang, 9*, 78–93.
16. Schneider K, Pauly KD, Gossen A, Mevissen L, Michel TM, Gur RC, et al. (2013). Neural correlates of moral reasoning in autism spectrum disorder. *Soc Cogn Affect Neurosci, 8*(6), 702–710.
17. Matsuzawa J, Matsui M, Konishi T, Noguchi K, Gur RC, Bilker W, Miyawaki T. (2001). Age-related volumetric changes of brain gray and white matter in healthy infants and children. *Cerebral Cortex, 11*(4), 335–342.
18. Gur RC. (2005). Brain maturation and its relevance to understanding criminal culpability of juveniles. *Curr Psychiatry Rept, 7*(4), 292–296.
19. Giedd JN, & Rapoport JL. (2010). Structural MRI of pediatric brain development: What have we learned and where are we going? *Neuron, 67*(5), 728–734.
20. *U.S. v. Montgomery* (2007). W.D.Mo. [Available on request].
21. Gur RC, Gur RE, Resnick SM, Skolnick BE, Alavi A, & Reivich M. (1987). The effect of anxiety on cortical cerebral blood flow and metabolism. *J Cerebr Blood Flow Metab, 7*, 173–177.
22. Gur RC, Mozley LH, Mozley PD, Resnick SM, Karp JS, Alavi A, et al. (1995). Sex differences in regional cerebral glucose metabolism during a resting state. *Science, 267*, 528–531.
23. State of Florida (2014). Department of Corrections Website Active Inmates: Long, Robert J (DC Number: 494041). http://www.dc.state.fl.us/ActiveInmates/. Accessed May 28, 2014.
24. *Long v. Florida* (1996). Initial brief of appellant. http://www.law.fsu.edu/library/flsupct/83593/83593ini.pdf. Accessed May 28, 2014.
25. Rosen J. (March 11, 2007). The brain on the stand. *New York Times*. http://www.nytimes.com/2007/03/11/magazine/11Neurolaw.t.html?pagewanted=print&_r=1&. Accessed May 28, 2014.
26. *Roper v. Simmons* (2005). 543 U.S. 551.
26a. Anderson JA, & Heaton P. (2013). Measuring the effect of defense counsel on homicide case outcomes. A report submitted to the National Institute of Justice, Washington, DC. https://www.ncjrs.gov/pdffiles1/nij/grants/241158.pdf. Accessed May 28, 2014.
27. Blume JH, & Paavola EC. (2011). Life, death, and neuroimaging: The advantages of the defense's use of neuroimaging in capital cases—lessons from the front. *Mercer Law Rev, 62*(3), 909.
27a. Bigler ED. (2013). Neuroimaging biomarkers in mild traumatic brain injury (mTBI). *Neuropsychol Rev, 23*(3), 169–209.
27b. Faigman DL, Monahan J, & Slobogin C. (2014). Group to individual (G2i) inference in scientific expert testimony. *Univ Chicago Law Rev, 81*(2), 417–480.
28. Gur RC, Ragland JD, Moberg PJ, Turner TH, Bilker WB, Kohler C, et al. (2001a). Computerized neurocognitive scanning: I. Methodology and validation in healthy people. *Neuropsychopharmacology, 25*, 766–776.
29. Gur RC, Richard J, Hughett P, Calkins ME, Macy L, Bilker WB, et al. (2010). A cognitive neuroscience-based computerized battery for efficient measurement of individual differences: Standardization and initial construct validation. *J Neurosci Meth, 187*, 254–262.
30. Roalf DR, Gur RC, Almasy L, Richard J, Gallagher S, Prasad K, et al. (2013). Neurocognitive performance stability in a multiplex multigenerational study of schizophrenia. *Schizophr Bull, 39*(5), 1008–1017.
31. Kitsuse JI, & Cicourel AV. (1963). A note on the use of official statistics. *Soc Problems, 11*(2), 131–139.
31a. Miller G. (December 12, 2013). Did brain scans just save a convicted murderer from the death penalty? *Wired*. http://www.wired.com/2013/12/murder-law-brain/. Accessed May 28, 2014.
32. Gur RC, Trivedi SS, Saykin AJ, & Gur RE. (1988). "Behavioral imaging"—a procedure for analysis and display of neuropsychological test scores: I. Construction of algorithm and initial clinical evaluation. *Neuropsychiatry, Neuropsychol Behav Neurol, 1*, 53–60.
33. Gur RC, Saykin AJ, Blonder LX, & Gur RE. (1988). "Behavioral imaging": II. Application of the quantitative algorithm to hypothesis testing in a population of hemiparkinsonian patients. *Neuropsychiatry, Neuropsychol Behav Neurol, 1*, 87–96.
34. Blonder LX, Gur RE, Gur RC, Saykin AJ, Hurtig HI. (1989). Neuropsychological functioning in hemiparkinsonism. *Brain Cogn, 9*, 177–190.

35. Gur RC, Saykin AJ, Benton A, Kaplan E, Levin H, Kester DB, & Gur RE. (1990). "Behavioral imaging": III. Inter-rater agreement and reliability of weightings. *Neuropsychiatry, Neuropsychol Behav Neurol, 3*, 113–124.
36. Shen D, & Davatzikos C. (2002). HAMMER: Hierarchical attribute matching mechanism for elastic registration. *IEEE Trans Med Imag, 21*(11), 1421–1439.
37. Gur RC, Erwin RJ, & Gur RE. (1992). Neurobehavioral probes for physiologic neuroimaging studies. *Arch Gen Psychiatry, 49*, 409–414.
38. Gur RC, Ragland JD, Moberg PJ, Bilker WB, Kohler C, Siegel SJ, & Gur RE. (2001b). Computerized neurocognitive scanning II: The profile of schizophrenia. *Neuropsychopharmacology, 25*, 777–788.
39. Hughes V. (2010). Head case. *Nature, 464*, 340–342.
40. Langleben DD, Schroeder L, Maldjian JA, Gur RC, McDonald S, Ragland JD, et al. (2002). Brain activity during simulated deception: An event-related functional magnetic resonance study. *NeuroImage, 15*, 727–732.
41. Langleben DD, Loughead JW, Bilker WB, Ruparel K, Childress AR, Busch S, & Gur RC. (2005). Telling truth from lie in individual subjects with fast event-related fMRI. *Hum Brain Map, 26*, 262–272.
42. Davatzikos C, Ruparel K, Fan Y, Shen DG, Acharyya M, Loughead JW, et al. (2005). Classifying spatial patterns of brain activity using machine learning methods: application to lie detection. *NeuroImage, 15*, 663–668.
43. *United States v. Scheffer* (1998). 523 U.S. 303.
44. Military Rule of Evidence 707 (2001, September). *156th officer basic course*. MAJ Charles H. Rose III. http://www.au.af.mil/au/awc/awcgate/law/mil-evidence-155.pdf. Accessed May 28, 2014.
45. National Research Council. (2003). The polygraph *and lie detection. Committee to review the scientific evidence on the polygraph*. http://www.ministryoftruth.me.uk/wp-content/uploads/2013/07/nas-polygraph.pdf. Accessed May 28, 2014.
46. Brown T, & Murphy E. (2010). Through a scanner darkly: Functional neuroimaging as evidence of a criminal defendant's past mental states. *Stanford Law Rev, 62*(4), 1119–1208.
47. Saks MJ, Schweitzer NJ, Aharoni E, & Kiehl K. (Forthcoming). The impact of neuroimages in the sentencing phase of capital trials. *J Empir Leg Stud*. http://papers.ssrn.com/sol3/papers.cfm?abstract_id=2274527. Accessed June 7, 2014.

29

Neurocriminology

Applications for Forensic Psychiatry

Robert A. Schug, Adrian Raine,
Yu Gao, Andrea Glenn, and
Yaling Yang

Essential to forensic psychiatry is an empirical understanding of the initiation, maintenance, and potential desistance from criminal behavior. Moreover, neurobiological crime research (i.e., neurocriminology)—with its extensive contributions to criminological study dating back more than a century[1]—has offered a unique understanding of the etiological mechanisms underlying antisocial behavior. As such, criminal justice systems in general and forensic psychiatry in particular stand to benefit tremendously from its application. Neuroimaging research has identified structural and functional deficits in frontal, temporal, and subcortical regions in antisocial children and adults, and these findings are largely supported by neurological studies of brain trauma in antisocial populations. Neuropsychological investigations have reported verbal, spatial, and executive dysfunction in antisocial adults and children. This neurobiological evidence base has currently begun to impact various aspects of criminal justice systems, including lie detection and judicial process applications; and may enhance forensic psychological assessment and inform policies and procedures regarding the identification, management, and treatment of various types of adult and juvenile offenders.

This chapter serves as an integrative review of findings from key areas of neurobiological research on criminal, violent, and antisocial behavior. Additionally, it provides an overview of current and potential application of this research within forensic arenas—which may be of value in informing the forensic clinical practitioner.

Neuroimaging

The past decade has been marked by an increase in neuroimaging research, and accumulating evidence continues to support a plausible relationship between brain dysfunction and antisocial behavior. Evidence implicating the prefrontal cortex is strongest—not surprising given the multiple functions associated with this region (including inhibiting behavioral impulses and regulating emotion generated by the amygdala and other subcortical components). In terms of structural imaging findings, several studies have noted significant gray matter volume reduction in the prefrontal cortex in individuals characterized by antisociality and aggression.[2] In terms of functional imaging findings, earlier studies reported decreased functioning (e.g., glucose metabolism and regional cerebral blood flow—or rCBF) in this region in antisocial individuals.[3,4]

Two prefrontal subregions—the orbitofrontal cortex (OFC) and dorsolateral prefrontal cortex (DLPFC) have been most consistently found to be impaired in individuals characterized by antisocial and violent behavior. The OFC plays an important role in ethical decision making and emotion regulation, whereas the DLPFC is critical in behavioral control and executive functioning. To date, structural imaging studies have shown volumetric/thickness reductions in the frontal cortex, particularly in the OFC and DLPFC, in antisocial and psychopathic individuals.[5–12] These findings are consistent with those from functional imaging studies, which have found abnormal OFC and DLPFC functioning during cognitive and emotional tasks in antisocial individuals. For example, Raine et al. found decreased glucose metabolism in OFC and DLPFC areas in murderers during a task involving attention and vigilance (the continuous performance task).[13] On balance, antisocial and violent individuals demonstrated increased neural activation in OFC and DLPFC regions during an emotional task (i.e., the viewing of affective images) compared to controls in subsequent studies[14,15]—although other investigators found psychopathic individuals were characterized by reduced OFC activation during an empathic processing task.[16] Other recent studies have reported altered structural and functional connectivity in frontal networks in antisocial individuals compared to normal controls.[17,18] Together, findings from these studies suggest that prefrontal impairments, particularly those found in OFC and DLPFC regions, may make crucial contributions to the neurobiological pathology in antisocial and violent persons.

Other brain structures have also been linked to violent criminal behavior. It has been known for several decades that damage to the temporal lobe may lead to dampened emotional responses, similar to those seen in individuals characterized by violence and antisociality.[19] To that end, several studies that have reported prefrontal deficits in their antisocial and violent participants have also reported deficits in temporal functioning. Soderstrom and colleagues, for example, found reduced rCBF in both frontal and temporal cortices in violent perpetrators relative to controls.[20] Hirono et al. similarly found reductions in rCBF in both the left anterior temporal cortex and bilateral dorsofrontal cortex in impulsive violent criminal offenders.[21] Similar structural and functional deficits have been reported in studies of children characterized by early-onset conduct disorder and aggression.[22,23]

Deficits in the amygdala-hippocampal complex—which lies within the temporal region—have been particularly associated with violence and antisociality. The amygdala is critically involved in the reception and production of emotion and the processing of fear conditioning, whereas the hippocampus plays a crucial role in emotional memory. Several studies have reported functional abnormalities in the amygdala-hippocampal complex in antisocial and aggressive individuals. For example, Kiehl et al. found criminal psychopaths showed reduced amygdala-hippocampal activations while viewing negative affective images,[24] and Soderstrom et al. found decreased hippocampal rCBF in violent offenders compared to controls.[20] Sterzer and colleagues reported reduced activation in the right dorsal anterior cingulate cortex in aggressive children with conduct disorders while viewing negative affective images.[25] Other recent studies of children characterized by conduct problems and psychopathic traits have reported reduced activation in similar regions (including the anterior cingulate cortex, inferior frontal gyrus, and amygdala) during empathic processing tasks,[26,27] as well as altered amygdala-prefrontal functional connectivity.[28] In aggregate, findings suggest that temporal lobe abnormalities, particularly associated with the amygdala and hippocampus, may lead to a lack of fear of punishment, and—in turn—a disruption of normal moral development (see the following).

Neurology

An empirical understanding of the pathogenesis of antisocial behavior has been greatly enhanced by neurological studies of brain trauma in antisocial individuals. Interestingly, there is a substantial overlap between age groups at highest risk for traumatic brain injury (adolescents, young adults, those over 75, males)[29] and increased antisocial behavior.[30] Unusually high prevalence rates of adult and childhood brain injury have been noted in some adult antisocial populations.[31,32] Case descriptions of frontally damaged patients who subsequently developed marked antisociality (Phineus Gage, patient E.V.R., and others) have provided even more-striking evidence.[33–36] In fact, this condition has been referred to as *acquired psychopathy*.[37]

Although injury to different brain regions may lead to a variety of impairments in cognitive and emotional functioning, studies indicate that aggressive behavior is more often associated with damage to the frontal and temporal regions. For example, Vietnam War veterans who suffered orbitofrontal lesions have demonstrated increased aggressive and violent attitudes compared to those with lesions to other brain regions, while those with temporal injuries reported more feelings of rage and hostility.[38] In fact, it has been suggested that damage to these two regions may lead to impairments in cognitive and emotion-regulation capabilities, and result in an individual using aggression and violence rather than more socially acceptable means (e.g., negotiation) to achieve his or her goals.[39]

Increased rates of brain injury history have also been reported in studies of juvenile criminals and delinquents,[40–42] at rates higher than nondelinquents,[43] and with head injuries often predating violent behavior and law-enforcement contact.[32,44] Other studies have reported antisocial and externalizing behavioral sequelae commonly following head injury in children,[45] and that these are often more persistent and severe when damage is incurred very early in life (i.e., before age 16 months).[46] However, it is worth noting that head injury—even frontal or temporal damage—does not automatically predispose one to delinquency. Rather, criminal behavior (and violence in particular) likely results from a complex interaction of risk factors such as genetic predisposition, emotional distress, poverty, substance abuse, child abuse, academic underachievement, learning disabilities, and school behavioral problems.[39,47] In fact, in some cases, brain injury has not only not resulted in behavioral changes, but has actually *reduced* aggression in previously aggressive individuals,[48–50] although this may have been associated with concomitant dorsolateral prefrontal damage (a region spared in the cases of Gage and E.V.R.[50] An alternative explanation may be that frontal lobe damage, particularly in the orbitofrontal cortex, is merely a *risk factor*, which does not necessarily result in antisociality in all cases. Furthermore, brain trauma (and acquired psychopathy in particular) may be a risk factor for subsequent neurodegenerative disorders, which may exacerbate antisocial tendencies.[37] In aggregate, studies to date suggest that neurological factors related to head injury may be significant in the understanding of the etiology of crime and violence, and have important implications in the practice of forensic psychiatry.

Neuropsychology

Research over the past several decades indicates an increasing interest in the relationship between neuropsychological functioning and the forensic aspects of behavior.[51] To date, studies of the neuropsychological correlates of violence, aggression, and antisociality have focused predominantly on verbal and spatial intelligence and executive abilities.

Verbal and Spatial Intelligence

Although deficits in general intellectual functioning (i.e., IQ or Full Scale IQ) are the best-replicated correlates of antisociality, violence, and criminality among individuals without mental illness, the identification of intelligence deficits in separate verbal versus spatial/performance components has also proved useful in the understanding of the etiology of antisocial behavior.[52] Decreased verbal as opposed to spatial/performance IQ (thought to represent left-hemispheric dysfunction) has commonly been noted in antisocial adults,[53] children and adolescents.[53–57] In fact, a recent meta-analysis showed that reduced verbal IQ is characteristic of antisocial males and females across different age groups.[58] Longitudinal data have shown early verbal deficits (i.e., at age 13) predict later delinquency (i.e., at age 18) for persistent, high-level criminality beginning before adolescence.[59] It has been proposed that verbal dysfunction leads to socialization failure by affecting the development of language-based self-control mechanisms[60,61]; although juvenile offenders characterized by verbal deficits may have a more positive prognosis with therapy and environmental modifications.[56] Some studies, however, have not identified general or verbal intelligence deficits in individuals with antisocial personality disorder (ASPD) and psychopathy,[63,62] although some specific traits of psychopathy (i.e., criminal versatility and violence) may be associated with verbal dysfunction.[51] Additionally, evidence from studies of youths with psychopathic-like traits (itself a controversial topic)[64] has been mixed.[65–67] Thus, while global and/or verbal intellectual dysfunction may characterize adult antisocials in general, they may not characterize specific constellations of antisocial traits.

Other longitudinal community-based studies[68,69] have reported both verbal and spatial deficits in youths characterized by different trajectories of antisocial behavior (in fact, Raine et al. found spatial but not verbal deficits at age 3)[68]—challenging the classic view of verbal but not performance intelligence deficits in antisocial individuals. Raine and colleagues propose early visuospatial deficits may interfere with mother–infant bonding, and may indicate right hemisphere dysfunction that interferes with emotional processing and regulation—subsequently leading to life-course antisocial behavior.

Executive Functioning

Executive functioning (EF) refers to the cognitive processes that facilitate goal-oriented, contextually appropriate behavior and effective self-serving conduct.[61,70] Deficits in EF are believed to represent frontal lobe impairment, and are indicated by poor performance on specific neuropsychological tasks (i.e., category, maze-tracing, Stroop interference, card sorting, verbal fluency and tower tests, and go/no-go and gambling tasks) that measure strategy formation, cognitive flexibility, or impulsivity.

Neuropsychological studies of EF and antisociality have commonly focused on categorical clinical diagnoses (i.e., ASPD, conduct disorder, and psychopathy) and legal/judicial concepts such as criminality and delinquency. Morgan and Lilienfeld's classic meta-analysis of 39 studies found overall reduced EF in antisocial individuals relative to controls, and strongest effect sizes for the Porteus Maze test and antisocial behavior defined by judicial status.[71] Executive dysfunction has more recently been associated with individuals characterized by aggression (e.g., male batterers), violence, and ASPD,[72–76] property crimes,[54] child molesters with and without pedophilia,[77] suicidality,[78] single compared to multiple homicide victims in death row inmates and indigent murder defendants,[79] murderers with schizophrenia compared to nonviolent men with schizophrenia,[80] forensic hospital patients with mental challenges compared to those without,[81] and reactive versus instrumental violent offenders.[82] Executive function has also been shown to be a predictor of responsivity to anti-aggression treatment in patients with schizophrenia.[83]

General EF deficits have not shown consistent associations with adult psychopathy,[63,84–86] and more recent evidence suggests that psychopathy may be characterized more by dysfunction in the OFC.[87] Additionally, increased performance on neuropsychological measures of DLPFC functioning has been demonstrated in successful, uncaught psychopaths compared to unsuccessful psychopaths and controls[88]; and white collar criminals have shown better EF performance relative to offender controls.[89] Furthermore, violent ASPD offenders with and without psychopathy have shown similar deficits related to "cool EF" (top-down processes that are distinctly cognitive in nature, such as working memory, response inhibition, planning, sustained attention, and attentional set-shifting—thought to be subsumed by the DLPFC and ventrolateral PFC) and "hot EF" (process subsumed by ventromedial connections between the mesolimbic reward pathway and the ventromedial PFC, which have an affective, motivational, or incentive/reward component—such as appraisal of the motivational significance of a stimulus in emotional decision making).[90]

Similar variability is found in results from studies measuring EF in children and adolescents with CD, depending upon sample characteristics, type of control group, method of assessment, operational definitions of EF, and methodology.[56,91] Executive dysfunction has been shown to characterize some youths[69,92–95] and not others.[59,94] Differential patterns of EF deficits among children and adults may be explained in part by the development of EF, which occurs with the ongoing myelination of the frontal cortex into adolescence and beyond.[94,96] This phenomenon has been reflected in several research reports. For example, Nestor found EF deficits in older (i.e., middle-aged) but not younger (i.e., early adulthood) maximum security hospital patients.[97] Blair found more pronounced EF impairments on a neuropsychological measure of OFC functioning in psychopathic adults relative to psychopathic children.[98] Furthermore, neuropsychological performance can be compromised by comorbid hyperactivity and aggression,[96,99] which may be present in varying levels throughout the developmental process. Overall, findings from neuropsychological studies continue to suggest an association between specific domains of cognitive functioning and antisocial, criminal, and violent behavior; and EF remains among the most promising foci of empirical inquiry among these studies, with particular relevance to forensic psychiatric practice.

Forensic Applications of Neurocriminological Research

The potential importance of neurocriminological research within criminal justice systems in general and forensic psychiatry in particular is significant. Although advances in technology have brought about new and exciting neurobiological approaches to antisocial behavioral research, forensic applications of biological risk factors for crime are not a novel concept and have their roots in the writings of early positivist criminology.[1] As such, it is important that the forensic clinical practitioner have an understanding of how neurobiological research to date has affected criminal justice systems in various areas, and how forensic practice in the future may depend more heavily on neurobiological assessment—which can inform policies and procedures involved in the identification, management, and treatment of various types of criminal offenders from different age groups. More critical, however, is a comprehensive understanding and appreciation of the philosophical, ethical, and political dilemmas surrounding its use in the furtherance of justice.

Lie Detection

The first practical applications of neurobiological measures in the criminal justice system involved the detection of deception. The polygraph ("lie detector") is the earliest and most widely known physiological measure of lie detection[100] and is based on the assumption that autonomic responses (e.g., increased heart rate, blood pressure, respiration rate, and skin conductance response) occurring during questioning indicate anxiety and therefore deception. Among the polygraph techniques are the control question technique, directed lie technique, and guilty knowledge test (GKT). Although the psychophysiological indicators of lying are often presumed to be unfalsifiable, and vehement proponents of the use of polygraph lie detection are found among law enforcement and national security policy makers, scientists generally consider this technique to be fraught with conceptual and methodological weaknesses, and polygraph evidence has largely been excluded from the courts.[101,102]

More recently, an interest in detecting deception using brain-based methods has developed. The most promising line of inquiry has focused on components of event-related potentials (ERPs—which refer to averaged changes in the electrical activity of the brain in response to specific stimuli); in particular, the P300 (a positive-going waveform occurring approximately 300 milliseconds after a stimulus)[103] response to significant, infrequent (i.e., "oddball") stimuli. In a GKT procedure based on the P300, crime-relevant information keys constitute the oddball stimuli. The effectiveness of ERP-GKT procedures has been demonstrated in several validation studies, and its potential utility in courtroom applications has been noted.[102] It is also worth noting that a sizeable body of literature has been developed on the psychophysiological correlates of antisocial behavior (i.e., peripheral physiological processes representing indirect measures of brain functioning, which may be characteristically different in criminal, violent, and antisocial individuals), particularly in the areas of EEG[104,105]—including the ERP,[106–108] skin conductance,[109–111] and heart rate measures.[104,112,113]

Recent interest in neuroimaging approaches to lie detection has also become apparent,[114,115] and such approaches could potentially have tremendous value in forensic assessment. For example, in criminal responsibility applications, Sadoff and Dattilio[116] propose the use of (functional) neuroimaging to evaluate the truthfulness of a defendant reporting amnesia for a criminal act—with sodium amytal interviewing or hypnosis subsequently applied to recover lost memories when bona fide amnesia is present. However, the structural and functional correlates of deception are complex and must be considered with caution. As an example, although initial evidence for structural brain deficits in pathological liars (i.e., reductions in prefrontal grey matter and *increases* in inferior, middle, and orbitofrontal white matter) has been reported,[117,118] a review of 15 functional imaging studies indicates activations in multiple cortical and subcortical regions during deception—although activation in the DLPFC appeared in 9 out of 15 studies.[119] This, along with the conceptual and methodological weaknesses that plagued the old technology, must be still be rectified before neuroimaging becomes a viable option for lie detection.[119]

Tests of neuropsychological functioning have also proved useful in the detection of another form of deception—malingering. Specific components of intelligence tests can indicate malingering, such as an unusual scatter of scores, failing/passing items that legitimate responders would tend to pass/fail, and "approximately correct" answers. Malingerers do not appear able to mimic the performance of brain-injured patients on memory assessments, and often score significantly below the level of chance on "forced choice" tests. Furthermore, the detection of malingering may be accomplished via the evaluation of consistency across measures of common constructs and/or across repeated administrations[119a] In aggregate, these methods demonstrate how neurobiological techniques may have much to contribute in the way of deception detection for forensic purposes in the near future.

Legal and Judicial Process

The legal system has already begun to be impacted by structural and functional brain imaging.[120] In 2006, Feigenson reported that approximately 130 court cases had admitted brain imaging data into evidence—a large number considering that the technique had only recently become more accessible, and possibly reflecting the belief that brain imaging is an objective measure of a defendant's mental functioning.[121] For the most part, brain abnormalities identified via brain imaging methods have been used to argue for reduced criminal responsibility, and outcomes of homicide cases utilizing this tactic have been mixed, ranging from successful NGRI defenses, to mitigation in sentencing (i.e., life imprisonment versus capital punishment), to failure resulting in guilty verdicts and the death sentence. While brain imaging methods may seem to have potentially significant implications within the legal system, there remain numerous limitations—including the inability of these methods to acquire functional data that are retrospective in nature (i.e., speaking to brain functioning at the time of the crime), and the subjectivity of the interpretation of structural findings.[120]

Measures of neuropsychological functioning may also have utility in the criminal justice system. For example, a diagnosis of mental retardation—determined predominantly by sub-average intellectual functioning (i.e., IQ <70; although current DSM 5 conceptualizations of intellectual disability no longer rely solely upon IQ levels) can markedly mitigate sentencing outcomes for murder defendants in general (and death penalty candidates in particular), and could potentially become a key component of pretrial evaluations of competency to stand trial.[122] Moreover, neurotransmitter functioning has been introduced as evidence to support an NGRI defense.[123] In summary, the practical application of neurocriminological research in informing legal and judicial processes remains in its incipient stages. Although the need remains for replication of current research findings to facilitate more widespread acceptance and implementation, these techniques nonetheless demonstrate significant potential.

Forensic Assessment

Finally, initial evidence suggests that neurobiological techniques may enhance specificity and efficacy in key areas of forensic assessment in the future—particularly in areas of diagnostic identification, providing treatment options, dangerousness and risk prediction, and treatment program evaluation.[124] Neurobiological factors may help extend the available range of diagnostic possibilities, assist in identifying difficult-to-assess psychobiological dysfunction (e.g., using blunted heart rate reactivity rather than self-report inventories to identify psychopathic traits, or brain imaging to identify pathological lying or malingering), and increase diagnostic specificity by decreasing group heterogeneity occurring within forensic-related psychopathologies. Neurobiological assessment methods that reduce diagnostic heterogeneity may also contribute to improved forensic pharmacological interventions,[125–127] and novel nonpharmacological interventions that consider and even alter biological vulnerabilities to juvenile antisocial behavior also have shown promise.[128–134] Neurobiological parameters may also be useful in predicting the risk of future antisocial behavior.[124] For example, reduced IQ and increased antisociality have been described as components of dangerousness, and these factors have differentiated death-row from life-sentence male murderers.[135] Other patterns of neuropsychological dysfunction associated with psychopathy[86] could be utilized as indices of risk, as elevated psychopathy ratings (i.e, *Psychopathy Checklist—Revised*)[136] are the most robust known actuarial predictors of criminal recidivism.[137] Reduced cerebrospinal 5-HIAA levels (a serotonin metabolite) have differentiated violent offenders who recidivate from non-recidivists,[138] whereas other neurobiological techniques, such as penile plethysmography, have demonstrated some effectiveness in differentiating child molesters from other sex offenders and nonoffenders, nonfamilial child molesters from incest offenders, and homicidal child molesters from nonhomicidal child molesters and nonoffenders—although this technique has been criticized by the scientific community.[139] The assessment of risk and prediction of dangerousness is among the gravest and most imperative roles of the forensic practitioner, and neurocriminological research may soon assist in increasing the capabilities of those called upon to do so.

Although the contributions of neurocriminological research to forensic assessment remain largely hypothetical, first evidence shows promise, and additional research is both feasible and warranted. Herculean efforts must, however, be undertaken to comprehend and address the significant philosophical, ethical, and political issues—largely focused on arguments of biological determinism versus free will—inherent to neurocriminological applications within criminal justice systems,[120,126] particularly because forensic psychiatry may one day be faced with issues such as government-sanctioned pre-emptive interventions that deny individual civil liberties, and even surgically implanted behavior-controlling neurotechnologies. However, beneath these legitimate concerns lies what may be an antiquated notion of the biological nature of crime. For although Lombroso's legacy carries on, its foundation has been rattled—we have since learned through neurocriminological research that biology is not destiny, and that physical properties of mind and body in the criminal may in fact be altered.

Conclusion

Key areas of neurocriminological research have contributed to a greater empirical understanding of the initiation, maintenance, and potential desistance from criminal behavior. This body of research has also served to inform prominent developmental perspectives of crime. In turn, applications of neurobiological crime research have become essential to the field of forensic psychiatry. As such, the two—neurobiological research and forensic psychiatric applications—are inextricably bound, each serving both to inform and benefit from the other. It is hoped that this interdependence of research and practice will contribute to a growing base of evidence from which the causes and cures of criminality will eventually be revealed.

References

1. Lombroso C. (1876). *Criminal man*. Milan: Hoepli.
2. Raine A, Lencz T, Bihrle S, LaCasse L, & Colletti P. (2000). Reduced prefrontal gray matter volume and reduced autonomic activity in antisocial personality disorder. *Arch Gen Psychiat, 57*, 119–127.

3. Volkow N, & Tancredi LR. (1987). Neural substrates of violent behavior. A preliminary study with positron emission tomography. *Br J Psychiat, 151*, 668–673.
4. Volkow ND, Tancredi LR, Grant C, Gillespie H, Valentine A, Mullani N, et al. (1995). Brain glucose metabolism in violent psychiatric patients: A preliminary study. *Psychiat Res, 61*, 243–253.
5. Aoki Y, Inokuchi R, Nakao T, & Yamasue H. (2013). Neural bases of antisocial behavior: A voxel-based meta-analysis. *Soc Cog Affect Neur, 9*, 1223–1231.
6. Bertsch K, Grothe M, Prehn K, Vohs K, Berger C, Hauenstein K, et al. (2013). Brain volumes differ between diagnostic groups of violent criminal offenders. *Eur Arch Psy Clin N, 263*, 593–606.
7 Howner, K., Eskildsen, S. F., Fischer, H., Dierks, T., Wahlund, L. O., Jonsson, T., Wiberg, M. K., & Kristiansson, M. (2012). Thinner cortex in the frontal lobes in mentally disordered offenders. *Psychiat Res-Neuroim, 203*, 126–131.
8. Laakso MP, Gunning-Dixon F, Vaurio O, Repo E, Soininen H, & Tiihonen J. (2002). Prefrontal volume in habitually violent subjects with antisocial personality disorder and type 2 alcoholism. *Psychiat Res-Neuroim, 114*, 95–102.
9. Ly M, Motzkin JC, Philippi CL, Kirk GR, Newman JP, Kiehl KA, et al. (2012). Cortical thinning in psychopathy. *Am J Psychiat, 169*, 743–749.
10. Yang Y, & Raine A. (2009). Prefrontal structural and functional brain imaging findings in antisocial, violent, and psychopathic individuals: a meta-analysis. *Psychiatry Res, 174*, 81–88.
11. Yang Y, Raine A, Colletti P, Toga AW, & Narr K.L. (2009). Abnormal temporal and prefrontal cortical gray matter thinning in psychopaths. *Mol Psychiatry, 14*, 561–562, 555.
12. Yang Y, Raine A, Colletti P, Toga AW, & Narr KL. (2010). Morphological alterations in the prefrontal cortex and the amygdala in unsuccessful psychopaths. *J Abnorm Psychol, 119*, 546–554.
13. Raine A, Buchsbau M, Stanley J, Lottenberg S, Abel L, & Stoddard J. (1994). Selective reductions in prefrontal glucose metabolism in murderers. *Biol Psychiatry, 36*, 365–373.
14. Müller JL, Sommer M, Wagner V, Lange K, Taschler H, Roder C., et al. (2003). Abnormalities in emotion processing within cortical and subcortical regions in criminal psychopaths: Evidence from a functional magnetic resonance imaging study using pictures with emotional content. *Psychiat Res-Neuroim, 54*, 152–162.
15. Schneider F, Habel U, Kessler C, Posse S, Grodd W, & Müller-Gartner H. (2000). functional imaging of conditioned aversive emotional responses in antisocial personality disorder. *Neuropsychobiol, 42*, 192–201.
16. Decety J, Skelly LR, & Kiehl KA. (2013). Brain response to empathy-eliciting scenarios involving pain in incarcerated individuals with psychopathy. *JAMA Psychiatry, 70*, 638–645.
17. Tang Y, Liu W, Chen J, Liao J, Hu D, & Wang W. (2013). Altered spontaneous activity in antisocial personality disorder revealed by regional homogeneity. *Neuroreport 24*, 590–595.
18. Yang Y, Raine A, Joshi AA, Joshi S, Chang YT, Schug RA, et al. (2012). Frontal information flow and connectivity in psychopathy. *Br J Psychiatry, 201*, 408–409.
19. Klüver H, & Bucy PC. (1939). Preliminary analysis of functions of the temporal lobes in monkeys. *Arch Neuro Psychiatry, 42*, 979–100.
20. Soderstrom H, Tullberg M, Wikkelsoe C, Ekholm S, & Forsman A. (2000). Reduced regional cerebral blood flow in non-psychotic violent offenders. *Psychiatry Res-Neuroim, 98*, 29–41.
21. Hirono N, Mega MS, Dinov ID, Mishkin F, & Cummings JL. (2000). Left frontaltemporal hypoperfusion is associated with aggression in patient with dementia. *Arch Neurol, 57*, 861–866.
22. Kruesi, M.J.P., Casanova, M.F., Mannheim, G. & Jonson-Bilder, A. (2004). Reduced temporal lobe volume in early onset conduct disorder. *Psychiat Res-Neuroim, 132*, 1–11.
23. Juhasz, C., Behen, M.E., Muzik, O., Chugani, D.C. & Chugani, H.T. (2001). Bilateral medial prefrontal and temporal neocortical hypometabolism in children with epilepsy and aggression. *Epilepsia, 42*, 991–1001.
24. Kiehl KA, Smith AM, Hare RD, Mendrek A, Forster BB., Brink J, et al. (2001). Limbic abnormalities in affective processing by criminal psychopaths as revealed by functional magnetic resonance imaging. *Biol Psychiat, 50*, 677–684.

25. Sterzer P, Stadler C, Krebs A, Kleinschmidt A, & Poustka, F. (2005). Abnormal neural responses to emotional visual stimuli in adolescents with conduct disorder. *Biol Psychiat, 57,* 7–15.
26. Lockwood PL, Sebastian CL, McCrory EJ, Hyde ZH, Gu X, De Brito SA, et al. (2013). Association of callous traits with reduced neural response to others' pain in children with conduct problems. *Curr Biol, 23,* 901–905.
27. Marsh AA, Finger EC, Fowler KA, Adalio CJ, Jurkowitz IT, Schechter JC, et al. (2013). Empathic responsiveness in amygdala and anterior cingulate cortex in youths with psychopathic traits. *J Child Psychol Psychiatry, 54,* 900–910.
28. Finger EC, Marsh A, Blair KS, Majestic C, Evangelou I, Gupta K, et al. (2012). Impaired functional but preserved structural connectivity in limbic white matter tracts in youth with conduct disorder or oppositional defiant disorder plus psychopathic traits. *Psychiat Res, 202,* 239–244.
29. Ehrenreich H, Krampe H, & Sirén, AL. (2007). Brain trauma. In AR Felthous, & H Saß (Eds.), *International handbook of psychopathic disorders and the law: Vol. 1* (pp.217–236). Chichester: John Wiley & Sons.
30. Moffitt, T.E. (1993). Adolescence-limited and life-course-persistent antisocial behavior: A developmental taxonomy. *Psychol Rev, 100,* 674–701.
31. Blake PY, Pincus, J.H. & Buckner, C. (1995). Neurologic abnormalities in murderers. *Neurology, 45,* 1641–1647.
32. Lewis DO, Pincus JH, Feldman M, Jackson L, & Bard B. (1986). Psychiatric, neurological, and psychoeducational characteristics of 15 death row inmates in the United States. *Am J Psychiat, 143,* 838–845.
33. Harlow JM. (1848). Passage of an iron bar through the head. *Boston Med Surg J, 13,* 389–393.
34. Saver JL, & Damasio AR. (1991). Preserved access and processing of social knowledge in a patient with acquired sociopathy due to ventromedial frontal damage. *Neuropsychologia, 29,* 1241–1249.
35. Damasio AR. (1994). *Descartes' error: Emotion, reason, and the human brain.* New York: GP Putnam's Sons.
36. Damasio AR, Tranel D, & Damasio H. (1990). Individuals with sociopathic behavior caused by frontal damage fail to respond autonomically to social stimuli. *Behav Brain Res, 41,* 81–94.
37. Granacher RP, & Fozdar MA. (2007). Acquired psychopathy and the assessment of traumatic brain injury. In AR Felthous, & H Saß (Eds.), *International handbook of psychopathic disorders and the law: Vol. 1* (pp.237–250). Chichester: John Wiley & Sons.
38. Grafman J, Schwab K, Warden D, Pridgen A, Brown, HR, & Salazar AM. (1996). Frontal lobe injuries, violence, and aggression: A report of the Vietnam Head Injury Study. *Neurology, 46,* 1231–1238.
39. León-Carrión J, & Ramos FJ. (2003). Blows to the head during development can predispose to violent criminal behaviour: Rehabilitation of consequences of head injury is a measure for crime prevention. *Brain Inj, 17,* 207–216.
40. Andrews TK, Rose FD, & Johnson DA. (1998). Social and behavioural effects of traumatic brain injury in children. *Brain Inj, 12,* 133–138.
41. Lewis DO, Pincus JH, Bard B, Richardson E, Prichep LS, Feldman M, et al. (1988). Neuropsychiatric, psychoeducational, and family characteristics of 14 juveniles condemned to death in the United States. *Am J Psychiat, 145,* 584–589.
42. Pincus HJ, & Lewis OD. (1991). Episodic violence. *Sem Neurol, 11,* 146–154.
43. Lewis DO, Pincus JH, Lovely R, Spitzer E, & Moy E. (1987). Biopsychosocial characteristics of matched samples of delinquents and nondelinquents. *J Am Acad Child Adolesct Psychiatry, 26,* 744–752.
44. Sarapata M, Hermann D, Johnson T, & Aycock R. (2008). The role of head injury in cognitive functioning, emotional adjustment and criminal behavior. *Brain Inj, 12,* 821–842.
45. Raine A. (2002a). Annotation: The role of prefrontal deficits, low autonomic arousal, and early health factors in the development of antisocial and aggressive behavior in children. *J Child Psychol Psychiatry, 43,* 417–434.
46. Anderson SW, Bechara A, Damasio H., Tranel D, & Damasio AR. (1999). Impairment of social and moral behavior related to early damage in human prefrontal cortex. *Nat Neurosci, 2,* 1031–1037.
47. Filley CM, Price BH, Nell V, Antoinette T, Morgan AS, Bresnahan JF, et al. (2001). Toward an understanding of violence: Neurobehavioral aspects of unwarranted physical aggression: Aspen

Neurobehavioral Conference consensus statement. *Neuropsychiatry Neuropsychol Behav Neurol, 14*, 1–14.

48. Bigler ED. (2001). Frontal lobe pathology and antisocial personality disorder. *Arch Gen Psychiatry, 58*, 609–611.
49. Ellenbogen JM. Hurford MO, Liebskind DS, Neimark GB, & Weiss, D. (2005). Ventromedial frontal lobe trauma. *Neurology, 64*, 757.
50. Mataró M, Jurado MA, García-Sánchez C, Barraquer L, Costa-Jussá FR, & Junqué, C. (2001). Long-term effects of bilateral frontal brain lesion: 60 years after injury with an iron bar. *Arch Neurol, 58*, 1139–1142.
51. Rasmussen K, Almvik R, & Levander S. (2001). Performance and strategy indices of neuropsychological tests: Relations with personality, criminality and violence. *J Forensic Neuropsychol, 2*(2), 29–43.
52. Wilson JQ, & Herrnstein R. (1985). *Crime and human nature*. New York: Simon & Schuster.
53. Raine A. (1993). *The psychopathology of crime: Criminal behavior as a clinical disorder*. San Diego, CA: Academic Press.
54. Barker ED, Séguin JR, White HR, Bates ME, Lacourse E, Carbonneau R, et al. (2007). Developmental trajectories of male physical violence and theft: Relations to neurocognitive performance. *Arch Gen Psychiatry, 64*, 592–599.
55. Brennan PA, Hall J, Bor W, Najman JM, & Williams, G. (2003). Integrating biological and social processes in relation to early-onset persistent aggression in boys and girls. *Dev Psychol, 39*, 309–323.
56. Teichner G, & Golden, CJ. (2000). The relationship of neuropsychological impairment to conduct disorder in adolescence: A conceptual review. *Aggression Violent Behav, 5*, 509–528.
57. Vermeiren R, De Clippele A, Schwab-Stone M, Ruchkin V, & Deboutte D. (2002). Neuropsychological characteristics of three subgroups of Flemish delinquent adolescents. *Neuropsychology, 16*, 49–55.
58. Isen, J. (2010). A meta-analytic assessment of Wechsler's P>V sign in antisocial populations. *Clin Psychol Rev, 30*, 423–435.
59. Moffitt TE, Lynam DR, & Silva PA. (1994). Neuropsychological tests predicting persistent male delinquency. *Criminology, 32*, 277–300.
60. Eriksson Å, Hodgins S, & Tengström A. (2005). Verbal intelligence and criminal offending among men with schizophrenia. *Int J Forensic Mental Health, 4*, 191–200.
61. Luria A. (1980). *Higher cortical functions in man* (2nd ed). New York: Basic Books.
62. Barkataki I, Kumari V, Das M, Taylor P, & Sharma T. (2006). Volumetric structural brain abnormalities in men with schizophrenia or antisocial personality disorder. *Behav Brain Res, 169*, 239–247.
63. Kosson DH, Miller SK, Byrnes, KA, & Leveroni CL. (2007). Testing neuropsychological hypotheses for cognitive deficits in psychopathic criminals: A study of global-local processing. *J Int Neuropsychol Soc, 13*, 267–276.
64. Salekin RT. (2006). Psychopathy in children and adults: Key issues in conceptualization and assessment. In C J Patrick (Ed.), *Handbook of psychopathy* (pp. 389–414). New York: Guilford Press.
65. Frick PJ, Cornell AH, Bodin SD, Dane HE, Barry CT, & Loney BR. (2003). Callous-unemotional traits and developmental pathways to severe conduct problems. *Dev Psychol, 39*, 372–378.
66. Loney BR, Frick PJ, Ellis ML, & McCoy MG. (1998). Intelligence, psychopathy, and antisocial behavior. *J Psychopathol Behav Assess, 20*, 231–247.
67. Salekin RT, Neumann CS, Leistico AR, & Zalot AA. (2004). Psychopathy in youth and intelligence: An investigation of Cleckley's hypothesis. *J Clin Child Adolesc Psychol, 33*, 731–742.
68. Raine A, Yaralian PS, Reynolds C, Venables PH, & Mednick SA. (2002). Spatial but not verbal cognitive deficits at age 3 in persistently antisocial individuals. *Dev Psychopathol, 14*, 25–44.
69. Raine A, Moffitt TE, Caspi A, Loeber R, Stouthamer-Loeber M, & Lynam, D. (2005). Neurocognitive impairments in boys on the life-course persistent antisocial path. *J Abnorm Psychol, 114*, 38–49.
70. Lezak MD, Howieson DB, Loring DW, Hannay HJ, & Fischer JS. (2004). *Neuropsychol Assess* (4th ed). New York: Oxford University Press.
71. Morgan AB, & Lilienfel SO. (2000). A meta-analytic review of the relationship between antisocial behavior and neuropsychological measures of executive function. *Clin Psychol Rev, 20*, 113–136.

72. Dolan M. (2012). The neuropsychology of prefrontal function in antisocial personality disordered offenders with varying degrees of psychopathy. *Psychol Med, 42*(8), 1715–1725.
73. Dolan M, & Park I. (2002). The neuropsychology of antisocial personality disorder. *Psychol Med, 32*, 417–427.
74. Hancock M, Tapscott JL, & Hoaken PNS. (2012). Role of executive dysfunction in predicting frequency and severity of violence. *Aggress Behav, 36*, 338–349.
75. Stanford MS, Conklin SM, Helfritz LE, & Kockler TR. (2007). P3 amplitude reduction and executive function deficits in men convicted of spousal/partner abuse. *Pers Indiv Differ, 43*, 365–375.
76. Teichner G, Golden CJ, Van Hasselt VB, & Peterson A. (2001). Assessment of cognitive functioning in men who batter. *Int J Neurosci, 111*, 241–253.
77. Schiffer B, & Vonlaufen C. (2011). Executive dysfunctions in pedophilic and nonpedophilic child molesters. *J Sex Med, 8*, 1975–1984.
78. Keilp JG, Gorlyn M, Russell M, Oquendo MA, Burke AK, Harkavy-Friedman J, et al. (2013). Neuropsychological function and suicidal behaviour: Attention control, memory and executive dysfunction in suicide attempt. *Psychol Med, 43*(3), 539–551.
79. Hanlon RE, Rubin LH, Jensen M, & Daoust, S. (2010). Neuropsychological features of indigent murder defendants and death row inmates in relation to homicidal aspects of their crimes. *Arch Clin Neuropsychol, 25*, 1–13.
80. Hanlon RE, Coda JJ, Cobia D, & Rubin LH. (2012). Psychotic domestic murder: Neuropsychological differences between homicidal and nonhomicidal schizophrenic men. *J Fam Viol, 27*, 105–113.
81. Bastert E, Schläfke D, Pein A, Kupke F, & Fegert J. (2012). Mentally challenged patients in a forensic hospital: A feasibility study concerning the executive functions of forensic patients with organic brain disorder, learning disability, or mental retardation. *Int J Law Psychiat, 35*, 207–212.
82. Broomhall L. (2005). Acquired sociopathy: A neuropsychological study of executive dysfunction in violent offenders. *Psychiat Psychol Law, 12*, 367–387.
83. Krakowski MI, & Czobor P. (2012). Executive function predicts response to antiaggression treatment in schizophrenia: A randomized control trial. *J Clin Psychiat, 73*(1), 74-80.
84. Blair RJ, & Frith U. (2000). Neurocognitive explanations of the antisocial personality disorders. *Crim Behav Mental Health, 10*, S66–S81.
85. Dinn WM, & Harris CL. (2000). Neurocognitive function in antisocial personality disorder. *Psychiat Res, 97*, 173–190.
86. Hiatt KD, & Newman JP. (2006). Understanding psychopathy: The cognitive side. In CJ Patrick (Ed.), *Handbook of psychopathy* (pp. 334–352). New York: Guilford Press.
87. Blair KS, Newman C, Mitchell DGV, Richell RA, Leonard A, Morton J, et al. (2006). Differentiating among prefrontal substrates in psychopathy: Neuropsychological test findings. *Neuropsychology, 20*, 153–165.
88. Ishikawa SS, Raine A, Lencz T, Bihrle S, & Lacasse L. (2001). Autonomic stress reactivity and executive functions in successful and unsuccessful criminal psychopaths from the community. *J Abnorm Psychol, 110*, 423–432.
89. Raine A, Laufer WS, Yang Y, Narr KL, Thompson P, & Toga AW. (2012). Increased executive functioning, attention, and cortical thickness in white-collar criminals. *Hum Brain Mapp, 33*, 2932–2940.
90. De Brito SA, Viding E, Kumari V, Blackwood N, & Hodgins S. (2013). Cool and hot executive function impairments in violent offenders with antisocial personality disorder with and without psychopathy. *PLOS One, 8*(6): e65566. doi:10.1371/journal.pone.0065566
91. Moffitt TE, & Henry B. (1989). Neuropsychological assessment of executive functions in self-reported delinquents. *Dev Psychopathol, 1*, 105–118.
92. Cauffman E, Steinberg L, & Piquero AR. (2005). Psychological, neuropsychological and physiological correlates of serious antisocial behavior in adolescence: The role of self-control. *Criminology, 43*(1), 133–176.
93. Kronenberger WG, Mathews VP, Dunn DW, Wang Y, Wood EA, Giauque AL, et al. (2005). Media violence exposure and executive functioning in aggressive and control adolescents. *J Clin Psychol, 61*(6), 725–737.

94. Nigg JT, Glass JM, Wong MM, Poon E, Jester J, Fitzgerald, HE, et al. (2004). Neuropsychological executive functioning in children at elevated risk for alcoholism: Findings in early adolescence. *J Abnorm Psychol, 113*, 302–314.
95. White JL, Moffitt TE, Caspi A, Jeglum D, Needles DJ, & Stouthamer-Loeber M. (1994). Measuring impulsivity and examining its relationship to delinquency. *J Abnorm Psychol, 103*, 192–205.
96. Raine A. (2002b). Biosocial studies of antisocial and violent behavior in children and adults: A review. *J Abnorm Child Psychol, 30*, 311–326.
97. Nestor PG. (1992). Neuropsychological and clinical correlates of murder and other forms of extreme violence in a forensic psychiatric population. *J Nerv Ment Dis, 180*, 418–423.
98. Blair RJR. (2006). The emergence of psychopathy: Implications for the neuropsychological approach to developmental disorders. *Cognition, 101*, 414–442.
99. Séguin JR, Nagin D, Assad JM, & Tremblay R. (2004). Cognitive-neuropsychological function in chronic physical aggression and hyperactivity. *J Abnorm Psychol, 113*, 603–613.
100. Trovillo PV. (1939). A history in lie detection. *J Crim Law Criminol, 29*, 848–881.
101. Iacono WG. (2007). Detection of deception. In JT Cacioppo, LG Tassinary, & GG Berntson (Eds.), *Handbook of psychophysiology* (3rd ed, pp.688–703). Cambridge: Cambridge University Press.
102. Iacono WG, & Patrick C. (2006). Polygraph ('lie detector') testing: Current status and emerging trends. In IB Weiner, & AK Hess (Eds.), *Handbook of forensic psychology* (3rd ed, pp.552–588). Hoboken, NJ: John Wiley & Sons.
103. Ishikawa, S. S., & Raine, A. (2002). Psychophysiological correlates of antisocial behavior: A central control hypothesis. In J. Glicksohn (Ed.), *The neurobiology of criminal behavior 8* (pp. 187–229). Norwell: Kluwer Academic Publishers.
104. Herpertz SC. (2007). Electrophysiology. In AR Felthous, & H Saß (Eds.), *International handbook of psychopathic disorders and the law: Vol. 1* (pp.187–198). Chichester: John Wiley & Sons.
105. Schug, RA, Yang Y, Raine A, Han C, Liu J, & Li L. (2011). Resting EEG deficits in accused murderers with schizophrenia. *Psychiat Res-Neuroim, 194*, 85–94.
106. Bernat EM, Hall JR, Steffen BV, & Patrick CJ. (2007). Violent offending predicts P300 amplitude. *Int J Psychophysiol, 66*, 161–167.
107. Gao, Y. & Raine, A. (2009). P3 event-related potential impairments in antisocial and psychopathic individuals: A meta-analysis. *Biol Psychol, 82*, 199–210.
108. Racer KH, Gilbert TT, Luu P, Felver-Gant J, Abdullaev Y, & Dishion TJ. (2011). Attention network performance and psychopathic symptoms in early adolescence: An ERP Study. *J Abnorm Child Psychol, 39*(7), 1001–1012.
109. Baker E, Shelton KH, Baibazarova E, Hay DF, & van Goozen SH. (2013). Low skin conductance activity in infancy predicts aggression in toddlers 2 years later. *Psychol Sci, 24*(6), 1051–1056.
110. Herpertz SC, Mueller B, Qunaibi M, et al. (2005). Emotional responses in boys with conduct disorder. *Am J Psychiat, 162*, 1100–1107.
111. Schug RA, Raine A, & Wilcox RR. (2007). Psychophysiological and behavioural characteristics of individuals with both antisocial personality disorder and schizophrenia-spectrum personality disorder. *Br J Psychiatry, 191*, 408–414.
112. Lorber MF. (2004). Psychophysiology of aggression, psychopathy, and conduct problems: A meta-analysis. *Psychol Bull, 130*, 531–552.
113. Stanford, MS, Houston RJ, & Barratt ES. (2007). Psychophysiological correlates of psychopathic disorders. In AR Felthous & H Saß (Eds.), *International handbook of psychopathic disorders and the law: Vol. 1* (pp. 83–101). Chichester: John Wiley & Sons.
114. Langleben DD, & Moriarty JC. (2013). Using brain imaging for lie detection: Where science, law, and policy collide. *Psychol Public Pol L, 19*(2), 222–234.
115. McCabe DP. (2011). The influence of fMRI lie detection evidence on juror decision-making. *Behav Sci Law, 29*, 566–577.
116. Sadoff RL, & Dattilio FM. (2011). Criminal responsibility. In EY Drogin, FM Dattilio, RL Sadoff, & TG Gutheil (Eds.), *Handbook of forensic assessment: Psychological and psychiatric perspectives* (pp. 121-144). Hoboken, NJ: John Wiley & Sons, Inc.

117. Yang Y, Raine A, Lencz T, Bihrle S, Lacasse L, & Colletti P. (2005). Prefrontal white matter in pathological liars. *Br J Psychiatry, 187,* 320–325.
118. Yang Y, Raine A, Narr KL, Lencz T, LaCasse L, Colletti P, et al. (2007). Localisation of increased prefrontal white matter in pathological liars. *Br J Psychiatry, 190,* 174–175.
119. Sip KE, Roepstorff A, McGregor W, & Frith CD. (2007). Detecting deception: The scope and limits. *Trends Cog Sci, 12,* 48–53.
119a. Ackerman, MJ. (1999). *Essentials of forensic psychological assessment.* New York: John Wiley & Sons.
120. Yang, Y, Glenn AL, & Raine A. (2008). Brain abnormalities in antisocial individuals: Implications for the law. *Behav Sci Law, 26,* 65–83.
121. Feigenson, N. (2006). Brain imaging and courtroom evidence; on the admissibility and persuasiveness of fMRI. *Int J Law Context, 2,* 233–255.
122. Dwyer RG, & Frierson RL. (2006). The presence of low IQ and mental retardation among murder defendants referred for pretrial evaluation. *J Foren Sci, 51,* 678–682.
123. Berman ME, & Coccaro EF. (1998). Neurobiologic correlates of violence: Relevance to criminal responsibility. *Behav Sci Law, 16,* 303–318.
124. Popma A, & Raine A. (2006). Will future forensic assessment be neurobiologic? *Child Adolesct Psychiat Clin North Am, 15,* 429–444.
125. Connor DF. (2002). *Aggression and antisocial behavior in children and adolescents.* New York: Guilford Press.
126. Moeller FG, & Swann AC. (2007). Pharmacotherapy of clinical aggression in individuals with psychopathic disorders. In AR Felthous, & H Saß (Eds.), *International handbook on psychopathic disorders and the law* (pp. 397–416). Chichester, UK: John Wiley & Sons.
127. Van de Wiel NMH., Van Goozen SMH, Matthys W, Snoek H, & Van Engeland H. (2004). Cortisol and treatment effect in children with disruptive behavior disorders: A preliminary study. *J Am Acad Child Adolesc Psychiatry, 43,* 1011–1018.
128. Fisher PA, Stoolmiller M, Gunnar MR, & Burraston BO. (2007). Effects of a therapeutic intervention for foster preschoolers on diurnal cortisol activity. *Psychoneuroendocrinology, 32,* 892–905.
129. Monastra VJ. (2008). Electroencephalographic feedback in the treatment of ADHD: A model for clinical practice. In VJ Monastra (Ed.), *Unlocking the potential of patients with ADHD: A model for clinical practice* (pp. 147–159). Washington, DC: American Psychological Association.
130. Murray-Close D, Han G, Cicchetti D, Crick NR, & Rogosch FA. (2008). Neuroendocrine regulation and physical and relational aggression: The moderating roles of child maltreatment and gender. *Dev Psychol, 44,* 1160–1176.
131. Olds D, Henderson CRJ, Cole R, Eckenrode J, Kitzman H, Luckey D, et al. (1998). Long-term effects of nurse home visitation on children's criminal and antisocial behavior: 15-year follow-up of a randomized controlled trial. *JAMA, 280,* 1238–1244.
132. Raine A, Mellingen K, Liu JH, Venables PH, & Mednick SA. (2003b). Effects of environmental enrichment at 3–5 years on schizotypal personality and antisocial behavior at ages 17 and 23 years. *Am J Psychiat, 160,* 1627–1635.
133. Schoenthaler SJ, & Bier ID. (2000). The effect of vitamin-mineral supplementation on juvenile delinquency among American schoolchildren: A randomized, doubleblind placebo-controlled trial. *J Altern CompMed, 6,* 19–29.
134. Stevens L, Zhang W, Peck L, Kuczek T, Grevstad N, Mahon A, et al. (2003). EFA supplementation in children with inattention, hyperactivity, and other disruptive behaviors. *Lipids, 38,* 1007–1021.
135. Heilbrun AB. (1990). Differentiation of death-row murderers and life-sentence murderers by antisociality and intelligence measures. *J Persona Assess, 54,* 617–627.
136. Hare RD. (2003). *The Hare psychopathy checklist—revised* (2nd ed). Toronto, ON: Multi-Health Systems.
137. Quinsey VL, Harris GT, Rice ME, & Cormier CA. (1999). *Violent offenders: Appraising and managing risk.* Washington, DC: American Psychological Association.

138. Virkkunen ME, DeJong J, Bartko J, Goodwin FK, & Linnoila M. (1989). Relationship of psychological variables to recidivism in violent offenders and impulsive fire setters. *Arch Gen Psychiatry, 46*, 600–603.
139. Bourget D, & Bradford JMW. (2008). Evidential basis for the assessment and treatment of sex offenders. *Brief Treat Crisis Intervent, 8*, 130–146.

30

How Can the Neuroscience of Memory Inform Our Understanding of Amnesia in Criminal Settings?

Alisa R. Gutman

Forensic psychiatrists are often confronted with issues of memory for criminal behavior. Given the prevalence of claims of crime-related amnesia, the forensic psychiatrist needs to have a basic understanding of our current views on memory systems and circuitry. With this knowledge, one can better apply a critical forensic lens to interviews with individuals who proclaim that they forget their crime. The content described herein is an overview and introduction to several different literatures, as each subtopic could easily be expanded into its own chapter or even textbook.

The neuroscience of memory has advanced to where our understanding of the impact of stress on memory is well understood. In general, stress impairs memory retrieval but enhances the consolidation of memory via action of the sympathetic nervous system and hypothalamic-pituitary-adrenal axis effects on the hippocampus, amygdala, and other memory structures. This chapter presents background to consider how the underlying neuroscience may impact our understanding for claims of crime-related amnesia and how we should integrate this updated understanding of stress and memory into our work in forensic psychiatry.

Crime-Related Amnesia

Claims of amnesia are common in criminal populations, making this a significant subject for consideration by forensic psychiatrists. This summary provides an epidemiological framework for how recent advances in neuroscience can inform our understanding of memory in criminal settings.

As early as 1948, Leitch found that 16 out of 51 individuals (31%) convicted of murder or manslaughter claimed amnesia.[1] In 1955, Guttmacher published that approximately 30% of individuals in his series of 36 individuals convicted of murder claimed amnesia for their crime.[2] Similarly, O'Connell found that 20 of 50 murderers (40%) in his sample claimed total or partial amnesia for their crime at some point. O'Connell went on to compare individuals who did and did not claim amnesia and found that these populations differed in several ways, including intelligence, personality, and precipitating factors to the crime. He found that the group claiming amnesia had lower average intelligence and higher rates of hysterical personality, and more associated factors (intoxication, sexual excitement, rage reaction). He suggests that those of lower intelligence may have a "naïve hope that guilt will not be attached if memory is absent."[3] However, subsequent studies did not find a similar connection between claims of amnesia and intelligence, instead finding generally average intelligence in their study populations.[4,5] Estimates from later samples vary, but confirm that reported partial or total amnesia for criminal offenses is relatively common.[4,6–10] Furthermore, there is an association between level of violence involved in the crime and subsequent claims of amnesia.[6,11]

Some psychiatric diagnoses have been associated with claims of amnesia for criminal activities, including psychosis, alcohol abuse, and personality disorders. Active psychotic disorders are present in some mentally ill individuals who claim amnesia for crimes, which is consistent with the idea that the presence of psychosis can impair attention and other important aspects of memory formation.[6,12,13] Alcohol intoxication and abuse can cause cognitive impairment that disrupts memory formation.[14,15] However, given that alcoholic blackout is a commonly accepted phenomenon, individuals may make false claims for alcohol-related amnesia. For example, Lynch and Bradford found using polygraph that individuals with longer histories of substance abuse were more likely to be truthful in claims of amnesia.[5] This suggests that there are cases in which intoxication is used as an excuse without evidence for physiological amnesia.

Given the traits implicit in psychopathy, it is not surprising that many studies have found a significant correlation between psychopathy and crime-related amnesia. In one study using polygraph as a tool for evaluating the validity of amnesia claims, personality disorders were associated with a higher rate of deception than other psychiatric diagnoses or individuals without major psychiatric diagnoses.[5] In a recent study, Cima and Van Oorsouw found that impulsive and antisocial characteristics of psychopathy were predictive for claims of crime-related amnesia. Further, they noted that offenders who claimed amnesia exhibit a greater tendency to malinger amnesia as well as general psychiatric symptoms.[16]

Some authors use the epidemiology and relatively high prevalence of crime-related amnesia as evidence for its validity. In their analysis of life sentenced prisoners, Pyszora et al. suggest that, "Amnesia in the context of these crimes of passion is almost invariably psychogenic in origin.... It is likely to have been caused either by dissociation or impaired memory encoding at the time of the offence (secondary to intense emotional arousal) or as a result of suppression/repression of the painful memory and/or avoidance of rehearsal, resulting in a failure of memory retrieval."[8] In contrast, Cima and colleagues call for a more skeptical approach to these amnesia claims, highlighting in their study that 53% of their sample failed a screen for malingering. In their sample, they found that individuals with reported crime-related amnesia were older than controls, had more prior convictions, and higher rates of substance abuse.[4]

Of particular importance in interpretation of crime-related amnesia is a recent study by Woodworth and colleagues in which they compared memory in the same individuals for homicide, non-homicidal violence, and positive life experiences. They found that individuals reported higher rates of amnesia for homicide (32.7%) as compared with non-homicidal violence (11.5%), or positive life events (13.5%). However, subjective and objective ratings of these same individuals' narratives indicated that memories for homicide were superior. In fact, homicide narratives were, on average, more than three times more detailed than the other memories assessed. The authors conclude that this may represent a failure of "meta-memory" in which people believe their memories are worse for these stressful events when, in fact, their memories are actually better.[11]

Memory Basics

Before describing how stress impacts learning and memory, it is necessary to give an overview of our current understanding of basic memory processes. Early theories for memory predicted that repetition of information has an important role in memory formation. Muller and Pilzecker are credited with introducing the concept of memory consolidation in their 1900 monograph "Experimentelle Beiträge zur Lehre vom Gedächtnis" (Experimental Contributions to the Science of Memory).[17] Taking from their memory studies using paired syllables, they observed that their subjects had a tendency to repeat syllables in their mind between tests. They suggested that "the perseverative tendencies of syllables... might also serve to consolidate the associations between these syllables." Further, they noted that disruption of this repetition by distraction or new learning interfered with later ability to recall the information.[18]

A series of mid-century studies in cognitive science supported this idea that memories are vulnerable in proximity to initial learning.[19] Amnesia can be induced with post-learning manipulations such as electroconvulsive shock[20] or protein synthesis inhibitors.[21] Further, performance on memory tasks is impaired with exposure to competitive learning.[22] In contrast, retention can be enhanced with post-learning treatments.[23,24]

Hebb's dual-trace memory theory postulated that new memories are stabilized by recurrent neural activity of the network representing the new experience.[25] His theory is commonly referenced as the idea that "neurons that fire together, wire together." Decades of neuroscience research have clarified the processes involved in synaptic consolidation of memories. The basic memory trace from an electrophysiological standpoint is termed long term potentiation (LTP). Long term potentiation was discovered in by Terje Lømo in 1966 while doing his doctoral work in Per Anderson's lab in Oslo.[26] Although it took many years for the scientific community to understand the significance of their findings, Lømo, Anderson, and Tim Bliss published the first manuscript documenting the process wherein they presented the idea that frequency potentiation in the hippocampus may be related to learning processes.[27] These findings confirmed Hebb's earlier learning model predicting that timing is an essential component of the neuronal trace for learning.

Studies examining biological mechanisms underlying LTP identified that neurotransmission via NMDA (*N*-methyl-D-aspartate) glutamate receptors is necessary for learning. An NMDA receptor antagonist, R-2-amino-5-phosphonopentanoate (D-AP5), was found to block the formation of LTP in hippocampal slices without impacting normal synaptic transmission.[28] This finding spurred 30 years of exploration into how NMDA receptors function and how this relates to memory encoding.[29] *N*-methyl-D-aspartate receptors are both ligand-gated and voltage-dependent. They act as coincidence detectors, requiring both glutamate and depolarization from another source to open and flux calcium and other cations.

In terms of definitions for the phases of memory, acquisition refers to the initial time period in which information is presented and registered for later recall. *Consolidation* is a term used multiply, but generally referencing the time period between acquisition and recall during which the memory trace is transferred from present information to information that can later be accessed as a memory. Herein, consolidation will refer to the process wherein synaptic changes lead to a memory of the event; sometimes called *encoding*, and follows the acquisition phase of whatever memory test is used. Memory tests with human subjects typically assess semantic memory, or concept-based knowledge, as this is easier to test in a laboratory setting than other types of memory.

Reconsolidation of Memory

In reviewing the current status of the neuroscience of memory systems, it is essential to next consider the phenomena of reconsolidation. Reconsolidation is a process wherein information is made vulnerable when recalled. Although this idea was controversial when reintroduced to the field by Przybyslawski and Sara (1997)[30] and Nader et al. (2000),[31] reconsolidation is now a well-established and important aspect of memory maintenance and potential modification. In fact, the seeds for reconsolidation were present in some of the earliest memory studies and the same basic evidence for consolidation of memories stands true for reconsolidation.[19] Namely, reactivation of memory results in (1) performance impairment with amnestic treatments,[32] (2) performance impairments with new competitive learning,[22] and (3) enhancement by administration of compounds.[33]

Pryzbyslawski and Sara showed that administration of an NMDA antagonist within 2 hours of testing resulted in later amnesia for a learned task in rats. When testing was delayed for 2 hours or more after treatment, there was no effect on later recall.[30] The authors published these findings as support for memory as a dynamic process, in contrast to the prevailing consensus at the time that memory was stable following consolidation.

Nader and colleagues demonstrated that infusion of anisomycin, a protein synthesis inhibitor, into the basolateral amygdala following retrieval of a consolidated fear memory produces amnesia for the memory on later testing. Importantly, they found that anisomycin had no effect on later retrieval without retrieval of the initial memory.[31] Over the last 15 years, this field has expanded and studies have repeatedly confirmed that retrieval of seemingly stable memories results in their entering an unstable state wherein they can be subject to manipulations.[34] Human studies have accumulated confirming that reconsolidation occurs for human memories and has potential implications for treatment of mental disorders such as post traumatic stress disorder and drug addiction.[35,36]

Stress and Memory

Early studies by Bruce McEwen and colleagues demonstrated higher uptake of radioactive glucocorticoid into the hippocampus.[37] Before this finding, studies of Henry Gustav Molaison (HM) had emerged implicating the hippocampus as a key structure for learning and memory in humans and launching decades of work in human cognitive science.[38] Further, animal studies were accumulating that demonstrated a relationship between stress and memory systems.[39] These and other findings cued researchers that stress may affect either the consolidation or expression of memories via glucocorticoid actions in the hippocampus and other brain regions.

Many studies clarifying stress effects on memory in humans employ the Trier Social Stress Test (TSST), which uses performance stress to induce a physiological response in subjects.[40] Making use of the TSST in conjunction with memory testing, researchers have been able to ask questions about how endogenous stress impacts both the consolidation and retrieval of memories. In early studies, both acquisition and testing for memory occurred after stress or glucocorticoid exposure, thereby limiting potential conclusions. In these studies, there was a strong inverse correlation between cortisol response and declarative memory for a word list. Administration of cortisol before learning led to the same memory impairment, suggesting endogenous release of cortisol was the causal factor in the observed stress-related memory deficit.[41] Similarly, in studies wherein items were learned before stress exposure, subjects exhibited poorer memory following stress exposure.[42,43] However, the timing between learning and stress exposure did not allow for conclusions about whether the observed stress effects were on memory formation or retrieval.

Later studies sought to disentangle the impact of stress and cortisol on memory formation and memory retrieval in order to develop a more nuanced understanding of the systems involved. Studies using a longer delay between learning and stress induction in rats clarified that poor memory recall in these studies is actually caused by an impairment in memory retrieval and not caused by an effect on the integrity of the initial memory.[44] Similar results were found in humans, with cortisone treatment resulting in impairment of retrieval for a word list but not affecting acquisition or consolidation of the memory.[45]

Kuhlmann et al. found that psychosocial stress exposure with the TSST led to impairment of memory retrieval in humans. This deficit was found for emotionally arousing words regardless of valence and no effect was observed for neutral words.[46]

In animal studies, these retrieval deficits are mediated by glucocorticoid receptors in the hippocampus and the effects are dependent on an intact basolateral amygdala.[47]

Given that, from an evolutionary standpoint, acute stress systems are designed for adaptive purposes, it would make far better biological sense for stress to facilitate memory for important events rather than to impair memory formation. It would be, for example, quite important to remember the events and circumstances surrounding where and in what circumstances a wild animal chased you. This is indeed the case, and in contrast to stress effects on memory retrieval, an extensive literature demonstrates that glucocorticoids actually enhance the acquisition and consolidation of memories.[48,49]

Buchanan and Lovallo found that cortisol administration to humans before incidental learning of pictures led to enhanced recall for more emotionally arousing (more salient) pictures.[50] In another study, stress-induced increases in cortisol prompted after slide presentation led to enhanced memory for emotionally arousing slides but did not affect memory for neutral slides.[51] Kuhlman and Wolf administered cortisol before viewing emotionally arousing or neutral pictures and found that cortisol treatment enhanced memory for emotionally charged pictures at the expense of neutral pictures. Interestingly, the cortisol and placebo groups did not differ on immediate recall, supporting the notion that cortisol impacts memory consolidation processes that occur after initial acquisition and even recall of information.[52] Notably, other studies have found glucocorticoid enhancement of memory consolidation independent of salience,[53,54] and even impairment of memory consolidation.

Maheu and colleagues looked at differential effects of propranolol (a beta-adrenergic blocker) and metyrapone (a corticosteroid synthesis inhibitor) on memory for neutral stories viewed after administration of the TSST. They found that propranolol treatment did not affect short- or long-term memory of the story, but metyrapone treatment impaired short-term memory for the story. They take these findings to suggest that the corticosteroid system plays a role in declarative memory after stress induction in humans.[55]

Taken in concert, these findings support a relationship between stress and arousal in memory consolidation, thereby suggesting that both stressful circumstances and salient content are important factors in how well information is encoded and maintained. This is further supported by literature showing a time-dependent relationship between norepinephrine and glucocorticoids in memory encoding.[56] Our basic stress response includes a rapid response from the sympathetic nervous system via epinephrine and norepinephrine and a slower response from the hypothalamic-pituitary-adrenal axis via glucocorticoids. Synthesizing data from his lab and others, Roozendaal has suggested a model wherein norepinephrine-dependent hypervigilance synergizes with the corticosteroid response, resulting in enhanced memory formation for stressful events.[56]

In addition to the important behavioral findings described in the preceding, molecular biology studies over the past decade have taken steps to identify the basic processes underlying these behavioral findings. For example, a series of elegant studies from Johannes Reul and colleagues has identified a rapid non-genomic mechanism wherein glucocorticoids facilitate signaling of the ERK-MAPK (extracellular signal-related kinases, mitogen-activated protein kinases) signaling pathway via glucocorticoid receptors. This leads to downstream effects on nuclear kinases MSK1 (mitogen- and stress-activated protein kinase) and Elk-1 in dentate gyrus granule neurons. These and other molecular mechanisms are critical for consolidation of memory.[57]

Implications for Forensic Psychiatry

How can we now reconcile the crime-related amnesia literature with the neuroscience of how stress impacts memory formation and retrieval?

Given our current understanding of stress and memory, it seems likely that a significant portion of crime-related amnesia claims can be explained either by retrieval deficits caused by stressful interviewing conditions or by frank malingering of amnesia with the hope of somehow reducing criminal responsibility. The notion, albeit popular, that the stressful nature of some crimes results in a deficit in memory encoding is highly unlikely given our current understanding that stress enhances memory consolidation. This type of amnesia, wherein circumstances surrounding a crime are forgotten, is more likely psychogenic in nature, and would fall under the category of dissociative amnesia in our current rubric.

Our present understanding of dissociative amnesia is largely phenomenological. Dissociative disorders are defined in DSM 5 as "a disruption of and/or discontinuity in the normal integration of consciousness, memory, identity, emotion, perception, body representation, motor control, and behavior." A diagnosis of dissociative amnesia requires that the inability to recall particular autobiographical information is "inconsistent with ordinary forgetting."[58] Functional neuroimaging of individuals with psychogenic memory impairment has identified disruption in anatomical regions important for memory.[59,60] Further research is necessary to better understand the neuroscientific underpinnings of dissociation and how it may relate to one's ability to access memory systems.[61]

It is certainly plausible that some individuals have psychological reasons for not wanting to access their memory for a crime. In his 1960 case series, O'Connell discusses differences in "hysterical" and malingered amnesia, offering that the consensus at the time was that differences in these phenomena were "one of degree rather than of kind." He goes on to point out that "the issue, so far as responsibility is concerned, is largely of academic interest."[3] We are still debating these same academic issues today and seem no closer to an understanding of how volition plays a role in claims of forgetting for such crimes.

Importantly, despite defendants' apparent hopes that amnesia will somehow diminish responsibility for an offense, the legal question of culpability does not rest on an individual's memory of the event. Unless amnesia is associated with legal insanity, such as may be the case with psychosis, forgetting in the present does not give any information as to an individual's state of mind at the time of the offense. In fact, amnesia in the present has the inherent consequence of impeding a potential insanity defense by making it impossible for an evaluator to comment on someone's reasoning and any other elements of the legal standard for insanity in a given jurisdiction.

This is not to suggest that claims for amnesia are never valid. There are certainly situations in which amnesia claims can be substantiated by further investigation. Alcohol intoxication, for instance, can lead to a well-accepted impairment of either memory formation or later ability to retrieve memories. Furthermore, the presence of structural or functional brain disorders can impair memory acquisition or consolidation and could therefore result in true amnesia. Without such structural impairments in memory acquisition or retrieval, we are left with either dissociative amnesia or malingering. The argument put forth here is that anatomical abnormalities are uncommon and, in fact, exceedingly rare in criminal settings, whereas malingering is common in individuals with antisocial traits.

These conclusions lead us to the important question of how one should proceed with an evaluation and opinion when claims of amnesia are made. Taken together, the crime-related amnesia and stress and memory research call for a high suspicion for either malingering or other alternative explanations to claims of amnesia. As always, evaluators should assess records and other collateral information for evidence of a neurological basis for memory impairment or intoxication sufficient to cause blackout. Without evidence for a medically valid reason for amnesia for an event, it is recommended to use formal testing for malingering as needed for an appropriate forensic assessment.

With regard to reconsolidation, it is essential for psychiatrists today to understand that memory systems are complex and, at times, more fluid than commonly thought. This touches on adjacent literatures in eyewitness testimony and false confessions that speak to what cognitive neuroscientists and psychotherapists have long understood: Human narratives can change over time. This leaves the ultimate issue as to how to execute the best clinical interview possible when confronted with a report of amnesia. As is always best practice in forensics, one should remain skeptical and consider alternative explanations before taking an amnesia claim at face value.

References

1. Leitch A. (1948). Notes on amnesia in crime for the general practitioner. *Med Press, 219*(21), 459–463.
2. Guttmacher MS. (1955). *Psychiatry and the law.* New York: Grune & Stratton.
3. O'Connell BA. (1960). Amnesia and homicide. *Br J Delinquency, 10*(4), 262–276.
4. Cima M, Nijman H, Merckelbach H, Kremer K, & Hollnack S. (2004). Claims of crime-related amnesia in forensic patients. *Int J Psychiatry, 27*(3), 215–221.
5. Lynch BE, & Bradford JM. (1980). Amnesia: Its detection by psychophysiological measures. *Bull Amer Acad Psychiatry Law, 8*(3), 288–297.
6. Taylor PJ, & Kopelman MD. (1984). Amnesia for criminal offences. *Psychol Med, 14*(3), 581–588.
7. Guojonsson GH, Petursson H, Skulason S, & Siguroardottir H. (1989). Psychiatric evidence: A study of psychological issues. *Acta Psychiatrica Scand, 80*(2), 165–169.
8. Pyszora NMB, & Kopelman MD. (2003). Amnesia for criminal offences: A study of life sentence prisoners. *J Forens Psychiatry Psychol, 14*(3), 475–490.
9. Bourget D, & Whitehurst L. (2007). Amnesia and crime. *J Amer Acad Psychiatry Law, 35*(4), 469–480.
10. Evans C, Mezey G, & Ehlers A. (2009). Amnesia for violent crime among young offenders. *J Forens Psychiatry Psychol, 20*(1), 85–106.
11. Woodworth M, Porter S, Ten Brinke L, Doucette NL, Peace K, & Campbell MA. (2009). A comparison of memory for homicide, non-homicidal violence, and positive life experiences. *Int J Psychiatry, 32*(5), 329–334.
12. Mafullul YM, Ogunlesi OA, & Sijuwola OA. (2001). Psychiatric aspects of criminal homicide in Nigeria. *East Afr Med J, 78*(1), 35–39.
13. Bourget D, & Gagne P. (2005). Paternal filicide in Quebec. *J Amer Acad Psychiatry Law, 33*(3), 354–360.

14. Zahr NM, Kaufman KL, Harper CG. (2011). Clinical and pathological features of alcohol-related brain damage. *Nat Rev Neurol, 7*(5), 284–294.
15. Lee H, Roh S, & Kim DJ. (2009). Alcohol-induced blackout. *Intl J Environ Res Public Health, 6*(11), 2783–2792.
16. Cima M, & Van Oorsouw K. (2013). The relationship between psychopathy and crime-related amnesia. *Int J Psychiatry, 36*(1), 23–29.
17. Müller GEPA. Experimentelle Beiträge zur Lehre vom Gedächtnis. (1990). *Leipzig: Zeitschrift für Psychologie und Physiologie der Sinnesorgane. Ergänzungsband*, 1, 1–300.
18. Lechner HA, Squire LR, & Byrne JH. (1999). 100 years of consolidation—remembering Muller and Pilzecker. *Learn Mem, 6*(2), 77–87.
19. Hardt O, Einarsson EO, & Nader K. (2010). A bridge over troubled water: Reconsolidation as a link between cognitive and neuroscientific memory research traditions. *Annu Rev Psychol, 61*, 141–167.
20. Duncan CP. (1949). The retroactive effect of electroshock on learning. *J Comp Phyysiol Psychol, 42*(1), 32–44.
21. Flexner LB, Flexner JB, Roberts RB, & Delahaba G. (1964). Loss of recent memory in mice as related to regional inhibition of cerebral protein synthesis. *Proc Natl Acad Sci USA, 52*, 1165–1169.
22. Gordon WC, & Spear NE. (1973). Effect of reactivation of a previously acquired memory on the interaction between memories in the rat. *J Exp Psychol, 99*(3), 349–355.
23. Krivanek J, & Hunt E. (1967). The effects of posttrial injections of pentylenetetrazole, strychnine and mephenesin on discrimination learning. *Psychopharmacologia, 10*(3), 189–195.
24. McGaugh JL, & Krivanek JA. (1970). Strychnine effects on discrimination learning in mice: Effects of dose and time of administration. *Physiol Behav, 5*(12), 1437–1442.
25. Hebb DO. (1949). *The organization of behavior: A neuropsychological theory*. New York: Wiley.
26. Lomo T. (2003). The discovery of long-term potentiation. *Philosph Trans R Soc London Biol Sci, 358*(1432), 617–620.
27. Bliss TV, & Lomo T. (1973). Long-lasting potentiation of synaptic transmission in the dentate area of the anaesthetized rabbit following stimulation of the perforant path. *J Physiol, 232*(2), 331–356.
28. Collingridge GL, Kehl SJ, & McLennan H. (1983). Excitatory amino acids in synaptic transmission in the Schaffer collateral-commissural pathway of the rat hippocampus. *J Physiol, 334*, 33–46.
29. Morris RG. (2013). NMDA receptors and memory encoding. *Neuropharmacology. 74*, 32–40.
30. Przybyslawski J, & Sara SJ. (1997). Reconsolidation of memory after its reactivation. *Behav Brain Res, 84*(1–2), 241–246.
31. Nader K, Schafe GE, & Le Doux JE. (2000). Fear memories require protein synthesis in the amygdala for reconsolidation after retrieval. *Nature, 406*(6797), 722–726.
32. Misanin JR, Miller RR, & Lewis DJ. (1968). Retrograde amnesia produced by electroconvulsive shock after reactivation of a consolidated memory trace. *Science, 160*(3827), 554–555.
33. Gordon WC. (1977). Susceptibility of a reactivated memory to the effects of strychnine: A time-dependent phenomenon. *Physiol Behav, 18*(1), 95–99.
34. Besnard A, Caboche J, & Laroche S. (2012). Reconsolidation of memory: A decade of debate. *Progr Neurobiol*, 99(1), 61–80.
35. Parsons RG, & Ressler KJ. (2013). Implications of memory modulation for post-traumatic stress and fear disorders. *Nat Neurosci, 16*(2), 146–153.
36. Schwabe L, Nader K, & Pruessner JC. (2014). Reconsolidation of human memory: Brain mechanisms and clinical relevance. *Biol Psychiatry, 76*(4), 274–280.
37. McEwen BS, Weiss JM, & Schwartz LS. (1968). Selective retention of corticosterone by limbic structures in rat brain. *Nature, 220*(5170), 911–912.
38. Scoville WB, & Milner B. (1957). Loss of recent memory after bilateral hippocampal lesions. *J Neurol, Neurosurg, Psychiatry, 20*(1), 11–21.
39. McEwen BS, & Sapolsky RM. (1995). Stress and cognitive function. *Curr Opin Neurobiol, 5*(2), 205–216.
40. Kirschbaum C, Pirke KM, & Hellhammer DH. (1993). The 'Trier Social Stress Test'—A tool for investigating psychobiological stress responses in a laboratory setting. *Neuropsychobiology, 28*(1–2), 76–81.

41. Kirschbaum C, Wolf OT, May M, Wippich W, & Hellhammer DH. (1996). Stress- and treatment-induced elevations of cortisol levels associated with impaired declarative memory in healthy adults. *Life Sci, 58*(17), 1475–1483.
42. Lupien SJ, Gaudreau S, Tchiteya BM, et al. (1997). Stress-induced declarative memory impairment in healthy elderly subjects: Relationship to cortisol reactivity. *J Clin Endocrinol Metab, 82*(7), 2070–2075.
43. Wolf OT, Kudielka BM, Hellhammer DH, Hellhammer J, & Kirschbaum C. (1998). Opposing effects of DHEA replacement in elderly subjects on declarative memory and attention after exposure to a laboratory stressor. *Psychoneuroendocrinology, 23*(6), 617–629.
44. de Quervain DJ, Roozendaal B, & McGaugh JL. (1998). Stress and glucocorticoids impair retrieval of long-term spatial memory. *Nature, 394*(6695), 787–790.
45. de Quervain DJ, Roozendaal B, Nitsch RM, McGaugh JL, & Hock C. (2000). Acute cortisone administration impairs retrieval of long-term declarative memory in humans. *Nat Neurosci, 3*(4), 313–314.
46. Kuhlmann S, Piel M, & Wolf OT. (2005). Impaired memory retrieval after psychosocial stress in healthy young men. *J Neurosci, 25*(11), 2977–2982.
47. Roozendaal B, Griffith QK, Buranday J, De Quervain DJ, & McGaugh JL. (2003). The hippocampus mediates glucocorticoid-induced impairment of spatial memory retrieval: Dependence on the basolateral amygdala. *Proc Natl Acad Sci USA, 100*(3), 1328–1333.
48. Wolf OT. (2009). Stress and memory in humans: Twelve years of progress? *Brain Res, 1293*, 142–154.
49. Diamond DM, Campbell AM, Park CR, Halonen J, & Zoladz PR. (2007). The temporal dynamics model of emotional memory processing: A synthesis on the neurobiological basis of stress-induced amnesia, flashbulb and traumatic memories, and the Yerkes-Dodson law. *Neural Plast*, 60803.
50. Buchanan TW, & Lovallo WR. (2001). Enhanced memory for emotional material following stress-level cortisol treatment in humans. *Psychoneuroendocrinology, 26*(3), 307–317.
51. Cahill L, Gorski L, & Le K. (2003). Enhanced human memory consolidation with post-learning stress: interaction with the degree of arousal at encoding. *Learn Mem, 10*(4), 270–274.
52. Kuhlmann S, & Wolf OT. (2006). Arousal and cortisol interact in modulating memory consolidation in healthy young men. *Behav Neurosci, 120*(1), 217–223.
53. Abercrombie HC, Kalin NH, Thurow ME, Rosenkranz MA, & Davidson RJ. (2003). Cortisol variation in humans affects memory for emotionally laden and neutral information. *Behav Neurosci, 117*(3), 505–516.
54. Maheu FS, Joober R, Beaulieu S, & Lupien SJ. (2004). Differential effects of adrenergic and corticosteroid hormonal systems on human short—and long-term declarative memory for emotionally arousing material. *Behav Neurosci, 118*(2), 420–428.
55. Maheu FS, Joober R, & Lupien SJ. (2005). Declarative memory after stress in humans: Differential involvement of the beta-adrenergic and corticosteroid systems. *J Clin Endocrinol Metab, 90*(3), 1697–1704.
56. Joels M, Fernandez G, & Roozendaal B. (2011). Stress and emotional memory: A matter of timing. *Trends Cogn Sci, 15*(6), 280–288.
57. Reul JM. (2014). Making memories of stressful events: A journey along epigenetic, gene transcription, and signaling pathways. *Frontiers Psychiatry, 5*, 5.
58. American Psychiatric Association. DSM-5 Task Force. (2013). *DSM V* (5th ed.). Washington, DC: American Psychiatric Association.
59. Arzy S, Collette S, Wissmeyer M, Lazeyras F, Kaplan PW, & Blanke O. (2011). Psychogenic amnesia and self-identity: A multimodal functional investigation. *Eur J Neurol, 18*(12), 1422–1425.
60. Markowitsch HJ. (1999). Functional neuroimaging correlates of functional amnesia. *Memory, 7*(5–6), 561–583.
61. Spiegel D, Loewenstein RJ, Lewis-Fernandez R, et al. (2011). Dissociative disorders in DSM-5. *Depression Anxiety, 28*(9), 824–852.

31

Indispensable Forensic Psychiatry and Psychology

The (Non) Challenge from Neuroscience

Stephen J. Morse

In a 2002 editorial published in *The Economist*, the following warning was given: "Genetics may yet threaten privacy, kill autonomy, make society homogeneous and gut the concept of human nature. But neuroscience could do all of these things first."[1] But neither genetics nor any other science that was predicted to revolutionize the law, including behavioral psychology, sociology, and psychodynamic psychology, to name but a few, has had this effect. This will also be true of neuroscience, which is simply the newest science on the block. Neuroscience is not going to do the terrible things *The Economist* fears, at least not in the foreseeable future. Neuroscience has many things to say, but not nearly as much as people who want to change the legal system would hope, especially in relation to criminal law. At most, in the near to intermediate term neuroscience may make modest contributions to legal policy and case adjudication. Nonetheless, there has been irrational exuberance about the potential contribution of neuroscience, an issue I have addressed previously and referred to as *brain overclaim syndrome*.[2]

The central thesis of this chapter is that forensic psychiatry and psychology (hereinafter FP for convenience) will remain indispensable contributors to criminal (and civil) law for the foreseeable future despite any likely advances from neuroscience or any other science. The reason is straightforward. The criminal law's criteria for responsibility and competence are acts and mental states and the law's model of the person is folk psychological, a being that can potentially be guided by reason and thus for whom mental states do play a partial causal explanatory role. Even when most relying on a scientific data base, FP is also resolutely folk psychological because it attempts to shed light on the subjects' acts and mental states. Even the most resolutely biologically oriented FP will have to translate its biological or other scientific data into the law's folk psychological criteria. A neuroscientist or geneticist, for example, cannot do this directly. At most, he or she can provide useful data. It is the FP that must explain the meaning of such data and clinical findings. As Phllip Resnick says generally about the work of the FP, "You need to understand why. And you can't see why on an fMRI."[3]

This chapter first addresses the law's motivation and the motivation of some advocates to turn to science to solve the very hard normative problems that law addresses. Next it discusses the law's psychology and its concepts of the person and responsibility. Then it considers the general relation of neuroscience to law, which I characterize as the issue of "translation." The following part canvasses various distractions that have bedeviled clear thinking about the relation of scientific, causal accounts of behavior to responsibility. Next, it examines the limits of neurolaw[4] and considers why neurolaw does not pose a genuinely radical challenge to the law's concepts of the person and responsibility. The penultimate part makes a case for cautious optimism about the contribution that neuroscience may make to law in the near and intermediate term. A brief conclusion follows. Throughout, I use the criminal law for my examples because the relation of neuroscience to criminal law, especially criminal responsibility, has most captured the public and legal imagination.

The Source of NeuroExuberance

Everyone understands that legal issues are normative, addressing how we should regulate our lives in a complex society. How do we live together? What are the duties we owe each other? For violations of those duties, when is the state justified in imposing the most afflictive—but sometimes justified—exercises of state power, criminal blame, and punishment?[5] When should we do this, to whom, and how much?

Virtually every legal issue is contested—consider criminal responsibility, for example—and there is always room for debate about policy, doctrine, and adjudication. In a recent book, Professor Robin Feldman has argued that law lacks the courage forthrightly to address the difficult normative issues that it faces.[6] The law therefore adopts what Feldman terms an "internalizing" and an "externalizing" strategy for using science to try to avoid the difficulties. In the internalizing strategy, the law adopts scientific criteria as legal criteria. A futuristic example might be using neural criteria for criminal responsibility. In the externalizing strategy, the law turns to scientific or clinical experts to make the decision. An example would be using forensic clinicians to decide whether a criminal defendant is competent to stand trial and then simply rubberstamping the clinician's opinion. Neither strategy is successful because each avoids facing the hard questions and impedes legal evolution and progress. Professor Feldman concludes, and I agree, that the law does not err by using science too little, as is commonly claimed. Rather, it errs by using it too much because the law is too insecure about its resources and capacities to do justice.

A fascinating question is why so many enthusiasts seem to have extravagant expectations about the contribution of neuroscience to law, especially criminal law. Here is my speculation about the source. Many people intensely dislike the concept and practice of retributive justice, thinking that they are prescientific and harsh. Their hope is that the new neuroscience will convince the law at last that determinism is true, no offender is genuinely responsible, and the only logical conclusion is that the law should adopt a consequentially based prediction/prevention system of social control guided by the knowledge of the neuroscientist-kings who will finally have supplanted the platonic philosopher-kings.[7] On a more modest level, many advocates think that neuroscience may not revolutionize criminal justice, but neuroscience will demonstrate that many more offenders should be excused and do not deserve the harsh punishments imposed by the United States criminal justice system. Four decades ago, our criminal justice system would have been using psychodynamic psychology for the same purpose. More recently, genetics has been employed in a similar manner. The impulse, however, is clear: jettison desert, or at least mitigate judgments of desert. As will be shown, however, these advocates often adopt an untenable theory of mitigation or an excuse that quickly collapses into the nihilistic conclusion that no one is really criminally responsible.

The Law's Psychology, Concept of the Person and Responsibility

Criminal law presupposes a "folk psychological" view of the person and behavior. This psychological theory explains behavior *in part* by mental states such as desires, beliefs, intentions, willings, and plans. Biological and other psychological and sociological variables also play a causal role, but folk psychology considers mental states fundamental to a full causal explanation and understanding of human action. Lawyers, philosophers, and scientists argue about the definitions of mental states and theories of action, but that does not undermine the general claim that mental states are fundamental.[8] Indeed, the arguments and evidence that disputants use to convince others presuppose the folk-psychological view of the person. Brains do not convince each other, people do. Folk psychology presupposes only that human action will at least be rationalizable by mental state explanations or will be responsive to reasons—including incentives—under the right conditions.

For example, the folk-psychological explanation for why you are reading this chapter is, roughly, that you desire to understand the relation of neuroscience to criminal responsibility or to law generally. You believe that reading the chapter will help fulfill that desire, so you formed the intention to read it. This is a practical, rather than a deductive, syllogism. Brief reflection should indicate that the law's psychology must be a folk-psychological theory, a view of the person as a conscious—and potentially self-conscious—creature who forms and acts on intentions that are the product of the person's other mental states. We are the sort of creatures who can act for and respond to reasons. The law treats persons generally as intentional creatures and not simply as mechanistic forces of nature.

Law is primarily action-guiding and is not able to guide people directly and indirectly unless people are capable of using rules as premises in their reasoning about how they should behave. Unless people could be guided by law, it would be useless (and perhaps incoherent) as an action-guiding system of rules. Legal rules are action-guiding primarily because these rules provide an agent with good moral or prudential reasons for forbearance or action. Human behavior can be modified by means other than influencing deliberation, and human beings do not always deliberate before they act. Nonetheless, the law presupposes folk psychology even when we most habitually follow the legal rules. Unless people are capable of understanding and then using legal rules to guide their conduct, the law is powerless to affect human behavior.

The legal view of the person does not hold that people must always reason or consistently behave rationally according to some preordained, normative notion of rationality. Rather, the law's view is that people are capable of acting for reasons and are capable of minimal rationality according to predominantly conventional, socially constructed standards. The type of rationality the law requires is the ordinary person's commonsense view of rationality, not the technical notion that might be acceptable within the disciplines of economics, philosophy, psychology, computer science, and the like.

Virtually everything for which agents deserve to be praised, blamed, rewarded, or punished is the product of mental causation and, in principle, is responsive to reasons, including incentives. Machines may cause harm, but they cannot do wrong, and they cannot violate expectations about how people ought to live together. Machines do not deserve praise, blame, reward, punishment, concern, or respect because they exist or because they cause results that change the world. Only people, intentional agents with the potential to act, can do wrong and violate expectations of what they owe each other.

Many scientists and some philosophers of mind and action might consider folk psychology to be a primitive or prescientific view of human behavior. For the foreseeable future, however, the law will be based on the folk-psychological model of the person and behavior described. Until and unless scientific discoveries convince us that our view of ourselves is radically wrong, the basic explanatory apparatus of folk psychology will remain central. It is vital that FP not lose sight of this model lest we fall into confusion when various claims based on neuroscience are made. If any science is to have appropriate influence on current criminal law and legal decision making, the science must be relevant to and translated into the law's folk-psychological framework.

All of the law's doctrinal criteria for criminal responsibility are folk-psychological. Begin with the definitional criteria, the "elements" of crime. The "voluntary" act requirement is defined, roughly, as an *intentional* bodily movement—or omission in cases in which the person has a duty to act—done in a reasonably integrated state of consciousness. Other than crimes of strict liability, all crimes also require a culpable mental state, such as purpose, knowledge, or recklessness. All affirmative defenses of justification and excuse involve an inquiry into the person's mental state, such as the belief that self-defensive force was necessary or the lack of knowledge of right from wrong.

Our folk-psychological concepts of criminal responsibility follow logically from the action-guiding nature of law itself, from its folk-psychological concept of the person and action, and from the aim of achieving retributive justice, which holds that no one should be punished unless they deserve it and no more than they deserve. The general capacity for rationality is the primary condition for responsibility, and the lack of that capacity is the primary condition for excusing a person. If human beings were not rational creatures who could understand the good reasons for action and were not capable of conforming to legal requirements through intentional action or forbearance, the law could not adequately guide action and would not be just. Legally responsible agents are therefore people who have the general capacity to grasp and be guided by good reason in particular legal contexts.[9]

In cases of excuse, the agent who has done something wrong acts for a reason but is either incapable of rationality generally or incapable on the specific occasion in question. This explains, for example, why young children and some people with mental disorders are not held responsible. The amount of lack of capacity for rationality that is necessary to find the agent not responsible is a moral, social, political and, ultimately, legal issue. It is not a scientific, neuroscientific, medical, psychological, or psychiatric issue.

Compulsion or coercion is also an excusing condition. Literal compulsion exists when the person's bodily movement is a pure mechanism that is not rationalizable by reference to the agent's mental states. These cases defeat the requirement of a "voluntary act." For example, a tremor or spasm produced by a neurological disorder is not an action because it is not intentional and, therefore, defeats the ascription of a voluntary act. Metaphorical compulsion exists when an agent acts intentionally but in response to some hard choice imposed on the agent through no fault of his or her own. For example, if a miscreant holds a gun to an agent's head and threatens to kill her unless she kills another innocent person, it would be wrong to kill under these circumstances. Nevertheless, the law may decide as a normative matter to excuse the act of intentional killing because the agent was motivated by a threat so great that it would be supremely difficult for most citizens to resist. Cases involving internal compulsive states are more difficult to conceptualize because it is difficult to define and assess "loss of control."[10] The cases that most fit this category are "disorders of desire," such as addictions and sexual disorders. The question is why these acting agents lack control, but other people with strong desires do not. If an agent frequently yields to his or her apparently very strong desires at great social, medical, occupational, financial, and legal cost, the agent will often say or observers will infer the agent was "out of control," and an excuse or mitigation is therefore warranted. But why mitigation or excuse should obtain is difficult to understand.

Lost in Translation? Legal Relevance and the Need for Translation

What in principle is the possible relation of neuroscience to law? We must begin with a distinction between internal relevance and external relevance. An internal contribution or critique accepts the general coherence and legitimacy of a set of legal doctrines, practices, or institutions and attempts to explain or alter them. For example, an internal contribution to criminal responsibility may suggest the need for doctrinal reform of, say, the insanity defense, but it would not suggest that the notion of criminal responsibility is itself incoherent or illegitimate. By contrast, an externally relevant critique suggests that the doctrines, practices, or institutions are incoherent, illegitimate, or unjustified. Because a radical, external critique has little possibility of success at present (as is explained in the following),

I make the simplifying assumption that the contributions of neuroscience will be internal and thus will need to be translated into the law's folk-psychological concepts.

The law's criteria for responsibility and competence are essentially behavioral acts and mental states. The criteria of neuroscience are mechanistic–neural structure and function. Is the apparent chasm between those two types of discourse bridgeable? This is a familiar question in the field of mental health law,[11] but there is even greater dissonance in neurolaw. Psychiatry and psychology sometimes treat behavior mechanistically, sometimes treat it folk-psychologically, and sometimes blend the two. In most cases properly understood, FP is quite close to folk psychology in approach. Neuroscience, in contrast, is purely mechanistic and eschews folk-psychological concepts and discourse. Neurons and neural networks do not act intentionally for reasons. They have no sense of past, present, and future, and no aspirations. They do not recognize that they will die. Thus, the gap will be harder to bridge.

The brain does enable the mind (even if we do not know how this occurs). Therefore, facts we learn about brains in general or about a specific brain could in principle provide useful information about mental states and about human capacities in general and in specific cases. Some believe that this conclusion is a category error.[12] This is a plausible view, and perhaps it is correct. If it is, then the whole subject of neurolaw is empty, and there was no point writing this chapter in the first place. Let us therefore bracket this pessimistic view and determine what follows from the more optimistic position that what we learn about the brain and nervous system can be potentially helpful to resolving questions of criminal responsibility if the findings are properly translated into the law's psychological framework.

The question is whether the new neuroscience is legally relevant because it makes a proposition about responsibility or competence more or less likely to be true. Any legal criterion must be established independently, and biological evidence must be translated into the criminal law's folk-psychological criteria. That is, the expert must be able to explain precisely how the neuroevidence bears on whether the agent acted, formed the required *mens rea*, or met the criteria for an excusing condition. In the context of competence evaluations, the expert must explain precisely how the neuroevidence bears on whether the subject was capable of meeting the law's functional criteria. If the evidence is not directly relevant, the expert should be able to explain the chain of inference from the indirect evidence to the law's criteria. At present, as I explain later, few such data exist, but neuroscience is advancing so rapidly that such data may exist in the near or medium term. Moreover, the argument is conceptual and does not depend on any particular neuroscience findings.

Dangerous Distractions Concerning Neuroscience and Criminal Responsibility and Competence

This section considers a number of related issues that are often thought to be relevant to criminal responsibility and competence but that are in fact irrelevant, confusing, and distracting: free will, causation as an excuse, causation as compulsion, prediction as an excuse, dualism, and the nonefficacy of mental states. It is important to correct these errors because much of the unjustified legal exuberance about the contributions of neurolaw flow from them and they incorrectly undermine the relevance and necessity of FP. The legal exuberance also flows, however, from unrealistic expectations about the scientific accomplishments of neuroscience. A later part of this article addresses the scientific exuberance.

Contrary to what many people believe and what judges and others sometimes say, free will is not a legal criterion that is part of any doctrine, and it is not even foundational for criminal responsibility.[13] Criminal law doctrines are fully consistent with the truth of determinism or universal causation that allegedly undermines the foundations of responsibility. Even if determinism is true, some people act and some people do not. Some people form prohibited mental states and some do not. Some people are legally insane or act under duress when they commit crimes, but most defendants are not legally insane or acting under duress. Moreover, these distinctions matter to moral and legal theories of responsibility and fairness that we have reason to endorse. Thus, law addresses problems genuinely related to responsibility, including consciousness, the formation of mental states such as intention and knowledge, the capacity for rationality, and compulsion. And note again that these are all folk psychological. The law, however, never addresses the presence or absence of free will.

When most people use the term *free will* in the context of legal responsibility, they are typically using it loosely as a synonym for the conclusion that the defendant was or was not criminally responsible. They typically have reached this conclusion for reasons that do not involve free will—for example, that the defendant was legally insane or acted under duress—but such use of the term *free will* only perpetuates misunderstanding and confusion. Once the legal criteria for excuse have been met—and no excuse includes lack of free will as a criterion—the defendant will be excused without any reference whatsoever to free will as an independent ground for excuse.

There is a genuine metaphysical problem regarding free will, which is whether human beings have the capacity to act uncaused by anything other than themselves, which is termed *metaphysical libertarianism*, and whether this capacity is a necessary foundation for holding anyone legally or morally accountable for criminal conduct. Philosophers and others have debated these issues in various forms for millennia. The majority of experts on this question are "compatibilists," people who think that responsibility is genuinely possible even if determinism is true.[14] But there is no resolution to the debate in sight. Indeed, some people might think that the problem is insoluble. This is a philosophical issue, but it is not a problem for the law, and neuroscience raises no new challenge to this conclusion. Solving the free will problem would have profound implications for responsibility doctrines and practices, such as blame and punishment, but having or lacking libertarian freedom is not a criterion of any civil or criminal law doctrine.

Neuroscience is simply the most recent, mechanistic causal science that appears deterministically to explain behavior. Neuroscience thus joins social structural variables, behaviorism, genetics, and other scientific explanations that have also been deterministic explanations for behavior. In principle, however, neuroscience adds nothing new, even if neuroscience is a better, more persuasive science than some of its predecessors. No science, including neuroscience, can demonstrate that libertarian free will does or does not exist. As long as free will in the strong sense is not foundational for just blame and punishment and is not a criterion at the doctrinal level—which it is not—the truth of determinism or universal causation poses no threat to legal responsibility. Neuroscience may help shed light on folk-psychological excusing conditions, such as automatism or legal insanity, but the truth of determinism is not an excusing condition. The law will be fundamentally challenged only if neuroscience or any other science can conclusively demonstrate that the law's psychology is wrong, and that we are not the type of creatures for whom mental states are causally effective. This is a different question from whether determinism undermines responsibility, however, and this chapter returns to the more radical challenge later.

A related confusion is that behavior is excused if it is caused, but causation per se is not a legal or moral mitigating or excusing condition. I termed this confusion the "fundamental psycholegal error."[15] At most, causal explanations can only provide evidence concerning whether a genuine excusing condition, such as lack of rational capacity, was present. For example, suppose a life marked by poverty and abuse played a predisposing causal role in a defendant's criminal behavior or that an alleged new mental syndrome played a causal role in explaining criminal conduct. The claim is often made that such causes—for which the agent is not responsible—should be an excusing or mitigating position per se, but this claim is false.

All behavior is the product of the necessary and sufficient causal conditions without which the behavior would not have occurred, including brain causation, which is always part of the causal explanation for any behavior. If causation were an excusing condition per se, then no one would be responsible for any behavior. Some people might welcome such a conclusion and believe that responsibility is impossible, but this is not the legal and moral world we inhabit. The law holds most adults responsible for most of their conduct, and genuine excusing conditions are limited. Thus, unless the person's history or mental condition, for example, provides evidence of an existing excusing or mitigating condition, such as lack of rational capacity, there is no reason for excuse or mitigation.

Even a genuinely abnormal cause is not per se an excusing condition. For example, imagine an armed robber who suffers from intermittent hypomania and who only robs when he is clinically hypomanic because only then does he feel sufficiently energetic and confident. In other words, the hypomania is a "but for" cause of his robberies. Nevertheless, he would not be excused for an armed robbery because hypomania seldom compromises rational capacity sufficiently to warrant an excuse. If he committed an armed robbery under the influence of a delusional belief his mania produced, then he might be excused by reason of legal insanity. In that case, the excusing condition would be compromised rationality and not the mania per se. In short, a neuroscientific causal explanation for criminal conduct, like any other type of causal explanation, does not per se mitigate or excuse. It only provides evidence that might help the law resolve whether a genuine excuse existed, or it may in the future provide data that might be a guide to prophylactic or rehabilitative measures.

Compulsion is a genuine mitigating or excusing condition, but causation—including brain causation—is not the equivalent of compulsion. Compulsion may be either literal or metaphorical and normative. It is crucial to recognize that most human action is not plausibly the result of either type of compulsion, but all human behavior is caused by its necessary and sufficient causes—including brain causation. Even abnormal causes are not necessarily compelling. To illustrate, suppose that a person has weak pedophilic urges and weak sexual urges in general. If this person molested a child there would be no ground for a compulsion excuse. If causation was the equivalent of compulsion, all behavior would be compelled and no one would be responsible. Once again, this is not a plausible account of the law's responsibility conditions. Causal information from neuroscience might help us resolve questions concerning whether legal compulsion existed, or it might be a guide to prophylactic or rehabilitative measures when dealing with plausible legal compulsion. Causation, however, is not per se compulsion.

Causal knowledge, whether from neuroscience or any other science, can enhance the accuracy of behavioral predictions, but predictability is also not a per se excusing or mitigating condition—even if the predictability of the behavior is perfect. To understand this, consider how many things we do that are perfectly predictable but for which there is no plausible excusing or mitigating condition. If the variables that enhance prediction also produce a genuine excusing or mitigating condition, then excuse or mitigation is justified for the latter reason and independent of the prediction.

For example, recent research demonstrates that a history of childhood abuse coupled with a specific, genetically caused enzyme abnormality that produces a neurotransmitter deficit vastly increases the risk that a person will behave antisocially as an adolescent or young adult.[16] Does this mean that an offender with this gene by environment interaction is not responsible or less responsible? No. The offender may not be fully responsible or responsible at all, but not because there is a causal explanation. What is the intermediary excusing or mitigating principle? Are these people, for instance, more impulsive? Are they lacking rationality? What is the actual excusing or mitigating condition?

Again, causation is not compulsion, and predictability is not an excuse. Just because an offender is caused to do something or is predictable does not mean that the offender was compelled to do the crime charged or is otherwise not responsible. Brain causation—or any other kind of causation—does not mean that we are automatons, not really acting agents at all, or otherwise excused.

Most informed people are not "dualists" concerning the relation between the mind and the brain. That is, they no longer think that our minds—or souls—are independent of our brains and bodies more generally and can somehow exert a causal influence over our bodies. It may seem as if law's emphasis on the importance of mental states as causing behavior is based on a prescientific, outmoded form of dualism, but this is not the case. Although the brain enables the mind, we have no idea how this occurs and have no idea how action is possible.[17] It is clear that, at the least, mental states are dependent upon or supervene on brain states, but neither neuroscience nor any other science has demonstrated that mental states do not play an independent and partial causal role.

Despite our lack of understanding of the mind-brain-action relation, some scientists and philosophers question whether mental states have any causal effect, thus treating mental states as "psychic appendixes" that evolution has created but that have no genuine function. These claims are not strawpersons. They are made by serious, thoughtful people.[18] As discussed later, if accepted, they would create a complete and revolutionary paradigm shift in the law of criminal responsibility and competence (and more widely). Thus, this claim is an external critique and must be understood as such. Moreover, given our current state of knowledge, there is little scientific or conceptual reason to accept it.[19]

In conclusion, legal actors concerned with criminal law policy, doctrine, and adjudication must always keep the folk-psychological view present in their minds when considering claims or evidence from neuroscience, and must always question how the science is legally relevant to the law's action and mental states criteria. The truth of determinism, causation, and predictability do not in themselves answer any doctrinal or policy issue. None of these claims cause any reason to doubt the relevance and necessity for FP, which aids courts and legislatures in making the crucial moral distinctions among differing acts and mental states.

The Limits of NeuroLaw: The Present Limits of Neuroscience

Most generally, the relation of brain, mind, and action is one of the hardest problems in all science. Again, we have no idea how the brain enables the mind or how action is possible.[20] The brain-mind-action relation is a mystery. For example, we would like to know the difference between a neuromuscular spasm and intentionally moving one's arm in exactly the same way. The former is a purely mechanical motion, whereas the latter is an action, but we cannot explain the difference between the two. We know that a functioning brain is a necessary condition for having mental states and for acting. After all, if your brain is dead, you have no mental states, are not acting, and indeed are not doing much of anything at all. Still, we do not know how mental states and action are caused.

Despite the astonishing advances in neuroimaging and other neuroscientific methods, we still do not have sophisticated causal knowledge of how the brain works generally and we have little information that is legally relevant. This is unsurprising. The scientific problems are fearsomely difficult. Only in the last 15 years have researchers begun to accumulate much data from functional magnetic resonance imaging (fMRI), which is the technology that has generated most of the legal interest. Moreover, virtually no studies have been performed to address specifically legal questions.

Before turning to the specific reasons for neuromodesty, a few preliminary points of general applicability must be addressed. The first and most important is contained in the previous message. Causation by biological variables, including abnormal biological variables, does not per se create an excusing or mitigating condition. Any excusing condition must be established independently. The goal is always to translate the biological evidence into the criminal law's folk-psychological criteria.

Assessing criminal responsibility involves a retrospective evaluation of the defendant's mental states at the time of the crime. No criminal wears a portable scanner or other neurodetection device that provides a measurement at the time of the crime, at least not yet. Further, neuroscience is insufficiently developed to detect specific, legally relevant mental content or to provide a sufficiently accurate diagnostic marker for even a severe mental disorder.[21] Nonetheless, certain aspects of neural structure and function that bear on legally relevant capacities, such as the capacity for rationality and control, may be temporally stable in general or in individual cases. If they are, neuroevidence may permit a reasonably valid retrospective inference about the defendant's rational and control capacities and their impact on criminal behavior. This will of course depend on the existence of adequate science to do this. We currently lack such science, but future research may provide the necessary data.

Questions concerning competence or predictions of future behavior are based on a subject's present condition. Thus, the problems besetting the retrospective responsibility analysis do not apply to such issues. The criteria for competence are functional. They ask whether the subject can perform some task—such as understanding the nature of a criminal proceeding or understanding a treatment option that is offered—at a level the law considers normatively acceptable to warrant respecting the subject's choice and autonomy.

Now, let us consider the specific grounds for neuromodesty in cognitive, affective, and social neuroscience, the subdisciplines most relevant to law. At present, most neuroscience studies on human beings involve very small numbers of subjects, although this phenomenon is starting to change. Most of the studies have been done on college and university students, who are hardly a random sample of the population generally and of criminal offenders specifically. There is also a serious question of whether findings based on subjects' behavior and brain activity in a scanner would apply to real-world situations (the issue of "ecological validity"). Further, most studies average the neurodata over the subjects, and the average finding may not accurately describe the brain structure or function of any actual subject in the study. Replications are few, which is especially important for law. Policy and adjudication should not be influenced by findings that are insufficiently established, and replications of findings are crucial to our confidence in a result. Finally, the neuroscience of cognition and interpersonal behavior is largely in its infancy and what is known is quite coarse-grained and correlational, rather than fine-grained and causal.[22] What is being investigated is an association between a condition or a task in the scanner and brain activity. These studies do not demonstrate that the brain activity is a sensitive diagnostic marker for the condition or either a necessary, sufficient, or predisposing causal condition for the behavioral task that is being done in the scanner. Any language that suggests otherwise—such as claiming that some brain region is the neural substrate for the behavior—is simply not justifiable based on the methodology of most studies. Moreover, activity in the same region may be associated with diametrically opposite behavioral phenomena—for example, love and hate.

There are also technical and research design difficulties. It takes many mathematical transformations to get from the raw fMRI data to the images of the brain that are increasingly familiar. Explaining these transformations is beyond me, but I do understand that the likelihood that an investigator will find a statistically significant result depends on how the researcher sets the threshold for significance. There is dispute about this, and the threshold levels are conventional. If the threshold changes, so does the outcome. I have been convinced by neuroscience colleagues that many such technical difficulties have largely been solved, but research design and potentially unjustified inferences from the studies are still an acute problem. It is extraordinarily difficult to control for all conceivable artifacts. Consequently, there are often problems of over-inference. Finally, it is also an open question whether accurate inferences or predictions about individuals are possible using group data when that group includes the individual.[23] This is a very controversial topic, but even if it is difficult or impossible now, it may become easier in the future. Over time, however, all these problems may ease as imaging and other techniques become less expensive and more accurate, research designs become more sophisticated, and the sophistication of the science increases generally.

Virtually all neuroscience studies of potential interest to the law involve some behavior that has already been identified as of interest, and the point of the study is to identify that behavior's neural correlates. Neuroscientists do not go on general "fishing" expeditions.[24] There is usually some bit of behavior—such as addiction, schizophrenia, or impulsivity—that investigators would like to understand better by investigating its neural correlates. To do this properly presupposes that the researchers have already identified and validated the behavior under neuroscientific investigation. Thus, neurodata can be no more valid than the behavior with which they are correlated.

On occasion, the neuroscience might suggest that the behavior is not well characterized or is neurally indistinguishable from other, seemingly different behavior. In general, however, the existence of legally relevant behavior will already be apparent before the neuroscientific investigation is begun. For example, some people are grossly out of touch with reality. If, as a result, they do not understand right from wrong, we excuse them because they lack such knowledge. We might learn a great deal about the neural correlates of such psychological abnormalities, but we already knew without neuroscientific data that these abnormalities existed, and we had a firm view of their normative significance. In the future, however, we may learn more about the causal link between the brain and behavior, and studies may be devised that are more directly legally relevant. I suspect that we are unlikely to make substantial progress with neural assessment of legally relevant mental content, but we are likely to learn more about capacities that will bear on excuse or mitigation. Again, however, the neurodata must be genuinely and not rhetorically relevant to the law's folk-psychological criteria.

The criteria for both responsibility and competence are behavioral; therefore, actions speak louder than images. This is a truism for all criminal responsibility and competence assessments. If the finding of any test or measurement of behavior is contradicted by actual behavioral evidence, then we must believe the behavioral evidence because it is more direct and probative of the law's behavioral criteria. For example, if the person behaves rationally in a wide variety of circumstances, the agent is rational even if the brain appears structurally or functionally abnormal. We also confidently knew that some people were behaviorally abnormal—such as being psychotic—long before there were any psychological or neurological tests for such abnormalities.

An analogy from physical medicine may be instructive. Suppose someone complains about back pain, a subjective symptom, and the question is whether the subject actually does have back pain. We know that many people with abnormal spines do not experience back pain, and many people who complain of back pain have normal spines. If the person is claiming a disability and the spine looks dreadful, evidence that the person regularly exercises on a trampoline without difficulty indicates that there is no disability caused by back pain. If there is reason to suspect malingering, however, and there is not clear behavioral evidence of lack of pain, then a completely normal spine might be of use in deciding whether the claimant is malingering. Unless the correlation between the image and the legally relevant behavior is very powerful, however, such evidence will be of limited help.

If actions speak louder than images, however, what room is there for introducing neuroevidence in legal cases? Is FP completely immune to neuroscientific findings? Let us begin with cases in which the behavioral evidence is clear and permits an equally clear inference about the defendant's mental state. For example, lay people may not know the technical term to apply to people who are manifestly out of touch with reality, but they will readily recognize this unfortunate condition. No further tests of any sort will be necessary to prove that the subject suffers from seriously impaired rationality. In such cases, neuroevidence will be at most convergent and increase our confidence in what we already had confidently concluded. Determining if it is worth collecting the neuroevidence will depend on whether the cost-benefit analysis justifies obtaining convergent evidence.

Roper v. Simmons is the most striking example of a case in which the behavioral evidence was clear.[25] In *Roper* the United States Supreme Court categorically excluded the death penalty for capital murderers who killed when they were 16 or 17 years old on the grounds that adolescents do not deserve the death penalty.[26] The amicus briefs were replete with neuroscience data showing that the brains of late adolescents are not fully biologically mature, and advocates used these data to suggest that adolescent killers could not fairly be put to death.[27] Now, we already knew from commonsense observation and from rigorous behavioral studies that juveniles are on average less rational than adults. What did the neuroscientific evidence about the juvenile brain add? It was consistent with the undeniable behavioral data and perhaps provided a partial causal explanation of the behavioral differences. The neuroscience data were therefore merely additive and only indirectly relevant, and the Supreme Court did not cite them, except perhaps by implication when it referred vaguely to "other" scientific evidence.[28]

Whether adolescents are sufficiently less rational on average than adults to exclude them categorically from the death penalty is a normative legal question and not a scientific or psychological question. Advocates claimed, however, that the neuroscience confirmed that adolescents are insufficiently responsible to be executed,[29] thus confusing the positive and the normative. The neuroscience evidence in no way independently confirms that adolescents are less responsible. If the behavioral differences between adolescents and adults were slight, it would not matter if their brains were quite different. Similarly, if the behavioral differences were sufficient for moral and constitutional differential treatment, then it would not matter if the brains were essentially indistinguishable.

If the behavioral data are not clear, then the potential contribution of neuroscience is large. Unfortunately, it is in just such cases that neuroscience at present is not likely to be of much help. I term the reason for this the "clear cut" problem.[30] Recall that neuroscientific studies usually start with clear cases of well-characterized behavior. In such cases, the neural markers might be quite sensitive to the already clearly identified behaviors precisely because the behavior is so clear. Less clear behavior is simply not studied, or the overlap in data about less clear behavior is greater between experimental and control subjects. Thus, the neural markers of clear cases will provide little guidance to resolve behaviorally ambiguous cases of legally relevant behavior and they are unnecessary if the behavior is sufficiently clear.

For example, suppose that in an insanity defense case the question is whether the defendant suffers from a major mental disorder, such as schizophrenia. In extreme cases, the behavior will be clear, and no neurodata will be necessary. Investigators have discovered various small but statistically significant differences in neural structure or function between people who are clearly suffering from schizophrenia and those who are not.[31] Nonetheless, in a behaviorally unclear case, the overlap between data on the brains of people with schizophrenia and people without the disorder are so great that a scan is insufficiently sensitive to be used for diagnostic purposes. In short, at present, in those cases in which the neuroscience would be most helpful, it has little to contribute. Again, this situation may change if neural markers become more diagnostically sensitive for legally relevant criteria.

Some people think that executive capacity—the congeries of cognitive and emotional capacities that help to plan and regulate human behavior—is going to be the Holy Grail to help the law determine an offender's true culpability. After all, there is an attractive moral case that people with a substantial lack of these capacities are less culpable, even if their conduct satisfied the prima facie case for the crime charged. Perhaps neuroscience can provide specific data previously unavailable to identify executive capacity differences more precisely.

There are two problems, however. First, significant problems with executive capacity are readily apparent without testing, and criminal law simply will not adopt fine-grained culpability criteria. Second, the correlation between neuropsychological tests of executive capacity and actual real-world behavior is not terribly strong.[32] Only a small fraction of the variance is accounted for, and the scanning studies will use the types of tasks the tests use. Consequently, we are far from able to use neuroscience accurately to assess nonobvious executive capacity differences that are valid in real-world contexts. Forensic psychology will be necessary, using the tools of interview and behavioral assessment that are the folk psychological bread and butter of the profession.

The Radical NeuroChallenge: Are We Victims of Neuronal Circumstances?

This part addresses the claim and hope alluded to earlier that neuroscience will cause a paradigm shift in criminal responsibility by demonstrating that we are "merely victims of neuronal circumstances" (or some similar claim that denies human agency). This claim holds that we are not the kinds of intentional creatures we think we are. If our mental states play no role in our behavior and are simply epiphenomenal, then traditional notions of responsibility based on mental states and on actions guided by mental states would be imperiled. But is the rich explanatory apparatus of intentionality simply a post hoc rationalization that the brains of hapless homo sapiens construct to explain what their brains have already done? Will the criminal justice system as we know it wither away as an outmoded relic of a prescientific and cruel age? If so, criminal law is not the only area of law in peril. What will be the fate of contracts, for example, when a biological machine that was formerly called a person claims that it should not be bound because it did not make a contract? The contract is also simply the outcome of various "neuronal circumstances."

Given how little we know about the brain–mind and brain–action connections, to claim that we should radically change our conceptions of ourselves and our legal doctrines and practices based on neuroscience is a form of neuroarrogance. Although I predict that we will see far more numerous attempts to introduce neuroevidence in the future, I have elsewhere argued that for conceptual and scientific reasons, there is no reason at present to believe that we are not agents.[33] It is possible that we are not agents, but the current science does not remotely demonstrate that this is true. The burden of persuasion is firmly on the proponents of the radical view.

What is more, the radical view entails no positive agenda. Suppose we are convinced by the mechanistic view that we are not intentional, rational agents after all.[34] What should we do now? We know that it is an illusion to think that our deliberations and intentions have any causal efficacy in the world. We also know, however, that we experience sensations—such as pleasure and pain—and care about what happens to us and to the world. We cannot just sit quietly and wait for our brains to activate, for determinism to happen. We must and will deliberate and act.

Even if we still thought that the radical view was correct and standard notions of genuine moral responsibility and desert were therefore impossible, we might still believe that the law would not necessarily have to give up the concept of incentives. Indeed, Greene and Cohen concede that we would have to keep punishing people for practical purposes.[35] Such an account would be consistent with "black box" accounts of economic incentives that simply depend on the relation between inputs and outputs without considering the mind as a mediator between the two. For those who believe that a thoroughly naturalized account of human behavior entails complete consequentialism, this conclusion might be welcomed.

On the other hand, this view seems to entail the same internal contradiction just explored. What is the nature of the agent that is discovering the laws governing how incentives shape behavior? Could understanding and providing incentives via social norms and legal rules simply be epiphenomenal interpretations of what the brain has already done? How do we decide which behaviors to reward or punish? What role does reason—a property of thoughts and agents, not a property of brains—play in this decision?

If the truth of pure mechanism is a premise in deciding what to do, no particular moral, legal or political conclusions follow from it.[36] The radical view provides no guide as to how one should live or how one should respond to the truth of reductive mechanism. Normativity depends on reason and, thus, the radical view is normatively inert. If reasons do not matter, then we have no reason to adopt any particular morals, politics, or legal rules, or to do anything at all.

Given what we know and have reason to do, the allegedly disappearing person remains fully visible and necessarily continues to act for good reasons, including the reasons currently to reject the radical view. We are not Pinocchios, and our brains are not Geppettos pulling the strings.

The Case for Cautious NeuroLaw Optimism

Despite having claimed that we should be exceptionally cautious about the current contributions that neuroscience can make to criminal law policy, doctrine, and adjudication, I am modestly optimistic about the near and intermediate term contributions neuroscience can potentially make to our ordinary, traditional, folk-psychological legal system. In other words, neuroscience may make a positive contribution even though there has been no paradigm shift in thinking about the nature of the person and the criteria for criminal responsibility. The legal regime to which neuroscience will contribute will continue to take people seriously as people—as autonomous agents who may fairly be blamed and punished based on their mental states and actions.

In general, my hope is that over time there will be feedback between the folk-psychological criteria and the neuroscientific data. Each might inform the other. Conceptual work on mental states might suggest new neuroscientific studies, for example, and the neuroscientific studies might help refine the folk-psychological categories. The ultimate goal would be a reflective, conceptual–empirical equilibrium.

More specifically, there are four types of situations in which neuroscience may be of assistance: (1) data indicating that the folk-psychological assumption underlying a legal rule is incorrect, (2) data suggesting the need for new or reformed legal doctrine, (3) evidence that helps adjudicate an individual case, and (4) data that help efficient adjudication or administration of criminal justice.

Many criminal law doctrines are based on folk-psychological assumptions about behavior that may prove to be incorrect. If so, the doctrine should change. For example, it is commonly assumed that agents intend the natural and probable consequences of their actions. In many or most cases it seems that they do, but neuroscience may help in the future to demonstrate that this assumption is true far less frequently than we think. In that case, the rebuttable presumption used to help the prosecution prove intent should be softened or used with more caution.

Second, neuroscientific data may suggest the need for new or reformed legal doctrine. For example, control tests for legal insanity have been disfavored for some decades because they are ill understood and hard to assess. It is at present impossible to distinguish "cannot" from "will not." Perhaps neuroscientific information will help to demonstrate and to prove the existence of control difficulties that are independent of cognitive incapacities. If so, then perhaps independent control tests are justified and can be rationally assessed after all. More generally, perhaps a larger percentage of offenders than we currently believe have such grave control difficulties that they deserve a generic mitigation claim that is not available in criminal law today. Neuroscience might help us discover that fact. If that were true, justice would be served by adopting a generic mitigating doctrine. On the other hand, if it turns out that such difficulties are not so common, we could be more confident of the justice of current doctrine.

Third, neuroscience might provide data to help adjudicate individual cases. Consider the insanity defense again. As in *United States v. Hinckley*,[37] there is often dispute about whether a defendant claiming legal insanity suffered from a mental disorder, which disorder the defendant suffered from, and how severe the disorder was.[38] At present, these questions must be resolved entirely behaviorally, and there is often room for considerable disagreement about inferences drawn from the defendant's actions, including utterances. In the future, neuroscience might help resolve such questions if the clear-cut problem difficulty can be solved. As mentioned previously, however, in the foreseeable future, I doubt that neuroscience will be able to help identify the presence or absence of specific *mens reas*.

Finally, neuroscience might help us to implement current policy more efficiently. For example, the criminal justice system makes predictions about future dangerous behavior for purposes of bail, sentencing, including capital sentencing, and parole. If we have already decided that it is justified to use dangerousness predictions to make such decisions, it is hard to imagine a rational argument for doing it less accurately if we are in fact able to do it more accurately. Validated behavioral prediction techniques already exist and should be used by FP because they are more accurate than pure clinical judgment.[39] The question is whether neuroscientific variables can add value by increasing the accuracy of such predictions considering the cost of gathering such data. Very recently, two studies have been published showing the potential usefulness of neural markers for enhancing the accuracy of predictions of antisocial conduct.[40] Although these must be considered preliminary, "proof of concept" studies,[41] it is perfectly plausible that in the future genuinely valid, cost-benefit justified neural markers will be identified, and thus, prediction decisions will be more accurate and just.

Conclusion

At present, neuroscience has little to contribute to more just and accurate criminal law decision making concerning policy, doctrine, and individual case adjudication. This was the conclusion reached when I tentatively identified "brain overclaim syndrome" 8 years ago, and it remains true today. In the future, however, as the philosophies of mind and action, and neuroscience mutually mature and inform one another, neuroscience will help us understand criminal behavior. Although no radical transformation of criminal justice is likely to occur, neuroscience can inform criminal justice as long as it is relevant to law and translated into the law's folk-psychological framework and criteria. For now and the foreseeable future, folk-psychological FP will be crucial to informing legal policy and adjudication about the relevance of mental abnormalities to legal criteria.

Acknowledgment

Jakob Elster and Michael Moore provided invaluable insights. Earlier versions of this chapter were originally published in different form as, (2011) Avoiding irrational neurolaw exuberance: A plea for neuromodesty, *Mercer Law* Review *62*, 837; (2011) The status of NeuroLaw: A plea for current modesty and future cautious optimism, *Journal of Psychiatry & Law, 39*, 595; Criminal law & neuroscience: Present and future, *Northern Ireland Law Quarterly*, in press. It is published here again in altered form. The overlap results from having achieved a settled understanding about the relation between law and neuroscience. Until there are conceptual or scientific breakthroughs that will cast doubt on this understanding—and there well may be such breakthroughs—for now this is my story and I am sticking to it.

References

1. (2002). The ethics of brain sciences: Open your mind. *Economist, 77.* www.economist.com/node/1143317/print Accessed October 5, 2011.
2. Morse SJ. (2006). Brain overclaim syndrome and criminal responsibility: A diagnostic note," *Ohio State J Crim Law, 3,* 397; Morse SJ. (2013). Brain overclaim redux. *Law Inequality, XXXI,* 509.
3. Doherty B. (2007). You can't see why on an FMRI: What science can and can't tell us about the insanity defense. *Reason* (quoting forensic psychiatrist, Phillip Resnick) Accessed online http://reason.com/archives/2007/06/19/you-cant-see-why-on-an-fmri. Of course, not all legal criteria involve "why" questions, but they all involve acts and mental content, and content cannot be inferred from brain structure or functional activity.
4. This is the term for the field that studies the relation of neuroscience to law that appears to have achieved almost universal acceptance. I will use it to follow the convention and because it is mellifluous, but strictly speaking there is no "neurolaw." There is simply law to which neuroscience may or may not be relevant and there may be specific regulation of the use of neuroscience in various contexts, but the latter, too, is simply law.
5. See for example, *In re Winship* 397 US 358, 364 (1970) (holding that due process requires that every conviction be supported by proof beyond reasonable doubt as to every element of the crime).
6. Feldman R. (2009). *The role of science in law.* New York: Oxford University Press.
7. Greene J, & Cohen J. (2006). For the law, neuroscience changes nothing and everything. In S Zeki, & O Goodenough (Eds.), *Law and the brain* (pp. 217–218, 224). New York: Oxford University Press.
8. I have emphasized "in part" so that no one confuses the view that folk psychological explanations are genuine explanations with metaphysical libertarianism. I discuss this issue elsewhere in this chapter.
9. I adapt the felicitous phrase 'to grasp and be guided by good reason' from Wallace J. (1994). *Responsibility and the moral sentiments* (p. 86). Cambridge, MA: Harvard University Press.
10. Morse SJ. (2002). Uncontrollable urges and irrational people. *VA Law Rev,* 88, 1025, 1035.
11. See for example, Stone AA. (1984). *Law, psychiatry, and morality* (pp. 95–96). Washington, DC: American Psychiatric Press.
12. See for example, Bennett MR, & Hacker PMS. (2003). *Philosophical foundations of neuroscience* (pp. 112, 270, 360, 381). New York: Blackwell; Pardo MS, & Patterson D. (2013). *Minds, brains and law: The conceptual foundations of law and neuroscience.* New York: Oxford University Press; (2010) Philosophical foundations of law and neuroscience. *Univ IL Law Rev,* 1211.
13. Morse SJ. (2007). The non-problem of free will in forensic psychiatry and psychology. *Behav Sci Law, 25,* 203, 204.
14. See, for example, Vihvelin K. (2013). *Causes, laws, and free will: Why determinism doesn't matter.* New York: Oxford University Press. Vihvelin provides a thorough metaphysical defense of the coherence and truth of compatibilism.
15. Morse SJ. (1994). Culpability and control. *Univ PA Law Rev,* 142, 1587, 1592–1694.
16. See, for example, Caspi A, et al. (2002). Role of genotype in the cycle of violence in maltreated children. *Science, 297,* 851. Indeed, the risk is nine times higher.
17. McHugh PR, & Slavney PR. (1998). *The perspectives of psychiatry* (2nd ed., pp. 11–12). Baltimore: Johns Hopkins University Press.
18. See for example Greene J, & Cohen J. (2006). For the law, neuroscience changes nothing and everything. In Zeki S, & Goodenough O (Eds.), *Law and the brain* (pp. 217–218, 224). New York: Oxford University Press.

19. Morse SJ. (2011). Lost in translation? An essay on law and neuroscience. In M Freeman (Ed.), *Law and neuroscience* (pp. 543–554). New York: Oxford University Press.
20. McHugh PR, & Slavney PR. (1998). *The perspectives of psychiatry* (2nd ed., pp. 11–12). Baltimore: Johns Hopkins University Press.
21. Frances A. (2009). Whither DSM-V? *Br J Psychiatry*, 195, 391. Many studies do find differences between patients with mental disorders and controls, but the differences are too small to be used diagnostically. But see generally, Ioannidis JPA. (2011). Excess significance bias in the literature on brain volume abnormalities. Arch Gen Psychiatry, 68, 773 (claiming, based on a meta-analysis of studies of brain volume abnormalities in patients with mental disorders, that many more studies than should be expected found statistically significant results and that this can be best explained by bias in the reporting of the data).
22. See for example, Miller GA. (2010). Mistreating psychology in the decades of the brain. *Perspect. Psychol Sci*, *5*, 716 (providing a cautious, thorough overview of the scientific and practical problems facing cognitive and social neuroscience).
23. Faigman DL, Monahan J, & Slobogin C. (2014) Group to individual inference (G2i) in scientific expert testimony. *Univ Chi Law Rev*, *81*, in press.
24. For an amusing exception, see Bennett CM, Baird AA, Miller MB, Wolford GL. (2009). Neural correlates of interspecies perspective taking in the post-mortem Atlantic Salmon: An argument for multiple comparisons correction. *J Serendipitous Unexpected Results*, *1*. Available at http://citeseerx.ist.psu.edu/viewdoc/download?doi=10.1.1.161.8384&rep=rep1&type=pdf. The study scanned a dead Atlantic salmon to demonstrate that significant results can be obtained from the most unpromising investigation unless the research design properly controls for chance findings (false positives).
25. *Roper v. Simmons* 543 US 551 (2005).
26. Ibid, 578–579.
27. Ibid, 569.
28. Ibid, 569, 573. The Supreme Court referred generally to other science, but it was not clear whether neuroscience played a specific role. The Supreme Court did cite neuroscientific findings in *Graham v. Florida*, 130 S. Ct. 2011 (2010), which categorically excluded juveniles from life without the possibility of parole in non-homicide cases (at 2034) and in *Miller v. Alabama*, 132 S. Ct. 2455 (2013), which held that the sentence of life without possibility of parole was constitutional for juveniles who committed homicide crimes, but that it was unconstitutional to impose this penalty mandatorily (at 2460). In both cases, the citation was conclusory and generally non-specific, and I believe it was dictum. The Supreme Court was responding in *Graham* to an argument that no party had seriously made, which was that the science of adolescent development had changed significantly since *Roper* was decided. Also in *Miller*, the Court drew a distinction between social science and "science" (at 2464, n. 5). Social science, like neuroscience, is science (and arguably more directly relevant to legal criteria for the reasons this chapter has discussed). The important distinctions are between good and bad science and legally relevant and legally irrelevant science.
29. *Roper v. Simmons* (n. 24) 569.
30. Morse SJ. (2011). Lost in translation? An essay on law and neuroscience. In M Freeman (Ed.), *Law and neuroscience* (p. 540). New York: Oxford University Press.
31. On the other hand, there may be reason to be cautious about such findings. See oannidis JPA. (2011). Excess significance bias in the literature on brain volume abnormalities. Arch Gen Psychiatry, 68, 773; see generally, Ioannides JPA. (2005). Why most published research findings are false. *PLoS Med*, 2, 696.
32. See for example, Barkley RA, & Murphy KR. (2010). Impairment in occupational functioning and adult ADHD: The predictive utility of executive function (EF) ratings versus EF tests. Arch Clin Neuropsychol, *25*, 157.
33. Morse SJ. (2011). Lost in translation? An essay on law and neuroscience. In M Freeman (Ed.), *Law and neuroscience* (pp. 543–554). New York: Oxford University Press; Morse SJ. (2008). Determinism and the death of folk psychology. *Minn J Law Sci Technol*, 9, 1.

34. Of course, the notion of being "convinced" would be an illusion too. Being convinced means that we are persuaded by evidence or argument, but a mechanism is not persuaded by anything. A mechanism is simply neurophysically transformed.
35. Greene J, & Cohen J. (2006). For the law, neuroscience changes nothing and everything. In S Zeki, & O Goodenough (Eds.), *Law and the brain* (p. 218). New York: Oxford University Press.
36. This line of thought was first suggested by Professor Mitchell Berman in the context of a discussion of determinism and normativity. Berman M. (2008). Punishment and justification. *Ethics 118*, 258, 271.
37. 525 F. Supp. 1342 (DDC 1981).
38. Ibid, 1346.
39. Skeem J, & Monahan J. (2011). Current directions in violence risk assessment. *Curr Dir Psychol Sci, 20*, 38.
40. Aharoni E, et al. (2013). Neuroprediction of future arrest. *PNAS*, 110, 6223; Pardini DA, et al. (2014). Lower amygdala volume in men is associated with childhood aggression, early psychopathic traits, and future violence. *Biol Psychiatry*, 75, 73.
41. For example, a re-analysis of the Aharoni et al. study (Zeki S, & Goodenough O (Eds.), *Law and the brain* (p. 218). New York: Oxford University Press) by Russell Poldrack, a noted "neuromethodologist" demonstrated that the effect size was tiny. http://www.russpoldrack.org/search?q=aharoni Also, the study used good but not use the best behavioral predictive methods for comparison.

APPENDIX

ACGME Program Requirements for Graduate Medical Education in Forensic Psychiatry

One-Year Common Program Requirements are in Bold

Introduction

Int. A. **Residency and fellowship programs are essential dimensions of the transformation of the medical student to the independent practitioner along the continuum of medical education. They are physically, emotionally, and intellectually demanding, and require longitudinally concentrated effort on the part of the resident or fellow.**

The specialty education of physicians to practice independently is experiential, and necessarily occurs within the context of the health care delivery system. Developing the skills, knowledge, and attitudes leading to proficiency in all the domains of clinical competency requires the resident and fellow physician to assume personal responsibility for the care of individual patients. For the resident and fellow, the essential learning activity is interaction with patients under the guidance and supervision of faculty members who give value, context, and meaning to those interactions. As residents and fellows gain experience and demonstrate growth in their ability to care for patients, they assume roles that permit them to exercise those skills with greater independence. This concept— graded and progressive responsibility—is one of the core tenets of American graduate medical education. Supervision in the setting of graduate medical education has the goals of assuring the provision of safe and effective care to the individual patient; assuring each resident's

and fellow's development of the skills, knowledge, and attitudes required to enter the unsupervised practice of medicine; and establishing a foundation for continued professional growth.

Int. B. Forensic psychiatry focuses on interrelationships between psychiatry and the law (civil, criminal, and administrative), including the psychiatric evaluation of individuals involved with the legal system, or consultations on behalf of the third parties such as employers or insurance companies; the specialized psychiatric treatment required by those who have been incarcerated in jails, prisons, or special forensic psychiatric hospitals; active involvement in the area of legal regulation of general psychiatric practice; and related education and research efforts.

Int. C. The education program in forensic psychiatry must be 12 months in length.

I. Institutions

I.A. Sponsoring Institution

One sponsoring institution must assume ultimate responsibility for the program, as described in the Institutional Requirements, and this responsibility extends to fellow assignments at all participating sites. The sponsoring institution and the program must ensure that the program director has sufficient protected time and financial support for his or her educational and administrative responsibilities to the program.

I.A.1. The sponsoring institution must also sponsor an Accreditation Council for Graduate Medical Education (ACGME)-accredited program in psychiatry.

I.B. Participating Sites

I.B.1. There must be a program letter of agreement (PLA) between the program and each participating site providing a required assignment. The PLA must be renewed at least every five years.

The PLA should:

I.B.1.a) identify the faculty who will assume both educational and supervisory responsibilities for fellows;

I.B.1.b) specify their responsibilities for teaching, supervision, and formal evaluation of fellows, as specified later in this document;

I.B.1.c) specify the duration and content of the educational experience; and,

I.B.1.d) state the policies and procedures that will govern fellow education during the assignment.

I.B.2. The program director must submit any additions or deletions of participating sites routinely providing an educational experience, required for all fellows, of one month full time equivalent or more through the ACGME Accreditation Data System (ADS).

I.B.3. The number of and distance between participating sites must allow for fellows' full participation in all organized educational aspects of the program.

I.B.4. Within at least one of the participating sites there should be an ACGME-accredited program in at least one of the following non-psychiatric specialties: family medicine, internal medicine, neurology, or physical medicine and rehabilitation.

II. Program Personnel and Resources

II.A. Program Director

II.A.1. There must be a single program director with authority and accountability for the operation of the program. The sponsoring institution's graduate medical education committee (GMEC) must approve a change in program director. After approval, the program director must submit this change to the ACGME via the ADS.

II.A.1.a) The program director must devote on average (over one month) at least 10 hours per week to the program with 1 or 2 fellows, or 15 hours per week to the program with 3 or more fellows. This must include activities related to administration, didactic teaching and fellow supervision outside of clinical activities, and time spent directly observing fellows or being observed in the clinical setting.

II.A.2. Qualifications of the program director must include:

II.A.2.a) requisite specialty expertise and documented educational and administrative experience acceptable to the Review Committee;

II.A.2.b) current certification in the subspecialty by the American Board of Psychiatry and Neurology (ABPN), or specialty qualifications that are acceptable to the Review Committee; and,

II.A.2.b).(1) The Review Committee accepts only ABPN certification in the subspecialty.

II.A.2.c) current medical licensure and appropriate medical staff appointment.

II.A.3. The program director must administer and maintain an educational environment conducive to educating the fellows in each of the ACGME competency areas. The program director must:

II.A.3.a) prepare and submit all information required and requested by the ACGME;

II.A.3.b) be familiar with and oversee compliance with ACGME and Review Committee policies and procedures as outlined in the ACGME Manual of Policies and Procedures;

II.A.3.c) obtain review and approval of the sponsoring institution's GMEC/DIO before submitting to the ACGME information or requests for the following:

II.A.3.c).(1) all applications for ACGME accreditation of new programs;

II.A.3.c).(2) **changes in fellow complement;**

II.A.3.c).(3) **major changes in program structure or length of training;**

II.A.3.c).(4) **progress reports requested by the Review Committee;**

II.A.3.c).(5) **responses to all proposed adverse actions;**

II.A.3.c).(6) **requests for increases or any change to fellow duty hours;**

II.A.3.c).(7) **voluntary withdrawals of ACGME-accredited programs;**

II.A.3.c).(8) **requests for appeal of an adverse action; and,**

II.A.3.c).(9) **appeal presentations to a Board of Appeal or the ACGME.**

II.A.3.d) **obtain DIO review and co-signature on all program information forms, as well as any correspondence or document submitted to the ACGME that addresses:**

II.A.3.d).(1) **program citations, and/or**

II.A.3.d).(2) **request for changes in the program that would have significant impact, including financial, on the program or institution.**

II.A.3,e) develop and implement a supervision policy that specifies lines of responsibility for program faculty members and fellows that is consistent with the supervision policy in the general psychiatry program; and,

II.A.3.f) participate in scholarly activities appropriate to the subspecialty, including local, regional, and national specialty societies, research, presentations, or publication.

II.B. Faculty

II.B.1. There must be a sufficient number of faculty with documented qualifications to instruct and supervise all fellows.

II.B.1.a) The faculty must include at least one certified child and adolescent psychiatrist.

II.B.1.b) In addition to the program director, there must be at least one faculty member certified by the ABPN in the subspecialty.

II.B.1.c) Each participating site must have a designated site director who is responsible for the day-to-day activities of the program at that site, with overall coordination by the program director.

II.B.2. The faculty must devote sufficient time to the educational program to fulfill their supervisory and teaching responsibilities and demonstrate a strong interest in the education of fellows.

II.B.3. The physician faculty must have current certification in the subspecialty by the American Board of Psychiatry and Neurology, or possess qualifications acceptable to the Review Committee.

II.B.4. The physician faculty must possess current medical licensure and appropriate medical staff appointment.

II.B.5. Faculty members must participate in scholarly activities appropriate to the subspecialty, including local, regional, and national specialty societies, research, presentations, or publications.

II.B.6. Faculty members must regularly participate in organized clinical discussions, rounds, journal clubs, and conferences.

II.C. Other Program Personnel

The institution and the program must jointly ensure the availability of all necessary professional, technical, and clerical personnel for the effective administration of the program.

II.C.1. In addition to the faculty psychiatrists, the faculty must include a lawyer and a forensic psychologist.

II.C.2. There must be a designated program coordinator.

II.D. Resources

The institution and the program must jointly ensure the availability of adequate resources for fellow education, as defined in the specialty program requirements.

II.D.1. Facilities must include at least one of the following: court clinics, inpatient forensic units, outpatient forensic clinics, or private practices; or inpatient and outpatient facilities, or specialized facilities that provide psychiatric care to correctional populations that include at least one of the following: prisons, jails, hospital-based correctional units, halfway facilities, rehabilitation programs, community probation programs, forensic clinics, juvenile detention facilities, or maximum security forensic hospital facilities.

II.D.1 .a) Support services at all participating sites must be available so that non-clinical duties do not adversely impact fellows' participation in the learning components of rotations and didactics, and to ensure a physically safe environment in which fellows may carry out their clinical and educational functions.

II.E. Medical Information Access

Fellows must have ready access to specialty-specific and other appropriate reference material in print or electronic format. Electronic medical literature databases with search capabilities should be available.

III. Fellow Appointments

III.A. Eligibility Criteria

Each fellow must successfully complete an ACGME-accredited specialty program and/or meet other eligibility criteria as specified by the Review Committee. The program must document that each fellow has met the eligibility criteria.

III.A.1. Prior to appointment in the program, fellows must have satisfactorily completed either an ACGME-accredited general psychiatry program or a general psychiatry program in Canada accredited by the Royal College of Physicians and Surgeons of Canada.

III.A.2. Prior to appointment in the program, each fellow must be notified in writing of the required length of education.

III.A.3. Prior to appointment to the program, the program director must receive documentation from the fellow's prior general psychiatry program verifying satisfactory completion of all educational and ethical requirements for graduation.

III.A.3.a) Agreements with applicants made prior to the completion of the general residency must be contingent on this requirement.

III.B. Number of Fellows

The program director may not appoint more fellows than approved by the Review Committee, unless otherwise stated in the specialty-specific requirements. The program's educational resources must be adequate to support the number of fellows appointed to the program.

III.B. 1. The presence of other learners must not interfere with the appointed fellows' education.

IV. Educational Program

IV.A. The curriculum must contain the following educational components:

IV.A. 1. Skills and competencies the fellow will be able to demonstrate at the conclusion of the program. The program must distribute these skills and competencies to fellows and faculty annually, in either written or electronic form. These skills and competencies should be reviewed by the fellow at the start of each rotation;

IV.A.2. ACGME Competencies

The program must integrate the following ACGME competencies into the curriculum:

IV.A.2.a) Patient Care

Fellows must be able to provide patient care that is compassionate, appropriate, and effective for the treatment of health problems and the promotion of health. Fellows:

IV.A.2.a).(1) must demonstrate proficiency in the psychiatric evaluation of individuals with a history of the following:

IV.A.2.a).(1).(a) criminal behavior;

IV.A.2.a).(1).(b) criminal responsibility and competency to stand trial;

IV.A.2.a).(1).(c) dangerousness; and,

IV.A.2.a).(1).(d) sexual misconduct.

IV.A.2.a).(2) must demonstrate proficiency in applying civil law and regulation of psychiatry issues when conducting a psychiatric evaluation of individuals with a history of the above.

IV.A.2.b) Medical Knowledge

Fellows must demonstrate knowledge of established and evolving biomedical, clinical, epidemiological, and social-behavioral sciences, as well as the application of this knowledge to patient care. Fellows:

IV.A.2.b).(1) must demonstrate competence in their knowledge of forensic psychiatry, including:

IV.A.2.b).(1).(a) assessment of competency to stand trial, criminal responsibility, amnesia, testamentary capacity, and civil competency;

IV.A.2.b).(1).(b) assessment of the accused sexual offender;

IV.A.2.b).(1).(c) ethical, administrative, and legal issues in forensic psychiatry;

IV.A.2.b).(1).(d) evaluation and treatment of incarcerated individuals;

IV.A.2.b).(1).(e) eyewitness testimony;

IV.A.2.b).(1).(f) history of forensic psychiatry;

IV.A.2.b).(1).(g) issues involved in the assessment of dangerousness;

IV.A.2.b).(1).(h) legal regulation of psychiatric practice;

IV.A.2.b).(1).(i) roles and responsibilities of forensic psychiatrists; and,

IV.A.2.b).(1).(j) writing of a forensic report.

IV.A.2.b).(2) must demonstrate competence in their knowledge of the legal system related to forensic psychiatry, including:

IV.A.2.b).(2).(a) **basic civil procedure;**
IV.A.2.b).(2).(b) **basic criminal procedure;**
IV.A.2.b).(2).(c) **children's rights;**
IV.A.2.b).(2).(d) **confessions;**
IV.A.2.b).(2).(e) **family law;**
IV.A.2.b).(2).(f) **fundamentals of law, statutes, and administrative regulations;**
IV.A.2.b).(2).(g) **jurisdiction;**
IV.A.2.b).(2).(h) **responsibility;**
IV.A.2.b).(2).(i) **structure and function of correctional systems;**
IV.A.2.b).(2).(j) **structure and function of juvenile systems;**
IV.A.2.b).(2).(k) **structure of federal and state court systems;**
IV.A.2.b).(2).(l) **theory and practice of sentencing of the convicted offender;**
IV.A.2.b).(2).(m) **tort law; and,**
IV.A.2.b).(2).(n) **use of a law library or online legal reference services.**

IV.A.2.b).(3) must demonstrate competence in their knowledge of civil law, including:

IV.A.2.b).(3).(a) **child abuse/neglect;**
IV.A.2.b).(3).(b) **child custody determinations;**
IV.A.2.b).(3).(c) **conservators and guardianships;**
IV.A.2.b).(3).(d) **developmental disability law, including individualized educational needs and the right to the least restrictive environment for education;**
IV.A.2.b).(3).(e) **parental competence and termination of parental rights;**
IV.A.2.b).(3).(f) **personal injury litigation;**
IV.A.2.b).(3).(g) **psychiatric disability determinations;**
IV.A.2.b).(3).(h) **psychiatric malpractice; and,**
IV.A.2.b).(3).(i) **testamentary capacity.**

IV.A.2.b).(4) must demonstrate competence in their knowledge of criminal law, including:

IV.A.2.b).(4).(a) **competence to be executed.**
IV.A.2.b).(4).(b) **competence to enter a plea;**
IV.A.2.b).(4).(c) **competence to stand trial;**
IV.A.2.b).(4).(d) **diminished capacity;**

IV.A.2.b).(4).(e) evaluations in aid of sentencing;
IV.A.2.b).(4).(f) insanity defense(s);
IV.A.2.b).(4).(g) safe release of persons acquitted by reason of insanity;
IV.A.2.b).(4).(h) testimonial capacity; and,
IV.A.2.b).(4).(i) voluntariness of confessions.

IV.A.2.b).(5) must demonstrate competence in their knowledge of the relevance of legal documents including:

IV.A.2.b).(5).(a) court testimony;
IV.A.2.b).(5).(b) hypnosis;
IV.A.2.b).(5).(c) imaging techniques;
IV.A.2.b).(5).(d) narcoanalysis;
IV.A.2.b).(5).(e) police reports;
IV.A.2.b).(5).(f) polygraphs;
IV.A.2.b).(5).(g) psychological and neuropsychological testing; and,
IV.A.2.b).(5).(h) any other evaluations or reports that are routinely encountered as part of forensic psychiatric evaluations.

IV.A.2.b).(6) must demonstrate proficiency in their knowledge of American culture and subcultures, including immigrant populations, particularly those found in the patient community associated with the educational program, with specific focus on the cultural elements of the relationship between the fellow and the patient including the dynamics of differences in cultural identity, values and preferences, and power.

IV.A.2.c) Practice-based Learning and Improvement

Fellows are expected to develop skills and habits to be able to meet the following goals:

IV.A.2.c).(1) Systematically analyze practice using quality improvement methods, and implement changes with the goal of practice improvement;

IV.A.2.c).(2) locate, appraise, and assimilate evidence from scientific studies related to their patients' health problems; and,

IV.A.2.c).(3) demonstrate administrative and teaching skills in the subspecialty.

IV.A.2.d) Interpersonal and Communication Skills

Fellows must demonstrate interpersonal and communication skills that result in the effective exchange of information and collaboration with patients, their families, and health professionals.

IV.A.2.d).(1) Fellows must demonstrate competence in interviewing socioculturally diverse patients and family in an effective manner, which may include those with limited English proficiency, health literacy, vision/sight, and hearing.

IV.A.2.e) Professionalism

Fellows must demonstrate a commitment to carrying out professional responsibilities and an adherence to ethical principles.

IV.A.2.e).(1) Fellows must demonstrate sensitivity and responsiveness to diverse patients, including but not limited to sex, age, culture, race, religion, disabilities, and sexual orientation.

IV.A.2.e).(2) Fellows must demonstrate competence in recognizing and appropriately addressing biases in themselves, others, and the health care delivery system.

IV.A.2.f) Systems-based Practice

Fellows must demonstrate an awareness of and responsiveness to the larger context and system of health care, as well as the ability to call effectively on other resources in the system to provide optimal health care.

IV.A.3. Curriculum Organization and Fellow Experiences

IV.A.3.a) The 12-month program must be completed within no more than a two-year period.

IV.A.3.b) Fellows must have at least six months of longitudinal experience in the management of patients in correctional systems.

IV.A.3.c) Clinical case conferences and seminars dealing with topics including law, ethics, the relevant basic and social sciences, and research must be conducted regularly and as scheduled.

IV.A.3.c).(1) Conferences in forensic psychiatry, including grand rounds, case conferences, seminars, and journal clubs, should be specifically designed to complement the clinical experiences.

IV.A.3.c).(2) Fellows must attend at least 70% of all required didactic components of the program. Attendance by fellows and faculty members should be documented.

IV.A.3.d) The didactic curriculum must include all topics for which fellows must demonstrate competence in knowledge.

IV.A.4. Fellow's experiences must include:

IV.A.4.a) evaluating and managing acutely- and chronically-ill patients in correctional systems;

IV.A.4. b) working with other professionals and personnel in both forensic and community settings;

IV.A.4c) treating a variety of patients, ranging from adolescence to old age and of diverse backgrounds;

IV.A.4.d) treating persons involved in the criminal justice system;

IV.A.4.e) reviewing written records, including clinical and legal documents, and preparing written reports and/or providing testimony in a diversity of cases, including:

IV.A.4.e).(1).(a) aiding the court in the sentencing of criminal offenders;

IV.A.4.e).(1).(b) allegations of sexual abuse;

IV.A.4.e).(1).(c) domestic relations cases;

IV.A.4.e).(1).(d) personal injury cases; and,

IV.A.4.e).(1).(e) other cases involving ethical issues and legal regulation.

IV.A.4.f) under supervision, testifying in court or in mock trial simulations; and,

IV.A.4.g) providing consultations to general psychiatric services on issues related to the legal regulation of psychiatric practice, including civil commitment and dangerousness, confidentiality, refusal of treatment, decision-making competence, and guardianship.

IV.A.4.g).(1) This should include consultations for patients from diverse socioeconomic, educational, ethnic, and cultural backgrounds, with a variety of diagnoses.

IV.A.5. There should be peer interaction among the fellows, organized around joint patient evaluation and/or care.

IV.A.6. Direct clinical work with children under the age of 14 years must only be provided by fellows who have previously completed ACGME-accredited education in child and adolescent psychiatry or by fellows who are under the supervision of a board-certified child and adolescent psychiatrist.

IV.A.7. Each fellow must have a minimum of two hours of faculty preceptorship weekly, one of which must be one-to-one preceptorship and one of which may be group preceptorship.

IV.A.8. Each fellow must maintain a patient log documenting all clinical experiences.

IV.B. Fellows' Scholarly Activities

IV.B.1. Fellows must participate in developing new knowledge or evaluating research findings.

V. Evaluation

V.A. Fellow Evaluation

V.A.1. Formative Evaluation

V.A.1.a) The faculty must evaluate fellow performance in a timely manner.

V.A.1.b) The program must:

V.A.1.b).(1) **provide objective assessments of competence in patient care, medical knowledge, practice-based learning and improvement, interpersonal and communication skills, professionalism, and systems-based practice;**

V.A.1.b).(2) **use multiple evaluators (e.g., faculty, peers, patients, self, and other professional staff); and,**

V.A.1.b).(3) **provide each fellow with documented semiannual evaluation of performance with feedback.**

V.A.1.b).(3).(a) **The evaluation must include review and discussion with each fellow of his or her education record documenting completion of all required components at the time of the evaluation of the program, evaluations of his or her clinical and didactic work by supervisors and teachers, and his or her patient log documenting all clinical experiences.**

V.A.1.c) **The evaluations of fellow performance must be accessible for review by the fellow, in accordance with institutional policy.**

V.A.1.d) Assessment should include quarterly written evaluations of all fellows by all supervisors and the directors of clinical components of the program.

V.A.2. **Summative Evaluation**

The program director must provide a summative evaluation for each fellow upon completion of the program. This evaluation must become part of the fellow's permanent record maintained by the institution, and must be accessible for review by the fellow in accordance with institutional policy. This evaluation must:

V.A.2.a) **document the fellow's performance during their education, and**

V.A.2.b) **verify that the fellow has demonstrated sufficient competence to enter practice without direct supervision.**

V.A.3. The final evaluation of each fellow must document proficiency in all required competency-based outcomes.

V.B. Faculty Evaluation

V.B.1. **At least annually, the program must evaluate faculty performance as it relates to the educational program.**

V.B.2. **These evaluations should include a review of the faculty's clinical teaching abilities, commitment to the educational program, clinical knowledge, professionalism, and scholarly activities.**

V.C. Program Evaluation and Improvement

V.C.1. **The program must document format, systematic evaluation of the curriculum at least annually. The program must monitor and track each of the following areas:**

V.C.1.a) **fellow performance,**

V.C.1.b) **faculty development, and,**

V.C.1.c) program goals and objectives, as well as program effectiveness in achieving them.

V.C.1.c).(1) At least one fellow representative and all faculty members should participate in these reviews.

V.C.2. **If deficiencies are found, the program should prepare a written plan of action to document initiatives to improve performance in the areas listed in section V.C.1. The action plan should be reviewed and approved by the teaching faculty and documented in meeting minutes.**

V.C.3. At least 80% of the program's eligible graduates from the preceding six years should have taken the ABPN certifying examination in forensic psychiatry.

V.C.4. At least 80% of the program's graduates from the preceding six years taking the ABPN certifying examination for forensic psychiatry for the first time must pass.

VI. Fellow Duty Hours in the Learning and Working Environment

VI.A. Professionalism, Personal Responsibility, and Patient Safety

VI.A.1. **Programs and sponsoring institutions must educate fellows and faculty members concerning the professional responsibilities of physicians to appear for duty appropriately rested and fit to provide the services required by their patients.**

VI.A.2. **The program must be committed to and responsible for promoting patient safety and fellow well-being in a supportive educational environment.**

VI.A.3. **The program director must ensure that fellows are integrated and actively participate in interdisciplinary clinical quality improvement and patient safety programs.**

VI.A.4. **The learning objectives of the program must:**

VI.A.4.a) **be accomplished through an appropriate blend of supervised patient care responsibilities, clinical teaching, and didactic educational events; and,**

VI.A.4.b) **not be compromised by excessive reliance on fellows to fulfill non-physician service obligations.**

VI.A.5. **The program director and sponsoring institution must ensure a culture of professionalism that supports patient safety and personal responsibility. Fellows and faculty members must demonstrate an understanding and acceptance of their personal role in the following:**

VI.A.5.a) assurance of the safety and welfare of patients entrusted to their care;

VI.A.5.b) provision of patient- and family-centered care;

VI.A.5.c) assurance of their fitness for duty;

VI.A.5.d) management of their time before, during, and after clinical assignments;

VI.A.5.e) recognition of impairment, including illness and fatigue, in themselves and in their peers;

VI.A.5.f) attention to lifelong learning;

VI.A.5.g) the monitoring of their patient care performance improvement indicators; and,

VI.A.5.h) honest and accurate reporting of duty hours, patient outcomes, and clinical experience data.

VI.A.6. All fellows and faculty members must demonstrate responsiveness to patient needs that supersedes self-interest Physicians must recognize that under certain circumstances, the best interests of the patient may be served by transitioning that patient's care to another qualified and rested provider.

VI.B. Transitions of Care

VI.B.1. Programs must design clinical assignments to minimize the number of transitions in patient care.

VI.B.2. Sponsoring institutions and programs must ensure and monitor effective, structured hand-over processes to facilitate both continuity of care and patient safety.

VI.B.3. Programs must ensure that fellows are competent in communicating with team members in the hand-over process.

VI.B.4. The sponsoring institution must ensure the availability of schedules that inform all members of the health care team of attending physicians and fellows currently responsible for each patient's care.

VI.C. Alertness Management/Fatigue Mitigation

VI.C.1. The program must:

VI.C.1.a) educate all faculty members and fellows to recognize the signs of fatigue and sleep deprivation;

VI.C.1.b) educate all faculty members and fellows in alertness management and fatigue mitigation processes; and,

VI.C.1.c) adopt fatigue mitigation processes to manage the potential negative effects of fatigue on patient care and learning, such as naps or back-up call schedules.

VI.C.2. Each program must have a process to ensure continuity of patient care in the event that a fellow may be unable to perform his/her patient care duties.

VI.C.3. The sponsoring institution must provide adequate sleep facilities and/or safe transportation options for fellows who may be too fatigued to safety return home.

VI.D. Supervision of Fellows

VI.D.1. In the clinical learning environment, each patient must have an identifiable, appropriately credentialed and privileged attending physician (or licensed independent practitioner as approved by each Review Committee) who is ultimately responsible for that patient's care.

Only licensed independent practitioners as consistent with state regulations and medical staff bylaws may have primary responsibility for a patient.

VI.D.1.a) This information should be available to fellows, faculty members, and patients.

VI.D.1.b) Fellows and faculty members should inform patients of their respective roles in each patient's care.

VI.D.2. The program must demonstrate that the appropriate level of supervision is in place for all fellows who care for patients.

Supervision may be exercised through a variety of methods. Some activities require the physical presence of the supervising faculty member. For many aspects of patient care, the supervising physician may be a more advanced fellow. Other portions of care provided by the fellow can be adequately supervised by the immediate availability of the supervising faculty member or fellow physician, either in the institution, or by means of telephonic and/or electronic modalities. In some circumstances, supervision may include post-hoc review of fellow-delivered care with feedback as to the appropriateness of that care.

VI.D.3. Levels of Supervision

To ensure oversight of fellow supervision and graded authority and responsibility, the program must use the following classification of supervision:

VI.D.3.a) Direct Supervision—the supervising physician is physically present with the fellow and patient.

VI.D.3.b) Indirect Supervision:

VI.D.3.b).(1) with direct supervision immediately available—the supervising physician is physically within the hospital or other site of patient care, and is immediately available to provide direct supervision.

VI.D.3.b).(2) with direct supervision available—the supervising physician is not physically present within the hospital or other site of patient care, but is immediately available by means of telephonic and/or electronic modalities, and is available to provide direct supervision.

VI.D.3.c) Oversight—The supervising physician is available to provide review of procedures/encounters with feedback provided after care is delivered.

VI.D.4. The privilege of progressive authority and responsibility, conditional independence, and a supervisory role in patient care delegated to each fellow must be assigned by the program director and faculty members.

VI.D.4.a) The program director must evaluate each fellow's abilities based on specific criteria. When available, evaluation should be guided by specific national standards-based criteria.

VI.D.4.b) Faculty members functioning as supervising physicians should delegate portions of care to fellows, based on the needs of the patient and the skills of the fellows.

VI.D.4.c) Fellows should serve in a supervisory role of residents or junior fellows in recognition of their progress toward independence, based on the needs of each patient and the skills of the individual fellow.

VI.D.5. Programs must set guidelines for circumstances and events in which fellows must communicate with appropriate supervising faculty members, such as the transfer of a patient to an intensive care unit, or end-of-life decisions.

VI.D.5.a) Each fellow must know the limits of his/her scope of authority, and the circumstances under which he/she is permitted to act with conditional independence.

VI.D.6. Faculty supervision assignments should be of sufficient duration to assess the knowledge and skills of each fellow and delegate to him/her the appropriate level of patient care authority and responsibility.

VI.E. Clinical Responsibilities

The clinical responsibilities for each fellow must be based on PGY level, patient safety, fellow education, severity and complexity of patient illness/condition, and available support services.

VI.F. Teamwork

Fellows must care for patients in an environment that maximizes effective communication. This must include the opportunity to work as a member of effective interprofessional teams that are appropriate to the delivery of care in the specialty.

VI.F.1. Contributors to effective interprofessional teams include consulting physicians, psychologists, psychiatric nurses, social workers, and other professional and paraprofessional mental health personnel involved in the evaluation and treatment of patients.

VI.G. Fellow Duty Hours

VI.G.1. Maximum Hours of Work per Week

Duty hours must be limited to 80 hours per week, averaged over a four-week period, inclusive of all in-house call activities and all moonlighting.

VI.G.1.a) Duty Hour Exceptions

A Review Committee may grant exceptions for up to 10% or a maximum of 88 hours to individual programs based on a sound educational rationale.

VI.G.1.a).(1) In preparing a request for an exception, the program director must follow the duty hour exception policy from the ACGME Manual on Policies and Procedures.

VI.G.1.a).(2) Prior to submitting the request to the Review Committee, the program director must obtain approval of the institution's GMEC and DIO.

VI.G.2. Moonlighting

VI.G.2.a) Moonlighting must not interfere with the ability of the fellow to achieve the goals and objectives of the educational program.

VI.G.2.b) Time spent by fellows in internal and external moonlighting (as defined in the ACGME Glossary of Terms) must be counted toward the 80-hour Maximum Weekly Hour Limit.

VI.G.3. Mandatory Time Free of Duty

Fellows must be scheduled for a minimum of one day free of duty every week (when averaged over four weeks). At-home call cannot be assigned on these free days.

VI.G.4. Maximum Duty Period Length

Duty periods of fellows may be scheduled to a maximum of 24 hours of continuous duty in the hospital. Programs must encourage fellows to use alertness management strategies in the context of patient care responsibilities. Strategic napping, especially after 16 hours of continuous duty and between the hours of 10:00 p.m. and 8:00 a.m., is strongly suggested.

VI.G.4.a) It is essential for patient safety and fellow education that effective transitions in care occur. Fellows may be allowed to remain on-site in order to accomplish these tasks; however, this period of time must be no longer than an additional four hours.

VI.G.4.b) Fellows must not be assigned additional clinical responsibilities after 24 hours of continuous in-house duty.

VI.G.4.c) In unusual circumstances, fellows, on their own initiative, may remain beyond their scheduled period of duty to continue to provide care to a single patient. Justifications for such extensions of

duty are limited to reasons of required continuity for a severely ill or unstable patient, academic importance of the events transpiring, or humanistic attention to the needs of a patient or family.

VI.G.4.c).(1) Under those circumstances, the fellow must:

VI.G.4.c).(1).(a) appropriately hand over the care of all other patients to the team responsible for their continuing care; and,

VI.G.4.c).(1).(b) document the reasons for remaining to care for the patient in question and submit that documentation in every circumstance to the program director.

VI.G.4.c).(2) The program director must review each submission of additional service, and track both individual fellow and program-wide episodes of additional duty.

VI.G.5. Minimum Time Off between Scheduled Duty Periods

VI.G.5.a) Fellows must be prepared to enter the unsupervised practice of medicine and care for patients over irregular or extended periods.

Forensic psychiatry fellows are considered to be in the final years of education.

VI.G.5.a).(1) This preparation must occur within the context of the 80-hour, maximum duty period length, and one-day-off-in-seven standards. Although it is desirable that fellows have eight hours free of duty between scheduled duty periods, there may be circumstances when these fellows must stay on duty to care for their patients or return to the hospital with fewer than eight hours free of duty.

VI.G.5.a).(1).(a) Circumstances of return-to-hospital activities with fewer than eight hours away from the hospital by fellows must be monitored by the program director.

VI.G.5.a).(1).(b) There are no circumstances under which fellows may stay on duty with fewer than eight hours off.

VI.G.6. Maximum Frequency of In-House Night Float

Fellows must not be scheduled for more than six consecutive nights of night float.

VI.G.7. Maximum In-House On-Call Frequency

Fellows must be scheduled for in-house call no more frequently than every third night (when averaged over a four-week period).

VI.G.8. At-Home Call

VI.G.8.a) Time spent in the hospital by fellows on at-home call must count toward the 80-hour maximum weekly hour limit The frequency of at-home call is not subject to the every-third-night limitation, but must satisfy the requirement for one-day-in-seven free of duty, when averaged over four weeks.

VI.G.8.a).(1) At-home call must not be so frequent or taxing as to preclude rest or reasonable personal time for each fellow.

VI.G.8.b) Fellows are permitted to return to the hospital while on at-home call to care for new or established patients. Each episode of this type of care, although it must be included in the 80-hour weekly maximum, will not initiate a new "off-duty period"

Suggested Readings

CLASSIC TEXTS

1. Cleckley H. (1941). *The mask of sanity.* St. Louis: CV Mosby.
2. East WN. (1927). *An introduction to forensic psychiatry in the criminal courts.* New York: William Wood & Company.
3. Foucault M. (1977). *Discipline and punish: The burden of the prison* (translated by E. Lean). New York: Penguin Viking Books.
4. Lindner RM. (1944). *Rebel without a cause: The hypnoanalysis of the criminal psychopath.* New York: Grune & Stratton.
5. Lombroso C. (1958). *The female offender.* New York: The Wisdom Library.
6. Mercier C. (1926). *Criminal responsibility.* New York: Physicians & Surgeons Book Company.
7. Ray I. (1838). *A treatise on the medical jurisprudence of insanity.* Boston: Little, Brown & Company.
8. Reik T. (1945). *The unknown murderer.* Englewood Cliffs, NJ: Prentice-Hall.
9. Rush B. (1812). *Medical inquiries and observations upon the diseases of the mind.* Philadelphia: Kimber & Richardson.
10. Stearns HP. (1883). *Insanity: Its causes and prevention.* New York: George Putnam & Sons.
11. Szasz TS. (1963). *Law, liberty and psychiatry.* New York: Macmillan.
12. Ward MJ. (1946). *The snake pit.* New York: Random House.
13. Whitlock FA. (1963). *Criminal responsibility and mental illness.* London: Butterworths.
14. Williams EH. (1931). *The insanity plea.* Baltimore: Williams & Wilkins.

GENERAL TEXTS

Law and Psychiatry

1. Allen IC, Ferster EZ, & Rubin JG. (1975). *Readings in law and psychiatry.* Baltimore: Johns Hopkins University Press.
2. Bluglass R, & Bowden P. (1990). *Principles and practice of forensic psychiatry.* Edinburgh: Churchill, Livingstone.
3. Brakel SJ, & Brock RS. (1971). *The mentally disabled and the law* (rev ed.). Chicago: University of Chicago Press.
4. Bromberg W. (1979). *The uses of psychiatry in the law: A clinical view of forensic psychiatry.* Westport, CT: Quorum Books.
5. Brooks AD. (1974). *Law, psychiatry, and the mental health system.* Boston: Little, Brown.

6. Curran WJ, McGarry AL, & Petty CS. (1980). *Modern legal medicine. Psychiatry and forensic science.* Philadelphia: FA Davis, 1980.
7. Curran WJ, McGarry AL, & Shah SA. (1986). *Forensic psychiatry and psychology.* Philadelphia: FA Davis.
8. Davidson H. (1965). *Forensic psychiatry* (2nd ed.). New York: Ronald Press.
9. Felthous AR, & Saab H. (2007). *International handbook on psychopathic disorders and the law.* New York: Wiley.
10. Gutheil TG, & Appelbaum PS. (2008). *Clinical handbook of psychiatry and the law* (3rd ed.). McGraw-Hill, New York.
11. Guttmacher MS. (1968). *A role of psychiatry in law.* Springfield, IL: Charles C Thomas.
12. Guttmacher MS, & Wiehofen H. (1952). *Psychiatry and the law.* New York: WW Norton.
13. Halleck SL. (1980). *Law in the practice of psychiatry: A handbook for clinicians.* New York: Plenum.
14. Hofling CK. (1980). *Law and ethics in the practice of psychiatry.* New York: Bruner-Mazel.
15. Katz J, Goldstein J, & Dershowitz AM. (1967). *A psychoanalysis, psychiatry and the law.* New York: Free Press.
16. Kolb LC. (1968). *Noyes' modern clinical psychiatry* (7th ed.). Philadelphia: Saunders.
17. Lifson LE, & Simon RI. (1998). *The mental health practitioner and the law: A comprehensive handbook.* Cambridge, MA: Harvard University Press.
18. Overholser W. (1953). *The psychiatrist and the law.* New York: Harcourt Brace.
19. Robitscher JB. (1966). *Pursuit of agreement, psychiatry and the law.* Philadelphia: Lippincott.
20. Rosner R. (1985). *Critical issues in american psychiatry and the law* (2nd ed.). New York: Plenum Press.
21. Rosner R. (1998). *Principles and practice of forensic psychiatry* (2nd ed.). London: Arnold Press.
22. Simon RI. (1992). Clinical psychiatry and the law (2nd ed.). Washington, DC: American Psychiatric Press.
23. Simon RI, & Gold L. (2010). *The American psychiatric textbook of forensic psychiatry* (2nd ed.). Washington, DC: American Psychiatric Press.
24. Stone AA. (1984). *Law, psychiatry, and morality: essays and analysis.* Washington, DC: American Psychiatric Press.
25. Watson AS. (1978). *Psychiatry for lawyers* (rev ed.). New York: International University Press.

Law and Psychology

1. Cooke G. (1980). *The role of the forensic psychologist.* Springfield, IL: Charles C Thomas.
2. Goldstein AM. (2007). *Forensic psychology: emerging topics and expanding roles.* Hoboken, NJ: Wiley.
3. Heibrun K. (2001). *Principles of forensic mental health assessment.* New York: Kluwer Academic/Plenum.
4. Kagehiro DK, & Laufer WS. (1992). *Handbook of psychology and law.* New York: Springer Science.
5. Sales BE. (1980). *Psychology in the legal process.* New York: Spectrum.
6. Schwitzgebel RL, & Schwitzgebel RK. (1980). *Law in psychological practice.* New York: Wiley.

Law and Mental Health

1. Barton WE, & Sanborn CJ. (1978). *Law and the mental health professions: friction and the interface.* New York: International University Press.

3. Heilbrun K, Grissl T, & Goldstein AM. (2009). *Foundations and forensic mental health assessment.* New York: Oxford University Press.

2. Heilbrun K, Marczyk GR, & DiMatteo D. (2002). *Forensic mental health assessment: A casebook.* New York: Oxford University Press.

4. Stone AA. (1975). *Mental health and law: A system in transition.* Washington, DC: National Institute of Mental Health.

Law and Nursing

1. Cazalas MW. (1978). *Nursing and the law.* Germantown, MD: Aspen.

SPECIALIZED TEXTS IN LAW AND MENTAL HEALTH AND LAW AND PSYCHIATRY

Involuntary Commitment and Patients' Rights

1. Asch SH. (1973). *Mental disability in civil practice.* Rochester, NY: The Lawyers Cooperative.
2. Brakel SJ, & Brock RS. (1971). The mentally disabled and the law (rev ed.). Chicago: University of Chicago Press.
3. Donaldson K. (1976). *Insanity inside out.* New York: Crown.
4. Kittrie N. (1971). *The right to be different.* Baltimore: Johns Hopkins University Press.
5. Polier JW. (1968). *The rule of law and the role of psychiatry.* Baltimore: Johns Hopkins Press.
6. Slovenko R. (1966). *Psychotherapy, confidentiality and privileged communication.* Springfield, IL: Charles C Thomas.

Child Psychiatry and the Law

1. Goldstein J, Freud A, & Solnit AJ. (1973). *Beyond the best interests of the child.* New York: The Free Press.
2. Goldzband MG. (1980). *Consulting in child custody: An introduction to the ugliest litigation for mental health professionals.* Lexington, MA: Lexington Books.
3. Schetky DJ, & Benedek EP. (1980). *Child psychiatry and the law.* New York, Bruner- Mazel.
4. Schetky DJ, & Benedek EP. (2002). *Principles in the practice of child and adolescent psychiatry.* Washington, DC: American Psychiatric Press.
5. Stuert IR, & Abt LE. (1981). *Children of separation and divorce: Management and treatment.* New York: Nostrand Reinhold.

Personal Injury Matters

1. Keiser L. (1968). *The traumatic neurosis.* Philadelphia: Lippincott.
2. Scrignar CB. (1984). *Posttraumatic stress disorder: Diagnosis, treatment, and legal issues.* New York: Praeger Publishers.

Criminal Law and Mental Illness

1. Fingarette H. (1972). *The meaning of criminal insanity.* Berkeley, CA: University of California Press.
2. Fingarette H, & Hasse AF. (1979). *Mental disabilities and criminal responsibility.* Berkeley: University of California Press.
3. Freedman LZ. (1983). *By reason of insanity: Essays on psychiatry and the law.* Wilmington, DE: Scholarly Resources.
4. Goldstein AS. (1967). *The insanity defense.* New Haven, CT: Yale University Press.
5. Group for the Advancement of Psychiatry. (1974). *Misuse of psychiatry in the criminal courts: Competency to stand trial.* New York. Group for the Advancement of Psychiatry.
6. Guttmacher MS. (1960). *The mind of the murderer.* New York: Farrar, Straus & Cudahy.
7. Halleck SL. (1967). *Psychiatry and the dilemmas of crime.* New York: Harper & Rowe.
8. Halleck SL, & Bromberg W. (1968). *Psychiatric aspects of criminology.* Springfield, IL: Charles C Thomas.
9. Lombroso C. (1958). *The female offender.* New York: The Wisdom Library.
10. MacDonald D. (1969). *Psychiatry and the criminal* (2nd ed). Springfield, IL: Charles C Thomas.
11. Malmquist CP. (2006). *Homicide: A psychiatric perspective* (2nd ed.). Washington, DC: American Psychiatric Publishing.
12. Morris N. (1982). *Madness and the criminal law.* Chicago: The University of Chicago Press.
13. National Institute of Mental Health. (1973). *Competency to stand trial and mental illness* (pamphlet). Rockville, MD: National Institute of Mental Health.
14. Roche PQ. (1958). *The criminal mind.* New York: Farrar, Straus & Cudahy.

15. Rosenberg CE. (1968). *The trial of the assassin Guiteau: Psychiatry and law in the gilded age.* Chicago: University of Chicago Press.
16. Slovenko R. (1966). *Crime, law and corrections.* Springfield, IL: Charles C Thomas.
17. Steadman H. (1979). *Beating a rap? Defendants found incompetent to stand trial.* Chicago: University of Chicago Press.
18. Weihofen H. (1933). *Insanity as a defense in criminal law.* New York: The Common World Fund.
19. Weihofen H. (1956). *The urge to punish.* New York: Farrar, Straus & Cudahy.
20. Wettstein RM. (1998). *Treatment of offenders with mental disorders.* New York: Guilford Press.
21. Whitlock FA. (1963). *Criminal responsibility and mental illness.* London: Butterworths.
22. Winslade WJ. (1983). *The insanity plea: The uses and abuses of the insanity defense.* New York: Charles Scribner's Sons.
23. Zilboorg G. (1954). *The psychology of the criminal act and punishment.* New York: Harcourt Brace.

Sex Offenders and Mental Illness

1. Karpman B. (1964). *The sexual offender and his offenses.* New York: Julian Press.
2. Mohr JW, Turner RE, & Jerry MB. (1964). *Pedophilia and exhibitionism.* Toronto: University of Toronto Press.
3. Rada RT. (1978). *Clinical aspects of the rapist.* New York: Grune & Stratton.
4. Resnick HLP, & Wolfgang ME. (1972). *Sexual behaviors: Social, clinical and legal aspects.* Boston: Little, Brown.
5. Slovenko R. (1965). *Sexual behavior and the law.* Springfield, IL: Charles C Thomas.

Violence and Dangerousness

1. American Psychiatric Association. (1974). Task Force Report No. 8: *Clinical aspects of the violent individual.* Washington, DC: American Psychiatric Association.
2. Monahan J. (1981). *The clinical prediction of violent behavior.* Rockville, MD: National Institute of Mental Health.
3. Rappeport JR. (1967). *The clinical evaluation of dangerousness of the mentally ill.* Springfield, IL: Charles C Thomas.
4. Tardiff K. (1999). Medical management of the violent patient: Medical assessment and therapy. New York: Marcel Dekker.

Malpractice Considerations

1. Cohen RJ. (1979). *Malpractice: A guide for mental health professionals.* New York: Free Press.
2. Dawidoff EJ. (1973). *The malpractice of psychiatrists.* Springfield, IL: Charles C Thomas.

Miscellaneous Texts

1. Brodsky SL. (1991). *Testifying in court: Guidelines and maxims for the expert witness.* Washington, DC: American Psychological Association Press.
2. Candilis PJ, Weinstock R, & Martinez R. (2007). *Forensic ethics and the expert witness.* New York: Springer.
3. Group for the Advancement of Psychiatry. (1991). *The mental health professional and the legal system.* New York: Brunner/Mazel.
4. Greenfield DP, Gottschalk JA. (2009). *Writing forensic reports: A guide for mental health professionals.* New York: Springer.
5. Gutheil TG. (1998). *The psychiatrist in court: A survival guide.* Washington, DC: American Psychiatric Press.
6. Gutheil TG. (2008). *The psychiatrist as expert witness.* Washington, DC: American Psychiatric Press.
7. Gutheil TG, & Dattilio FM. (2008). *Practical approaches to forensic mental health testimony.* Philadelphia: Wolters Kluwer/Lippincott Williams &Wilkins.
8. Perlin NL. (1989). *Mental disability law: Civil and criminal.* Charlottesville, VA: Michie Company.

9. Reid WH. (2013). *Developing a forensic practice: Operations and ethics for experts.* New York: Routledge, Taylor & Francis.
10. Robitscher J. (1980). *The powers of psychiatry.* Boston: Houghton Mifflin.
11. Wexler DB, & Winick BJ. (1991). *Essays in therapeutic jurisprudence.* Durham, NC: Carolina Academic Press.
12. Ziskin J, & Faust D. (1988). *Coping with psychiatric and psychological testimony* (4th ed.). Marina Del Rey, CA: Law and Psychology Press.

RELEVANT PUBLICATIONS BY ROBERT L. SADOFF, M.D., EDITOR

Educational Facilities in Forensic Psychiatry

1. Dattilio FM, Sadoff RL, & Gutheil TG. (2003). Board certification in forensic psychiatry and psychology: Separating the chaff from the wheat. *J Psychiatry Law, 31,* 5–19.
2. Jablon MC, Sadoff RL, & Heller MS. (1970). A unique forensic diagnostic hospital. *Am J Psychiatry, 126*(11), 1663–1667.
3. Heller NS, Sadoff RL, & Polsky S. (1968). Developing clinical facilities in forensic psychiatry. *Am J Psychiatry,* 124(11), 1562–1568.
4. Sadoff RL. (1974). Comprehensive training in forensic psychiatry. *Am J Psychiatry, 131*(2), 223–225.
5. Sadoff RL, & Dattilio FM. (2012). Formal training in forensic and mental health: Psychiatry and psychology. *Intl J Law Psychiatry, 35,* 343–347.
6. Sadoff RL, Polsky S, & Heller MS. (1969). *The forensic psychiatry clinic: Model for a new approach* (pp. 273–277). New York: Grune & Stratton.
7. Sadoff RL, Thornberry TP, Gottlieb DW, & Young J. (1980). Teaching forensic psychiatry. *Bull Amer Acad Psychiatry Law, 7*(3).

Books on Forensic Psychiatry

1. Dattilio FM, & Sadoff RL. (2007). *Mental health experts: Roles and qualifications for court* (2nd ed.). Mechanicsburg, PA: Pennsylvania Bar Institute.
2. Drogin EY, Dattilio FM, Sadoff RL, & Gutheil TG. (2011). *Handbook of forensic assessment: Psychological and psychiatric perspectives.* Hoboken, NJ: Wiley.
3. Sadoff RL. (1978). *Violence and responsibility.* New York: Specter Publications.
4. Sadoff RL. (1982). *Legal issues and the care of psychiatric patients: A guide for mental health professionals.* New York: Springer.
5. Sadoff RL. (1983). *Forensic psychiatry.* Philadelphia, Saunders.
6. Sadoff RL. (1988). *Forensic psychiatry: A practical guide for lawyers and psychiatrists* (2nd ed.). Springfield, IL: Charles C Thomas.
7. Sadoff RL. (2008). *Issues in pharmacy, law and ethics: The Max and Rose Sadoff Symposia.* Minneapolis, MN: University of Minnesota, College of Pharmacy, Bookmobile Publishing.
8. Sadoff RL. (2010). *Ethical issues in forensic psychiatry: Minimizing harm.* London: Wiley-Blackwell.
9. Sadoff RL, & Dattilio FM. (2008). *Crime and mental illness.* Mechanicsburg, PA: Pennsylvania Bar Institute.
10. Sadoff RL, & Lewis MB. (1975). *Psychic injuries.* New York: Matthew Bender.
11. Simon RI, & Sadoff RL. (1992). *Psychiatric malpractice: Cases and comments for clinicians.* Washington, DC: American Psychiatric Press.

Miscellaneous Articles

1. Accreditation Council for Graduate Medical Education. *ACGME Program Requirements for Graduate Medical Education in Forensic Psychiatry.* Retrieved from
2. Sadoff RL. (1977). Changing laws and ethics in psychiatry. *Bull Amer Acad Psychiatry Law, 5*(1).
3. Sadoff RL. (1978). Developing community mental health center-criminal justice system interactions. *Intl J Law Psychiatry, 1,* 427–436.
4. Sadoff RL. (1984). Practical, ethical problems of the forensic psychiatrist in dealing with attorneys. *Bull Amer Acad Psychiatry Law, 12*(3), 243–252.

Index